ANYWHERE

A MYTHOGEOGRAPHY OF SOUTH DEVON

AND HOW TO WALK IT

CECILE OAK

Published by:
Triarchy Press
Axminster, England

info@triarchypress.net
www.triarchypress.net

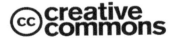 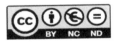

A catalogue record for this book is available from the British Library.

paperback ISBN: 978-1-911193-12-8

ePub ISBN: 978-1-911193-13-5

pdf ISBN: 978-1-911193-14-2

Note of guidance from the author:

Please feel free to read *Anywhere* in any way you want and take away from *Anywhere* whatever you wish; read it is as a novel, as a failed conference report, as travel writing, as a meandering guidebook, as a textbook written by a drunken geographer. Or all of these. I hope that everyone, whether on the ground or in their imaginations, will use this book as a guide to making their own journeys in their own 'South Devon'.

Additional images associated with each chapter of the book can be found at:
www.triarchypress.net/anyimages

The Stranger

Cecile Oak was born in Brianclose, Yorkshire. She was educated at the William Beveridge Community School and New College, Oxford. After graduating with a Double First in English, she worked in Paris as an independent curator and as creative director of the Les Nap gallery in the Chiaia district of Naples. After returning to the UK in 2005, she established herself as a leading agent and producer, notably with the Egalité agency. In 2013 she began full-time doctoral studies at Leeds University and was awarded a PhD for her thesis 'Heterotopian and chorastic trends in the progressive fatalism of Maeterlinck and Villiers De L'Isle Adam'. She presently lives in the south of Italy with her daughter, and lectures in Performance at the University of Tropea.

The Guide

A.J. Salmon was born in Coventry in the English West Midlands in the late 1980s. Despite a happy family background, he left school at 16 with few qualifications. Moving to Bristol he featured on the performance poetry scene and worked as the tutor of a poetry class in Horfield Jail. In 2009 he was found guilty of stealing over a thousand books from local bookshops and was jailed for six months, enrolling in his own poetry class. On release, he moved progressively westwards. After working as a freelance proof-reader, he dropped from view around 2009 having told a local film-maker in Exeter that he would be on permanent pilgrimage. Since then reports of him are sporadic at best, but he continues to publish work in various magazines and with Triarchy Press, mailing his work from public libraries in Devon.

"Most people at some time or other have wallowed in the Slough of Despond, some have fought fiercely with Apollyon. Almost all have known what it is to pass through the Valley of Humiliation.... All of us, unless we are hermits, must pass through Vanity Fair. A very few of us, rare souls, have talked with the Shepherds on the Delectable Mountains, and even rested in the trees in the Land of Beulah."

Mary P. Willcocks (*Bunyan Calling*)

"...immersion.... triggered as an embodied state, accessed from within the audience's interiorities and attuned-ness to twenty-first century global migration politics, enhanced by their first hand lived knowledge and/or second hand mediatised awareness of what is at stake for bodies at borders...."

Royona Mitra (*Decolonizing Immersion*)

"No one makes a mythogeography until they learn how to walk in more than one body; until they can walk in a place where they are at home as if they were a stranger, and in a place where they are a stranger as if they were at home."

Phil Smith (*I'm Walking Backwards for Quatermass*)

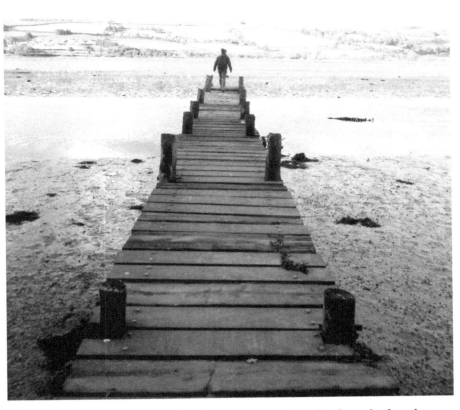

Additional images associated with each chapter of the book can be found at:
www.triarchypress.net/anyimages

Chapter One: A journey begins, Yorkshire to Devon

Leeds railway station is an odd place to begin a walk in Devon. Yet a walk in Devon can begin anywhere: in Saugor, Trinidad, Venus, R'lyeh or Z. Or all those places.

Setting off mid-morning from my home in Yorkshire in the spring of 2016, I catch the train down through Birmingham and Bristol. I plug in Philip Glass, then Gloria Coates, Belbury Poly, Delia Derbyshire and, around Bristol Parkway, the recently elevated David Bowie; covering the table with notes, slim volumes, A4 papers and printouts from online discussion forums. Spread before me like charts for a treasure hunt is everything I have gleaned about the subject of my adventure: the 'new walking movement'.

Until a moment two weeks ago, the only 'movement' walking had for me was the obvious one foot in front of the other. Now I am on my way to investigate a not quite secret, not quite public, obsession of folk for whom walking is at worst a work of art and at best a pilgrimage. I wish I shared the sincerity of their publications; but I am here to improve my chances of what Americans call "tenure".

On the train I have been distilling something from the rich jumble of threads and flashes of their books and blogs down to what I imagine, if this conference is halfway representative, will be its themes. All that despite a feeling that this walking movement's picture of itself is no clearer than a Polaroid taken in a blackout.

Rattling past the massive Morrisons' distribution depot on the fringes of Weston-super-Mare, a diminutive giant made of withies looms over a small pond. He is a little spiky around his pronounced buttocks. It strikes me, like a first sip of gin, that just maybe what I am working on is a lot of arse.

> *New cartographies: strategic information or gift wrapping?*
> *The activist's turn towards the spatial: after the Arab Spring, what now?*
> *Walking, sustainability and the Anthropocene: why are we pretending?*

Different jokes, but the same comic structure? These are not real papers! They are some kind of fake news, a satire on their own formalism. I dig into the doorstep of extraneous documents and find a rather more likely programme; far less funny, a mix of the startlingly mundane and the contrived unexpected; like a real conference programme. What I have been reading up until Highbridge is a list of fringe provocations written by some clever dick.

I was not expecting walking to be so tricksy.

We cross into Devon sometime after Taunton. *Country Life* has just declared the county the best place to live in Britain; one of their criteria is the number of entries in *Who's Who*.

I change trains at Exeter St David's in order to travel on the slow stopper service for the final part of my journey; so I can take in some of the smaller places along the way, referenced in a specially written guidebook supplied with the other conference papers.

Just after leaving the city, looking back on my left, I catch a glimpse of the faded Pussy Riot graffiti promised by the guidebook's author, A.J. Salmon. I know there will be no time for sightseeing for me; no sooner are the sessions over than I am going straight back to my desk in Yorkshire to get things down as freshly as I can. I write fast. I will complete a 20,000-word report in three days, click SEND and hope that someone remembers my gratuitous labours at a future interview; I am on my own now, already playing the game.

I window-shop the Devonian backdrop flashing by as best I can; the quirky detail of the substantial guidebook makes it clear that something rather more thorough is expected. And I am painfully aware that I should have travelled down much earlier. Two days of fringe activities have been arranged informally to precede the conference proper; details of which are supplied with the official papers. However, only yesterday I had the viva for my PhD – awarded with minor corrections, breathes huge sigh – and baulked at the option to travel immediately and sleep on the train.

What gets to me now is not so much the minor depression that I knew would descend around Wolverhampton, after the last fizz of sparkling wine finally left my body, but the prospect of arriving in Paignton at nightfall. Not that I have anything against Paignton, or think it super-sinister after sunset – I know nothing about the town – but I have a phobia about arriving in new places after dark. I fear darkness in new places.

I was a slow starter in academia; I was a 'mature' (they mean 'tardy') student; but once I got up steam I slid into a hyper-acceleration that everyone else seems to regard as their (and the world's) worst enemy. Perhaps because I began from a standing start, just to get up to 'pedestrian' has been an extraordinarily big bang for me. I love research: the speed of it, its forensic qualities, hunting across an index, eyes tuned. For this conference I must have flipped a hundred or more books, blogs and papers. I've read the recent stuff – Careri, Solnit, Richardson, Papadimitriou (I loved *Scarp*), and the Fife Psychogeographical Collective's *From Hill to Sea* – but it was the older things that have really stuck: Machen, Murray, Graham, Shepherd and Donald Maxwell's 'Detective In' books. This walking-as-art or walking-as-magic thing has been going on for decades; not quite conspiratorial, but always just below the radar.

And odd.

Like, just one example, *Walking with Fancy* by E.L. Grant Watson – published in the middle of blitz and war. A chapter begins, "The three of us sat on the step outside the kitchen door and watched the hermaphrodite copulation of slugs". One day I hope I get to write chapter openings like that. Or, at least, to speculate like Watson: "suppose that the pineal gland in a man's brain were a fully developed third eye, opening upward and directing its gaze into the heavens.... Would it be possible for him to be so exclusively occupied with commerce and war... when the infinity of space was extended always before that skyward-directed eyeball?"

Is that really 1942?

I feel a little raw today. The awkward ending of a brief relationship after the collapse of a long one. That. The most recent a bad call, followed by a lengthy extrication. All the while in thesis writing-up mode. Even so, none of that prepares me for the full body skinning that is shortly to come. In some of the articles the ambulatory authors write about a thing they call the "hyper-sensitization of the disrupted walker". It doesn't sound so bad, a mild attuning to the world; it is not like that, it is nerve surgery with aesthetics and without anaesthetics and I am on my way to an appointment at the operating theatre.

My daughter, Sophia, is safely away, and being spoiled rotten by her Zan and Granfer in Cheshire. I wonder if I should have brought Sophia along with me to the conference?

The train trundles through Starcross and Dawlish Warren. There are skeletal wrecks there in the estuary mud; the black cormorants indistinguishable from the crusty spars.

Another wreck, just before the Warren – Salmon's guidebook says it was full of coal – had broken its back fleeing a Nazi sub. A mast points darkly from the silhouette of deck and hull. The Warren stretches out beyond it, sand dunes is all, where once a republic of weekenders were sold ice cream by a schoolboy Tommy Cooper. Blown away by storms. Just like that.

After cup-like clods of rusty clinker mixed among rocky boulders, we pass the squat blancmange of Langstone Rock – a blasphemy, in more ways than one, the guidebooks (not Salmon's) call it "Devon's Ayers Rock" – and race along the sea wall. The waves are beating up high sheets of water that fall against the side of the carriage. I get up to stand by the window in the doorway, press my face to the glass to catch the cold sensation of the waves, when the pane is – bang! – rattled by a piece of shingle picked up in the water. I am shocked that such a thing is possible on a train and sit back down again, shamed. An elderly woman, 90 if she is a day, grabs my arm in her bony fingers: "isn't it exciting!"

The service stops at Dawlish, so I step off the train for a moment to savour the sight of the boiling water. Barely on the platform, I feel a thump run through the concrete. No time to retreat, the blanket of water descends over me. Scuttling inside, drenched to my underwear, the rest of the carriage refuses to hide their amusement and I am pestered all the way to Newton Abbot with offers of paper handkerchiefs.

I don't mind too much. Coursing through my nervous system is all that caffeine-borne reading; all the vicarious journeys I have been taking, and my growing addiction to the dull sting of ordinary ideas, traded over and over and over again –

site-specificity, atmospheres, looking-anew, emotional landscapes and embodied knowing – as if the same smart alec insights could be perpetually rearranged. I have taken my first field trip in Devon – one metre from the train and back – I almost feel an affinity with physical geographers.

The most sensible thing to do is change in the toilet, but Salmon writes about a Dream Church just the other side of Newton Abbot. Sense prevails and I rush to the cubicle to change my shirt. Someone has written on the towel dispenser, in a long and graceful hand, the single word "seraphinianus"; not the usual kind of lavatorial message, though it may still be obscene. Returning to my seat I see a church, or the top part of it, white and geometrical and disappointing; an air of green despondency hanging about its squatness. Then it is gone, hidden by tall concrete walls of road construction, their light grey surfaces spattered with mud from the red ground.

In the fields the sheep are stained pink; the colours of the old deserts and crumbled mountains. Ah, Salmon. Yes. I nod to Salmon. Whoever s/he is......

We stop at Torre, then Torquay and finally approach the station at the end of the line. As we are drawing in, there is an assembly of beach huts, shoulder to shoulder in a car park, like Emperor Penguins keeping warm. Later, on a long-abandoned airfield, high above the Teign, I will find a story of these same huts; how a writer and comedian, well-known on 1970s' TV, used them to block the runways against a sneak invasion by the Nazis.

Chapter Two: Paignton

I write up my reflections in a seaside-modernist café overhanging the ocean.

The colours in the water, greens and purples, are greying now. At first glance I am charmed by the poetic agency of the weathering on the prom wall:

OVER IN SECURITY P I T
CU T PAIN
KEEP O – POO
INSE RT PAIN

But I fancy the agency is human. Worried about it getting late, I scuttle down the promenade towards the grandly eccentric shape of my hotel. On the grass, landward of some beach huts, a group of young people are sporadically stamping their feet like herring gulls, as if trying to bring up worms from the ground.

There has been a 'mix up'. I don't have a room. Great.

Indeed, the hotel does not book rooms to individuals on a dance week. I explain that my room has been booked by the dance and theatre school of one of the conference's sponsoring universities. The staff are sympathetic; a room is vacant due to a 'no show' and if I don't mind putting up with this week's samba enthusiasts I am welcome to it. Relieved of the prospect of wandering a strange town, roomless, I would be happy to endure cha-cha-cha maniacs.

I deposit my bags, feeling buoyed up and confident, and brave the road, strung with coloured bulbs, towards the bars in town. I have decided not to go to the official launch, which anyway will be almost over by now, but try to catch a fringe drink flagged up on Facebook. There are no walkers there; two anglers waiting for an all-night fishing trip is all. I stride out to catch the launch but that has ended, no one there; the manager tells me the delegates have moved on to a restaurant. He doesn't know which one, just that it is not his.

I wander up a short bright street of amusement centres, shops, cafés, a tattoo parlour, and takeaways; this does not feel like conference delegate territory to me. A group, who I hope are walkers, turn out to be a gaggle of language students from Spain.

Next morning, at breakfast, I miss the sign about waiting to be seated and go straight to a table, making notes on my reading and losing track of time. By the time I am identified as still not served, I feel obliged to eat as a special effort has been made to rush me my food. The breakfast is far too big for me. The Polish waitress is keen to tell me about the dance floor, assuming that I'm here for the samba (a conference on walking seems hardly credible). Isadora Duncan danced here, she says, something about shenanigans under a piano and there is a secret tunnel and (lowering her voice very slightly) prayer steps oriented to Mecca.

On my way out I try not to delay at the paintings of the hotel when it was still a private house; there were minarets then, but when I look back on my dash into town they are missing. Infuriated with myself, I feel compelled to stop and check Salmon. Indeed, he does mention my hotel; how it and others were owned at various times by members of the sewing machine dynasty, the Singers. But mine was designed by its first resident, a Colonel Smith, who created an identical but pink version somewhere near Nice. Smith had been responsible for the conservation of Islamic monuments in India, hence the minarets and rumours of his secret Indian wife; the tunnel probably didn't help (but it was actually to link the house to a glass bathing pool sunk in the beach, long since washed away by storms – already, so much about storms!)

I wonder if I am reading of a genuine resistance within the established order, a cultivation of otherness and intrigue, of a radical and stubborn doubleness... or whether these are no more than fancy ornaments on a more familiar machine.

The sea wind, bursting through the gaps between the beach huts, blows right through me; I am surprised at how hollow and tender I am. As if all that I became while studying 'The Quest in Symbolist Theatre' has turned to air, and my new doctoral robes are no more resistance to the storm to come than a flimsy negligee. I laugh thinly in the face of the breeze. Under my panting, I repeat over and over again until it loses all meaning: "Negligee, negligee, negligee, negligee...."

I find the conference venue easily; arranged across two of those big Singer houses, now hotels. The universities have booked them cheap and out of season. I take a deep breath at the giant door, ready to take speed notes of everything I see and hear. But at the registration, the delegate badges are mostly still in their boxes and an apologetic volunteer is explaining to a group of academics that the conference has been abandoned. The organisers have gone to the railway station to see off the keynote speakers. I rush to the station, perhaps to catch some last words, a snatched interview, explanations from the organisers, something to justify the expenses I was granted to bring me here.

An hour later, I am back at the conference venue, hoovering up whatever papers and programmes I can find, collaring volunteers and scouring the hotel waste bins until I am asked to leave by hotel staff. I have what I need, and head back to my own hotel. The samba is in full swing in the oval ballroom. I find a space at the bar and begin to assemble my notes. I have an early gin and tonic.

Scribbling furiously, in a quieter part of my brain I get to thinking about what one of the organising committee has said at the station, upset because "this was our chance, our movement's chance to get the big names to notice we are here". The stars were less upset; perhaps relieved at missing out on their appropriation to resistance walking.

(Just as Colonel Smith might have avoided an invitation to join Salmon's weird and dissident Devon.) I had managed to get a word with one of them as their train was pulling in and she was excited: "Who do they think they are, these radical walkers? But then, what's the point of being radical if you don't... you know... well jolly good luck to them, I say! Who are they? Whoever we want to believe they are! I saw some of them going, you know? Which is what this is all about, really. The out there."

And she ran her hand down the cast iron pillar holding up the station canopy, overpainted so many times that its Victorian lumpiness had become flesh-like; clotted cream yellow and lipstick red.

At the station one of the organisers had explained to me that the star speakers had all addressed the official launch, along with their dialogue partners who had waited until then before setting off for the ambulatory conference. Then, conversations, between unlikely companions, had tendrilled off into beach walks and pub crawls, and perhaps I could still get some idea of what was discussed from the few remaining delegates?

I kick myself under the bar table for my tardiness.

Then I notice the tunnel doorway. Small, cream, unsigned, raised up above the floor of the bar; is it wonky in its frame? Or is that just me, cranky at the thought of what I missed? Still just morning, the dancers are already making abstract shapes and patterns in the sunlight bouncing off the sea and streaming through the glass. I contemplate trying the handle of the secret portal. Instead, I repack my shoulder bag and leave the hotel, setting off back over the long rectangle of grey grass and across a 'geoplay' park, a set of sandpits and climbing frames on geological themes, already itself becoming de-fabricated and fossilised, thick fingers of moss occupying letters cut in stone. A dry watercourse, representing flash floods three hundred million years ago, ends in a ring-a-roses of orange bollards and plastic hazard tape.

My hunch is a good one. I quickly find a delegate from Belgium, on his way to a rump conference that has been swiftly organised by the more institutionally-minded of the attendees; those with travel grants and accommodation expenses to justify (like me) and public impact targets to reach (thankfully not). A hotel where many of the delegates are staying has opened up its lounge, ballroom and bar; a rough, handwritten schedule of papers has been sellotaped to a mirror in the lobby. I find a group in session in the ballroom, 'The Business of Drifting', and sneak in.

A handful of miffed delegates are listening impatiently to an aggressive entrepreneur who is eager to have their advice on how to get tax breaks "for situationism" and the problems of monetising ambience. He concludes with a proposal to transform radical walking into an analytical business tool. The session moves quickly on; there are no questions.

The session closes with two short papers, one on the mis-telling of the Kinder Scout Mass Trespass story (how posterity was mugged by an adroit Communist Party, so other broader-based trespasses mobilising thousands at Winnats Pass and elsewhere, are rarely heard of), and another on 'the liminal space of coastline' (what

13

would a conference be without at least one 'liminal space'?) about the emerging significance of "the muddy and the uncertain".

I ask myself how I have been lured here, why I was driven to read so many books and websites in preparation, what un-earthed mania I am now a part of? And contributing to?

One of the fringe delegates produces a frame from her backpack, stained wood, three-sided only. She asks us to imagine what landscape might have just escaped it.

I feel a little woozy now, after yesterday's long journey, and retire to the bar where the spring water is complimentary. There is some strange talk there about traces found in the sand, ashes from intensely hot burning body shapes, a fire on a rock out at sea last night; wishful rumours that the long dead New York artist Ana Mendieta had not expired on a broken sidewalk, but is asking that delegates look back to the origins of their practice in her own 'Moffitt Building Piece' film, in which pedestrians pass by a pool of blood on a city street; that none of us are doing anything more than walking by the cracks in her sidewalk. That we are all still passing by 'on the other side'. I feel bad for not enjoying the wit of this messing with us.

The water doesn't help.

I go back to listen to the papers, but excuse myself to pursue a delegate who has presented a paper on 'refusing'; apparently there is a man in Swansea who stands in front of cars, causing traffic jams. He refuses to explain his actions. This ambusher has been found "mute of malice"; psychiatrists have failed to decide if he is sane. He bridges and traduces. He places an enigma at the head of the transport queue and will not let it move. The state has recently put him away for 36 weeks. The delegate who gives the paper does not address my fusillade of questions about motives and drives, but muddies the waters with stories about a woman on a mobility scooter squirting cars in Newquay with tomato ketchup.

A retired professor wanders by pondering aloud how far from Frankfurt we have really come. A quietly spoken poet, recently returned from a residency in Canada, confesses to us her personal healing while out walking in deep wilderness and her fear for its English equivalent under the strain of house building for two million immigrants. The young delegate who presented on the Swansea sabotage clumsily interrupts her, his voice trembling as he speaks angrily of microscopically polluted space, its image purified to return it to the idea of "untouched", the universal at the service of the elite, then leaves, embarrassed.

The wheels are starting to part company with the chassis.

On my way back to my hotel, I find a group of 'microgeographers' (artist-cum-microbiologist hybrids) obsessing over microbial blooms on signage at the geologically-themed playpark. They are dressed in an assortment of science modes: suit, overalls, mini skirt. They explain that they are interested in the mobility of microbial colonies in the built environment, asserting that they parallel human travel. They want to push pedestrians off their usual macroscopic paths and get them down on their hands and knees. So I spend a few minutes with them, down in the play park, while one of the microgeographers – a young woman, her hair trailing in the sand – speaks evangelically about the role microbiota will play in future architectures. When I get up, I look back to the town and in the midday gloom I see it as a blossoming slime mould, problem-solving and shimmering collectively. For some reason, this puts me in mind of Salmon's tale about an unfortunate addict who in the 1990s (these stories play on a difficult edge between public health interests and privacy) had infected a section of the town's teenage male population with Hepatitis B in exchange for their pocket money. While Salmon never groups such stories together, he relates a number of transformations, scares and catastrophes caused by the spread of tiny living organisms, claiming to have been out walking on a hill in Newton Abbot in 2005 with a GP who had just been issued with a list of local buildings designated for conversion to morgues in the event of an avian flu scare playing out. The authorities had planned for the deaths of up to one in three of the population. Salmon and his walking companions had looked strangely on the town and its passers-by as if they were already ghostly. I wonder if it is possible to find out which buildings were designated, and what that does to them: a morgue for dancing, a morgue for mending cars, a morgue for shopping, a morgue for watching movies.

Back at the door of my hotel, I meet another delegate – there *was* someone else from the conference staying here all along.... she has been suddenly alerted to the imminent death of her father and is rushing for the station. The hotel manager is driving her and he soon draws up and the woman is away. Later, she emails me to describe a journey leaping on and off multiple trains, crossing numerous train companies and networks, always with the wrong tickets, each time the guard helping, phoning ahead, arranging for the smooth execution of a two minute change of trains, always refusing to take any extra fare, of their union badges, of their 'railway family' loyalty, even of a guard who attempts to counsel her with the story of his own need – "it was a genuine sharing, he was lovely about his mother who was ill. Suddenly the system came alive, as if it was a human system, a system with a skeleton crew hidden inside the official one, improvising".

I imagine her running between platforms.

"It's like when they ban fishing and the fish come back in massive numbers; remove the neo-liberal crap for a second and human beings emerge out of nowhere."

She is able to hug her father before he dies.

A shadow biosphere, a Neanderthal recognition.

I collect a few things in my shoulder bag and set out again. I mooch about the pier for a few minutes. Outside the attractions are wrapped like artillery. Inside a sign on a simulator declaims: "ANXIETY, PANIC, TERROR, *breakthrough... the cycle never ends*".

Walking away from the sea, the 'main drag' is almost hypnotic; at the top a gate, with FUNLAND in cast iron, opens onto an in-between space with a strange booth; a barker is needling an unenthusiastic bunch of lads to bet their £2 against his £20 that they can hang on a pole for 2 minutes.

I feel as if I might spend the rest of my life exploring the parade's alternating stratigraphy of excess and absence. Maybe never ever leaving this stretch; there are enough cafés and the food will soon kill me. I am a referee for the different architectures wrestling each other; the Regency Palace has some ironwork that may even be Regency, then an Italianate Tower and a hoarding in the Chinese restaurant style. There is a scintillation of postmodern discourses in sugar, nationalism, exotic other, sentimentality: Fascism Street meets Poverty Row. Polished marble columns wrapped in a tsunami of anti-pigeon wire.

YOU THINK IT
WE PRINT IT!
Superman, Volkswagen, I Heart England.

Generalisations do not apply here: one failed anachronism (according to Salmon the longest continuously running movie house in the world until it closed) next to another (a steam-powered branch railway). Salmon promises a plastic chip-man, a humanoid cone of chips splashing vinegar on his own head; but he has been replaced by a flesh and blood Eastern European in a hand-made hat of giant yellow fabric chips, handing out samples from a Styrofoam punnet. His chips are as orange as Donald Trump! I eat one; it has that crispy fat thing that lures you in. I am tripping on animal grease.

The displays of T-shirts are like overpowering life choices: warriors or robotoid fans or fairy princesses, aggrieved parents or living sex dolls or improbable gangstas. Later, I pass young men sporting these shirts, rehearsing intimidating swaggers and poking their tats at the world; living USBs to a 'box set' gangland.

It would be easy to miss the gems under the awnings, to not raise your eyes to the terracotta mouldings above the drill-in shop signs. To not savour the fat on the air. Looking without sentimentality or cynicism, doing the best I can – and I am following instructions from Salmon here! – there is a poetry in the odd dynamics of new and old, and a kind of hyper-detailed and abstracted landscape of philosophical assumptions and ruling images condensed down onto kitchen magnets and sun hats. I do not need to buy anything to get their full value.

I wander across the railway lines and into a street called Hyde Road. Not much is designed here; there are so many layers – art deco, neo-neo-neoclassical, cheap temporary banners with childish fonts, pictograms, gothic (had to be in *Hyde* Road) – the whole is meaningless. No wonder the folk here are so reactionary; their clothes avoid any statement, nothing goes with anything else; with the exception of a few Goths they are terrified of uniforms. Even the man in a yellow two-piece has failed to find one to match the other. It's as if everyone were dressed from a jumble sale donated to by the upper middle classes. Not everyone is poor here, but there is a sort of poverty, not just of imagination, that pervades everything.

I find a really odd display of shop window dummies done up in wedding clothes; headless bridesmaids, bride with a painted face and a bridegroom with a fibreglass complexion. A poster advertises "health walks".

Around the corner in Torquay Road, a J.D. Wetherspoon pub, the Isaac Merritt (named after one of those sewing machine Singers), sets the bar for authenticity: a framed postcard showing a seafront of the 1960s, lit in New York neon. There is a humility too. There are no elders, only the old; weathering is the last remaining egalitarianism. The seagulls shriek in warning.

I play with the idea of getting the train straight home. I am not expected back for a couple of days; I am not even sure if I can swap my ticket. I dither before a heterotopian junk shop, shelves filled with a glorious concatenation of commercial icons: novelty bread bins, Stars Wars medievalism and Toby Juggery. What if we were to organise society more like a junk shop?

"Love the thing, hate the commodity" I had read that on a leaflet I had found in one of the conference bins.

I go back to the station to check the timetable, but cross to the wrong platform by mistake: a flaccid penis in spilled coffee on the floor of the footbridge, a steam locomotive pressuring up on the other side of a fence. I retrace my steps and wander aimlessly around the bus station for a while, then down the side of a church that is being converted into flats. Piles of broken slate. Where am I going? What am I doing? This feels like a very odd kind of 'conference report' to be wandering around in...

Opposite is an empty shop; among many things it has been, one faded sign reads "Internet Cafe". There is still some beauty in the building; its dimpled window, disembowelled security camera spilling guts like spaghetti, and a security grille like a piece of garden furniture.

I stand and look at the empty shop... at another limp dick splashed on a wall... at the buttocks of a stylish 'flat iron' building, its fine shape cluttered by layers of here today and mostly gone tomorrow entrepreneurs. What characterises these endless redundancies and barely recognisable adaptations is that they are all sites of connection – the 'flat iron' building is designed after something somewhere else, New York probably. I will find American colonial style houses with verandas and thin pillars hidden inside shells adopted like hermit crabs, I will find numerous Chinese characters, and neoclassical pillars hidden in more chicken wire.

What is in decline here is not simply economic, but connectivity, sense, weave; and rather than being torn apart, it is simply drooping.

The dull grey light eats up all the magic. Yet I am completely exhilarated.

A coat of arms so faded that none of its symbols nor any of its motto is legible. A scatter of sea-shells discarded in an alley. On a small ledge between two layers of limestone, differently worked, is a part of a charm, so perished that its plastic gems blend exactly with the fossilised crinoids in the stone ledge; another shell collection, this time junked into a giant puddle behind a den; a neatly dressed graffiti boy flying out of a yellow wall; more flaccid dicks in damp patches; two bricks like a ballsack strung for ballast beneath an A sign; a man with his world on his back yelling into a mobile "hello, Dave, I got rid of them"; a woman in a charity shop excited about "them doubling the thickness of Cup-a-Soup", her friend mourning the death of a budgie that caught influenza in a draught; those viruses again, even in the wind. I love the poetry of ordinary chat. Just as the wind emptied me out, now all these things have come rushing in and filling me up; I feel like a walking junkshop. Salmon's jumble of stories is dressing me differently.

I turn up an unnamed back way, beside the derelict internet café. On the side of a house near Winner Street ('Wynerde', vineyard) a reparative filler in the cracks on a sidewall has coalesced into a monstrous crinoid, like one of Cthulhu's inferiors found beneath the geology of madness. I can mention this so casually because one of the lounge bar papers has referenced the "sneaking up on reality" in what the philosopher Graham Harman calls "weird realism". Exploiting the imagination of H.P. Lovecraft, the writer of uncanny tales, Harman has found a dynamic gap in Lovecraft's writing, the refusal of the objects of his fiction to allow language to describe them, thus permitting Lovecraft to write at length of things that are always just out of the reach of his description, and yet this "absent thing-in-itself can have gravitational effects on the internal content of knowledge, just as Lovecraft can allude to the physical form of Cthulhu even while cancelling the literal terms of the description".

'A CENTURY Of Playtime' has shut for good. A bakery is selling intimidating marshmallow cones. In 'The Vinyl Frontier' – its logo incorporating a 33rpm disc into the body of the Starship Enterprise – a woman is singing as I enter: "you'll never walk aloooone.... you're a bit foreign, aren't you? There's good and bad in all races... I always say what I think, it's the quiet ones... know what I mean?" (Does she mean me? I hope she is too drunk – or is this an exaltation that would have made her a saint in another time? – to notice I am here.) "What's the clicking? Is that me – no! I've left my castanets in Cyprus!! Power to the people! Up the Revolution! They all complain, but they don't do anything..." God, is this what remains of Westcountry leftist radicalism? I feel quite warmed and heartened it could be so irrational; I wonder what things would be like if people like her were not tolerated, but in charge; maybe they soon will be. Salmon says that I will find an unlikely bust of the artist Robert Lenkiewicz in the window of a hairdressers, but I have no idea who he is. The faded word DUTY above a parking place. Torn tarpaulin flapping in noisy shreds from a roof crowned in scaffold.

This is a scarred body, but what would a body be if entirely composed of scars? Could it hold together?

A few days before, a woman lay in this street dying of stab wounds.

At the corner a mermaid is, without explanation, blowing a horn. Once I have found some wi-fi I look up mermaids playing horns and find only one, a twin-tailed one, like Starbucks' Melusine – though, to be precise, Melusine is a serpent not a fish – in an illustration in Richard de Fournival's 'Bestiaire d'Amour'. Or maybe Lasirn counts; a mermaid myth from Haiti, for she has a trumpet and a mirror; the mirror for the luminal/liminal region where sky and water meet, she blends opposites of storm and calm. Or maybe this is the horn-playing Arista, daughter of Disney's Triton; a story that could have started anywhere on the slave triangle linking Europe,

Africa and the Caribbean. Peeved hawks, a lion and possibly Cthulhu have been worked into the capitals on the pharmacy building.

Down Fisher Street a mediaeval cottage squats under a roof of moss. The pub sign of 'The Torbay Inn' is an old map, before the whole spa, health, romanticism thing happened to the English coastline. A house is being gutted.

At the end of the road, I pass a giant tree stump, part of a garden gobbled up. Sculpted in crazed faces that are cracking as the deadwood splits, winking through graffitied mascara; the seats in the base are howling mouths. Next door the flats have the feel of power stations that "rise like a surfacing whale from the sweeping landform". I scuttle round the rear of a strip of housing, through a communal drying area and salute its flying colours. I cross the road and walk behind the leisure centre, through derelict buildings, full of decades of tangled bramble, then ponds of rusty water, and tree stumps sporting shelves of fungi. I track the edge of a sports field and, in a corner, take a muddy path into the woods and on to a forbidding, crudely stencilled notice:

PRIVATE NATURE
RESERVE
KEEP OUT

I backtrack, skirt the woods, try to cross a stream, but I am too nervous to dare step into its soft bed, looking like stinking chocolate, and instead find another way in, struggling up a cloggy hill beside slipping dogs with invisible owners.

Near the top of the hill I get scared. The dogs are gone, the wind drops. The silence feels heavy. I can see the layout of the land below: a trailer camp, playing fields, the sea. I like dogs so I zoom in on some distant barking for company. I am torn between the exposed crown of the hill and its creepy paths. I meet no one, but I feel watched. Faces in trees. I imagine wolves dressed in North Face and jeans. Things made of mud with fingers and tongues. Eeee. I want to go back now, but came this way because it seemed the quickest way of going back. Why did I think there'd be anyone out here? Did I assume that radical walkers would make for the woods like ramblers?

Just as things can change from interesting to magical so quickly, and in the ruins of a palace or under a precarious tree you can raise your arms from your sides and waggle your hands with the angry leaves, become tree, well, just as quickly I am a little girl, head full of warnings and ugly fairy tales and stuff I should never have been allowed to watch by irresponsible parents....

A crazy spaniel runs up. I fuss it for a moment before it runs off; no owner appears.

A.J. Salmon has dredged up a letter about this place from the correspondence pages of the *Fortean Times* to add to some contemporary ugliness about cock fights and badger baiting. Although Salmon's narrative is largely an interpretative one, it is clear that he has walked these places, probably repeatedly. Published in the 1980s, the letter Salmon quotes claims to describe events in the woods I am becoming entangled in, fording its glutinous streams, misled by its paths to full stops and protected areas. The correspondent, a Neville Stanikk, writes of a second disused quarry in the woods "which could only be reached by climbing a cliff and forcing one's way through bramble and holly thicket". Stanikk "being of an artistic temperament" regarded the quarry floor as his "canvas" and decorated it with a pentagram of white pebbles, triggering rampant local 'foaftales' of Satanic kidnap and human sacrifice.

The Devil is always in this landscape. 'Dawlish', which I had passed through on the train, means 'devil water'. In 1855, people there had gone on an armed hunt for the cloven-hoofed one, and cornered him in a wood. Their hounds returned "baying and terrified". There are stones in the sea off Dawlish that are all that is left of a parson and his clerk, tricked into the waves by a partying Devil. Salmon has drawn on the work of local Forteans to lay out a plethora of interpretations for the "devil's footprints" that people found in 1855 in the snow, trailing from Exmouth to Totnes: kangaroos, otters, a grapple dangling from a balloon, ufos, and most extraordinarily, four or five hundred Romanies from "seven tribes" using 'measure stilts' made from step ladders, systematically marking the area to scare off rival Romanies.

Whatever 'it' was, it was not and never could be one thing – able to vault a 14-foot wall and yet pass through a tiny pipe. It was a mutability. In the same way as its route described a certain geographical territory, so it also appropriated an ideological territory. Claims were made by anti-Puseyites (those who objected to ritual in the Church of England) about the devilish qualities of their 'high church' neighbours, determined to drive the last hint of faith from their churches. "The hounds of homogeneity that Pan had sent scarpering" were back.

I turn around, drop down through the trees and the slippery steps in the grass, rewalk my path through the sports field and leisure centre. I am heading back to the train station, but on the Dartmouth Road I meet a student who I saw attending the papers in the improvised session earlier; she lives locally. I walk with her a way down Dartmouth Road, the wrong way for me now, till her turning. I tell her of my turning back in the woods and she speaks about fear, how it is fear that drives her interest in walking and geography; she fears everything, fear has become a language for her, she measures every place by panic and every person by their level of threat. I should have asked her how she assesses me; but it only strikes me later that she might have interpreted my Northern friendliness as a kind of aggression.

ANXIETY, PANIC, TERROR, breakthrough... the cycle never ends.

I'm trapped in that cycle. I had thought that my walking now might help. The student points me back up the main road, and describes the turning to the steam railway station. I can catch that train back to the main town station. Then the train north.

Torbay Road, Great Western Road, bus station, junction of Dartmouth Road and Totnes Road, unnamed service road behind New Street, unnamed road into Palace Avenue, Winner Street, Fisher Street, Dartmouth Road, Great Western Close, Dartmouth Road, service road behind Torbay Leisure centre, edge of playing field, various paths on Clennon Hill, Dartmouth Road.

Chapter Three: Goodrington

I somehow miss the turning for the steam railway and end up in a huge, empty car park. The sun comes out and turns a scree of compressed sandstone at the edge of the car park blood red. A branch, six metres long, has been torn from a tree and lies pointing to a set of wooden steps up a steep red mound. The steps are rotted a little, with few footprints, but muddy. For no reason, I decide to climb the stairs. To what? This is nothing, surely? A few trees. The attraction is across the other side of the car park; sets of water slides and pools, the beach, the trainline somewhere there.

It's a strange place I have chosen to explore. High up above the car park, I feel slightly vertiginous. I have only been walking for an hour or so; I can't have found *somewhere*. The place feels very intense, however. A tree grows precariously from a small cliff of red slate, half its roots undermined and exposed and the whole thing hanging above a deep, wide channel, unfeasibly spreading itself upwards like a spray of inverted tentacles. Someone has painted the trunk with bright yellow alien graffiti, a watery voice prompting me to see the eye and beak of a squid in it; though it is just as likely to represent a flying machine. Close by is half an archway, snapped sometime in two. On one side a person-sized 'human-carrot' has been graffitied.

I am struck by feelings of amputation and dismemberment, by a new set of steps that disappear into the ground.

On what remains of a wall, someone has left a sophisticated marijuana holder, on the lid it says AMSTERDAM and I can't help but think of Hamsterdam in 'The Wire'; a place of experimental solutions. The box sits on a small, heavily-thumbed paperback: *The King in Yellow* by Robert Chambers. I flick through it – one chapter is called 'The Yellow Sign'. I wouldn't want to get too stoned up here, with all these sheer drops. I am becoming unnecessarily sensitive, but I am strangely seized by the place. Totally distracted; it does not strike me until later that maybe the owner of the book and box might return, might want them back; or that he might even be here now, hidden.

I keep holding my arms up to the precarious octopus tree and its yellow jellyfish spaceship graffiti; as if I am inventing a new religion.

Something happened here. Time was truncated like the arch. Something is still held in mid-air, but all the oxygen is sucked out of it.

ANXIETY, PANIC, TERROR, breakthrough... the cycle never ends

But I am not scared. Imagination running away with me, for sure. What I am feeling is joy; away from having to analyse and to interpret, the images and the thick materials and solid stones and teetering tree are all running directly into me.

I flick through the book. "Have you found the Yellow Sign?" It seems to be a collection of interlinked tales, all connected by this mysterious Yellow Sign. Then it gets weird, because in one of the stories, the dope box I found here on the broken wall, or one very like it, appears in the writing. A character, an artist, opens it up, a gift from his model: "on the pink cotton inside lay a clasp of black onyx, on which was inlaid a curious symbol or letter in gold. It was neither Arabic or Chinese, nor, as I found afterwards, did it belong to any human script."

I am certain the enigmatic jelly saucer graffito is this Yellow Sign! The neither-this-nor-thatness of it! The artist's model, Tess, who finds it in the story, like me, came across it dropped or abandoned, "she had found it one day coming from the Aquarium at the Battery". And she explains that, "'That was last winter, the very day I had the first horrid dream about the hearse'"; a dream in which an elusive man they both keep seeing in the local churchyard drives the hearse.

The artist tries to dismiss their fears as no more than "a soft-shell crab dream", but The Yellow Sign calls forth the hearse driver from their reveries. When he arrives, he comes in as numinous a description as any in Lovecraft. A doctor finds the artist barely alive, Tess dead, and the driver who haunted them both "a horrible decomposed heap on the floor – the livid corpse of the watchman from the church: 'I have no theory, no explanation. That man must have been dead for months!'"

I took the paperback and put it in my backpack. Not for the horror, but for the possibility that if time was messing with me, then I could mess with time.

Online later, I found a brief mention of there having been a big house up here above the car park. Called SIMLA, it was another part of India appropriated to Devon. A gazette had one Samuel Slade, a grocer in Torquay, living there in the late 19th century; the same Samuel Slade perhaps as was digging up kists and other grave goods on Dartmoor at the same time? After his most significant find, this Slade went to fetch William Pengelly, the great Torbay palæontologist, but by the time they returned, Slade's helpers had deserted and "stolen his umbrella". Slade proceeded to thieve the five great slabs of the Thornworthy tomb for Torquay Museum. The stones have since been transferred to a museum on the moor. Stones that should be covered in earth, to make a mound. I would keep seeing them.... there would be one alongside Roselands Road; it was probably just builders' spoil, but even that might contain recycled parts of forgotten tombs.

SIMLA was bombed in World War II. Searching online for "Simla Paignton" takes me to a posting about wartime casualties, but no mention of victims. The interference of colonial echoes in waves of fascist bombers. The quiet up here is queasy.

From a break in the trees, I can see beyond the railway station across the bay to Brixham and Berry Head, where the key back story in director Clive Austin's feature 'The Great Walk' (2013) takes place: the disappearance of a radical walker that acrimoniously destroys 'The Nine' walking group and sends them splintering into abject dispersal, torn by suspicion. And where the southernmost colony of guillemots will be one of the first signals that climate change and temperature rise are pushing resilient species around.

According to a copy of the local rag I found in the bar of my hotel, four bodies have washed up this month in the bay; different times, different places, all middle-aged men. If there is a meaningful pattern, other than a common despair, the local media are not telling.

The thing about a mobile art is that it moves within other mobilities; there is no universe at rest, only the ongoing shipwreck that is our single opportunity.

Standing on the edge of the sheer drop to the car park, I can see below the horizon the oil tankers, motionless, waiting for the price of oil to shift on the markets before they can unload profitably. Turning time into money by immobility. I have no way of making sense of that. It turns my head into the kind of thought experiment that Einstein was famous for; a 'stand in' for the woman on the train travelling close to the speed of light being overtaken by constants. Except that I am not on the train, I am not going home, I am imagining being the woman on the train and wondering whether her imagination slides up the curve of attraction bent by that locomotive the same way as mine. Could I experience it right off its tracks?

Two young women surprise me, coming up the rotting wooden steps and making their way deep into the ruin of the site; I suppose they have come to talk, to somehow rearrange the ruins of their own lives in relation to these. Maybe smoke some dope and text their friends.

"'drunk alive!... the beak is the beast that enters into you, the sucker is what of you enters the beast, but far worse than the terror of being eaten alive is the indescribable ordeal of being drunk alive!'"

"That's quite something..."

"It's something like that. It's French..."

"Jules Verne?"

"No. I'll google it."

I've bumped into a group from the fringe conference – 'psychoswimographers' – they have come searching for a "crystal cave". I meet them clustered at an information board at the back of Goodrington Sands, next to a fake adobe Spanish-colonial café on the edge of a boating lake. The café looks like a badly iced cake. I am there to ask directions for the station. I found the bridge over the line, but got lost in a strange tangle of water slides, redundant go-kart track and disused offices, and distracted by a fabulous palimpsest of faded layers of advertisement that reads TAKE INFINITE PLEASURE WHEREVER YOU GO. I want to stop there. To savour the rhyme of PLEASURE WHEREVER.

"We're cheating," says the Irish one. "We shouldn't be psycho'ing until we're in the water."

"How can you 'drift' in water?" Then I realise just how stupid that question is.

The swimmers are very excited by the story of Peggy's Pool and want to test its bottomlessness. But Peggy's Pool's has been concreted over and filled with giant fibreglass swans.

According to the information board, the wall of the children's playground is the remnant of a huge 'cottage' owned by the 'Misses Brown', beyond which is a green space marked out by four stone bollards, the bounds of a burial ground – hundreds of Napoleonic French cadavers, former tenants of a 'hospital', now a BREWERS FAYRE pub, its tatty lettering gap-toothed. The corpses vibrate under the various games of football and Frisbee. A council plaque asks for "the appropriate degree of respect". Maybe it is better for one's grave to become a playground; the French playwright Jean Genet advocated that all performances be staged where the audience must first walk through graves to get to the auditorium. I think I agree. But for everything, not just theatre.

The hem of the ocean is glowing green with revived sea grasses. The offspring of huge fish, theoretically, swim in their shadows. Perhaps life is coming back.

We pass through the weird confabulation of structures; the hospital turned pub, the wriggling turquoise worm cast of a waterslide, a geological interpretation office that seems permanently shut, a bellowing mosaic Basking Shark protesting its missing pieces. This is where I got lost before! For a place of spectacle and holiday, the ruin in structure and details is striking: a metal gibbet in the play park, a row of beach huts in Smarties colours, a steam train reversing its Pullman observation carriages, hands waving to strangers, hopeful for reply.

And down onto the beach. My feet in the sand, at last.

In August 1998 on the beaches at Goodrington, Preston and Paignton, due to sustained high temperatures, a shoal of razorfish moved further inshore than is usual and at low tide a panic ensued among the holidaymakers as hundreds cut their feet on the shells resting just beneath the surface of the sand in shallow water. The behaviour of the animals was unusual, but explainable; a reminder that the predictability of nature is only part of the story, and that all sorts of different rhythms – colony collapse, tremors, drift, flocking – some with violent and sudden force, are interwoven with the more easily foreseen. The fact that this parable-like event (described by the local MP, a witness, as "like a scene from Jaws") was caused by a common shoreline sea creature is a pointer that the coming plagues will consist of 'simple creatures' rather than monsters.

At the end of the beach, we clamber over the rocks as they go through their geological phases, red and soft, hardened with razor-like barnacles, eroded pools of green slushy weed, breccias, mudstones, slates, pumice from a volcanic vent. The further we climb round the cliff base the further back in time we go, and the rock gets sharper.

After half an hour of clambering we find the cave. Stripped of its wonders by Victorians unable to restrain themselves from the plunder in their own land they had meted out to everyone else's. A weird self-wounding. A sign that there was a kind of atomism at the heart of their empire, what geologists call an "unconformity", a missing few hundred years of empathy. That all their obedience is in the name of doing whatever they liked to others. An empty yoni to Shag Rock's shrunken and disappearing lingam.

There are still some strange butterscotch crystals in the cave, splayed like a broken chocolate orange. Made in the same material, a tiny pyramid minus its benben stone; the egg-island of origins chipped from its base. Geometry without an artist, an immaculate annihilation. I have read of the horrors visited on those who remove stones from cairns; we return the butterscotch.

From the mouth of the Crystal Cave, we can see to Churston and its beach huts, like a necklace of cheap beads. And maybe I imagine it, because it does not make much sense on Google Maps, but I think I see the modernist shapes of the houses on Broadsands Road and Rock Close; the failed attempt to create a model modernist community there. The impetus had come from the Elmhirsts' experimental arts and design community at Dartington Hall, a few miles away, but it was scuppered by the ideology of individualism, and the fear and suspicion of neighbours: "I hope it will never be mentioned to those who may dwell at Churston that they are intended to become a community or that there would be any species of communal life".

ANY SPECIES OF COMMUNAL LIFE...

It is as if a theory of miscegenation were made universal; that any contact – other than Margaret Thatcher's individual and family – could not be 'natural', and certainly never to be mentioned; that anything else would take on species-qualities, leviathan, monstrous; why, with those unimpeded sea views thanks to the flat roofs, what fishy things might they become!

The architectural designs for the Churston houses were described by the local Planning Committee as like "Exeter jail, a sugar box with slits cut in it, or a Lancashire cotton factory". Political democracy failed the region then, as Salmon claims it is failing it now. Like the Lutyens experiment at Cockington, the Churston modernist community was an attempt to get ahead of history; so, this place had been modern once and been turned back by cold sabotage. Rubbish had been 'freely' chosen over elegance, the politicians and planners climbing over the ruins they were piling up at their own feet. Conservative populists condemned these spaces to passivity. And it worked, at the expense of retaining only the worst and most insular of identities, the invention of a localism completely at odds with the history of its historically multiplicitous and infected spaces.

Salmon describes exactly what they feared: a scene at Elbury Cove, just below Churston, from Michael Winner's 1964 movie 'The System' (aka 'The Girl-Getters'). Skull heads, a huge mask leaking from the nose, a party on the beach that turns into a ritual procession. All written by a Brixham author. Chanting "Down with the groom, down with the groom!" young men, who each year gather in Torquay and connive to seduce young female holidaymakers, burn dummies, not of high church

Anglicans like those burned on the cathedral fires, but of a marriage couple, bride and groom, echoes from Hyde Road; an incineration of holy matrimony.

In view too is Galmpton, where Robert Graves at Vale House wrote *The White Goddess*, about an essential three-fold muse-divinity within all divinities, for which he invented his own fundamental source: a tree calendar for which there is no equivalent in historical literature. 'Captain' Graves's thesis rests on his assumption that his intuition and the gathering of real trees could only mean that the poetic timetable he imagined must once have been real, but lost.

For my sake the psychoswimographers turn back where the rocks become sheer cliff. I want to swim with them, but I have all my things to carry. I do not see the attraction in wading barefoot across sharp underwater rocks. Am I ruining things for us? Perhaps I *should* cut up my feet, shed one skin to reveal the raw bone-pilgrim underneath? But the psychoswimographers are far more pragmatic and we scuttle back across the eras to a tiny beach at the bottom of a set of steps. When we first passed through it, the little cove had been empty, but now there is a genial professor-type, seated in a mudstone armchair, perusing a journal. He does not look up. When he looks, he does not speak. As if he expects us to ask him the question. He soon leaves.

The T-shirts worn by the psychoswimographers are stained with iron oxide from the rocks.

I gyrate under a borrowed towel to dress in a borrowed swimming costume. Despite occasional critical forays into the theatrical, it's never struck me before that one wears a *costume* to swim. Before I met these psychoswimographers I had not thought of how dance-like the whole swimming thing, with its balletic strokes, is.

The water is a partner, generous with its lifts.

No. The water is as icy as a critic. The sand is merciful. While the others move resolutely up to their necks I proceed a digit, and then a limb, at a time, feeling viscera shrink. The blood just under my skin is racing furiously. How can I be this stupid? it demands. The water is as clear as it is cold; like bathing in a Fox's Glacier Mint. It makes everything very 'now'; it sucks in and concentrates everything into the sharp point of its particular cold. I wonder what the 'professor' was reading; something obscure and interesting I hope, a poem by Blok perhaps, but it is more likely a back copy of *Lobster*, an account of tangles by someone enmeshed, tentacles critiquing tentacles, wrapping untruths inside conspiracies, enigmas in small clubs of men. I am so sick of them. Their worship of life-as-thriller. Their big boys' rules that run through everything like calcite; bright, invisible and hard.

The psychoswimographers swim out from the narrow end of the funnel of water into the open sea. Their goggles bump along above the surface and they call back encouragement. The cold is intimate with my hips. Goosebumps come rippling up my front and I press on through the water's thickness. I am surprised when a dark warmth comes back to me; as if I leapfrogged straight to the latter stages of hypothermia. I am aware now that walking is not enough; I have to step out of my depth and change.

Out at the edge where the rocks end their triangle in uneven sea, the psychoswimographers are turning somersaults and shouting something about ideas; but I am deep in the soft lozenge silence of the tiny cove. I slip off the sand and into the thick liquid, surprised at how buoyed I am. And how it changes everything; shocked at just how land-locked my usual way of seeing is. But this is like being inside a 3D model; with each stroke the two house-high walls of rock turn their masses lazily, opening up an orifice to my left. A fleshy stump of rock pushes up above the surface, and white flecks react. Everything is much bigger now. I have only swum a couple of tentative breast strokes from my shoreline mentality, but things have all gone jelly, Max Ernst unexpectedly animated.

Vanessa, one of the psychoswimographers, speaks about "jellies". She is a Jellyfish Whisperer. I had not thought much about stings; for sure, climate change had washed up some giant jelly things here the summer before; there were photos of them in the café I wrote my notes in. But I was more fixating on the four bodies washed up in the bay in a month, the swell of despair that had waterlogged them, and that being "drunk alive" may be a more genuine psychogeographical state of being than reading books about it.

Back on the shore I talk again to Ness. She swims with endurance swimmers, competitive swimmers, all-year-round swimmers; she swims weird places like ornamental ponds and the Trafalgar Square fountains (the battle where those dead, buried back there under Youngs Park, got their injuries) and lidos and the Liffey (*An Life*). There is a continuity between her swimming and a more sporty, ordinary, physical one; closer than that between radical walking and, say, rambling. But maybe that is unfair to radical walking; maybe it is necessary to push off from a number of shores?

As I turn back to the thinning strip of beach, four large black Labradors come bounding and slithering down the rocks from the direction of Goodrington and two black and one yellowy-white Labradors from the direction we have come. I wonder how we did not see any of them before. Did they swim round from Broadsands? They crash into the water around me. The seven dogs are a wonky chequerboard and I am a bobbing knight. I try to lure them deeper into the water, to swim with them, but they have gone as quickly as they arrived, heading off in opposite directions to those from which they came; no sign of owners.

We climb up a volcanic vent that Salmon calls 'Sugarloaf' and our ways part where the path junctions off down a little alley to the left, into Oyster Bend. They carry away my wet costume and towel.

There are tiny lion's heads on the semis here; African crystals. In one of the gardens is an antique cart once used for transporting holidaymakers' suitcases from the station to their lodgings. Some of the houses have the same Spanish Colonial look as the café. Once across the main road, past a huge amputated aircraft propeller, I feel a grid of missing and overridden roads, half roads and spirit roads, the ghost of a village green, a sign for 'Crystal Close', cul-de-sacs and roads to nowhere, roads covered in green moss and three odd grey-pink rock columns and an old faded-red pillar box. What is the meaning of these colour-coded combinations?

At the junction of Drake and Grange Roads I turn up the footpath called Roselands Road, but it is no Road; or maybe it was a very long time ago. It has the feel of something that predates other marks, it predates the stuckness of the suburbs, the path fades at times then lowers itself into the clear shape of a hollow way. In places fallen trees block the way through; a large section of fence has blown down, the part still standing sports a fading and untouched neo-Nazi graffito. It is easy to miss just how extreme the politics here are – the prettiness, the fun of holiday, the shapes of entertainment could all throw a glancing surveillance off their trail, but here walking shocks me. In the creases of lamp posts, scratched in the council paint of old benches, burned with lighters into the roofs of shelters – 'BNP' means almost nothing organisationally now, but here these letters are an untouched part of the backdrop. No one had attacked them or painted them out. Few people are so singular and narrow in their politics as these three letters; people move along continua and such letters stretch them towards genocide; it is an imprinting 'node'.

Large branches and thick trunks have crashed down across the path and repeatedly I have to lever myself under and over the broken trees; the path is flanked by a constricted stream that has all the bondage marks of a mill leat. The path peters out, but I follow its line across the field as if there were still something there. I mistake the screaming of children at play in a school playground for the zoo, which I know is somewhere nearby, a woman I ask for directions mentions it. The yelps and cries do not sound like those of a generation stitched to their phones; but of children loving being outside on a cold wet day and loving being with each other. A woman with a dog, which licks my hand, chats briefly.

A chequerboard is propped in the window of a house. I think of the seven dogs; of night and day and weaving.

Tanners Road, car park, Goodrington Sands South beach, Saltern Cove, Armchair Rock, Shell Cove, Crystal Cove, up the path at Armchair Rock, Coastal Path going north, Oyster Bend, Barn Road, left along Dartmouth Road, Hookhills Grove, right into Hookhills Road, Grange Road, at the junction with Drake Drive left down the Roselands Road footpath and then along path through hollow lane and fields and hollow lane/alley until Roselands Drive, cross over and down the footpath opposite to Brixham Road, turn right, Battersway Road, Claylands Drive, entrance to Paignton Zoo.

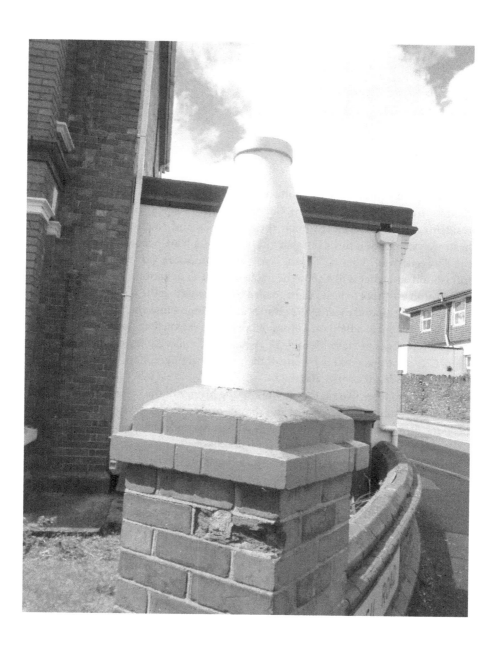

Chapter Four: Back into Paignton and on to Cockington Court

Paignton Zoo's giraffe house produces a fluctuating low-frequency drone which induces tremors, irritation, heart flutters and disturbance in the bodies of local residents, "waves passing through their buttocks and thighs". Folk blamed the heating system. But it turns out that giraffes hum; at least, according to biologists at the University of Vienna. Giraffes are communicators on the border between infrasound and what is just about hearable by us. The irritations and upsets suffered at Paignton are those of its giraffes; goaded by the refusal of the residents to interpret, translate and respond to what the giraffes are humming into their buttocks.

I take a room at a B&B on Totnes Road. Before exhaustion closes above my head I read a few pages of Steve Mentz's *Shipwreck Modernity: Ecologies of Globalization, 1550-1719*, lent/given to me by one of the psychoswimographers. I'd worried about extra luggage, but it's worth its weight.

Mentz proposes two motors at work in the history of the colonial period, which isn't over yet: theft (that's obvious) and composture (as in the work of a compost heap breaking down dead stuff into nutrients). Modernity, under the pretence of producing itself, was stolen, via the Renaissance, from antiquity; posing as a re-birth: "[T]he past, like the recycling, never goes away. A composting model recognizes multiple presences in multiple states of decay... a fertilizing combination of the living and the dead".

Rather than discovery, and more than conquest, what characterises globalisation best for Mentz is shipwreck "reinscribing onto vaster and less-known spaces classical and medieval tropes of doomed ships and misdirected sailors. Shipwreck becomes less the exception than the rule".

Then, coming right up to date, Mentz challenges the idea of an "Anthropocene", an era in which humans become an independent geological force. Even if it is the fault of humans that the climate is in such an awful state, that still doesn't make it *our* climate or *our* era. In place of the Anthropocene's tale of dominant human influence on the planet, Mentz proposes a 'salad' of forces. But that still doesn't mean things are going to be OK.

I am trying to get to sleep now, but I am just as spooked as Mentz is by the prospect of a "coming era" of jellies which "beheads Anthropos, but at a great cost. In a heat death of supercomposture, everything becomes the same as everything else".

Eeee.

I didn't know then how many wrecks I would encounter: the South Coaster between Dawlish Warren and Starcross, the imploded diving ship in Plymouth, even Lethbridge's pool in his garden was the scene of a kind of controlled shipwreck, the Venetian galley with its slaves on Church Rocks, another slave ship sunk at A la Ronde, Crowhurst's 'Teignmouth Electron', Simon Chalk's 'Spirit of Teignmouth' which wrecked before it even sailed, Pete Goss's catamaran 'Team Philips', the Pirate's Chest café at Coryton Cove, incinerated, and T-189 sunk on top of HMS Venerable's wreck at Roundham Head (the last are two of over 100 wrecks in Torbay gone under in the last 300 years). Each is a ruin of an ambition; described through the figure, thieved from antiquity by Osip Mandelstam, of Ulysses and his "unbridled thirst for space".

That night I dreamed of a door that moved around on its own. It reminded me of Gwenda in Agatha Christie's 'Sleeping Murder' who asks to put a new door through a wall in her home, only for the workmen to discover that there has been one there before; she orders new steps and new wallpaper and in both cases she has chosen what was there years before.

The following morning, I immediately pass a door in a tall high wall, bricked up. Next to it is an entrance between two stubby pillars to a park. I feel drawn, but nervous. I read the information board guiltily, like someone in a gallery who consults a painting's label rather than trust their own judgement. I like the sound of the meadow, but I will give the woods a miss.

Stepping through the pillars, I am shocked by the change of sound level; the engines from the road are suddenly and absurdly muffled. A wave of quietness comes surging over me. It does not make much sense physically, I have only taken a couple of steps. I am in a pleasingly cool, dark tunnel of trees. The day has started hot and I am enjoying a shady, quiet transition.

Ahead, a mouth of sun opens upon the meadow. Beyond are the deep woods. Two paths join a third and in the middle of the base of the triangle a woman is seated, head back, eyes closed, lapping up the sunlight. To the right of her is an odd-looking tree: a huge, thick and even cylinder of green, its trunk encased in geometrical ivy, and then at the top, a single bough of the tree has escaped and sprayed out a canopy. An absurdist tree. I take the path to my left, intending to head back to the road, but the path keeps leading me to locked gates labelled NO ENTRY and I lack the cheek to climb them. The path takes me into the woods I did not want to visit.

I pass another strange tree. An even huger trunk, but this one with massing branches split and crumpled to the ground, the limp arms of a defeated fighter. I wonder about climbing up to it, but keep to the path tracking the edge of the woods. All it does is bring me to another locked gate and NO ENTRY and then uphill deeper into the trees. I hear voices. I turn and begin to retrace my steps, but notice there is a quicker way back via the giant tree. I pick my way down carefully, foothold to foothold, root to rock to slope, noticing that this clamber is down some older path: rusted and twisted remnants of railings are not quite hidden in the leaves.

Back in the meadow, two spaniels are playing in the shadow of a tree so perfect in its canopy that the scene looks like the final shot from something gnostic directed by David Lynch. I pass the drive to Primley Lodge and turn into Waterleat Road, and there, up a turning to the right, are the marks of a mill leat; the tops of two arches in a red stone wall almost buried by a rising road surface. I follow the road in a spiral up and around the hill, with the meadow and the woods hidden within it. I am in a band of suburbia, now. A study in small front gardens: bleak and Zen, crazy-paved, riot of colour, mess of lavender and leafy shrubs, manicured mini-lawn, concrete gryphon and giant snail. Each garden united by the same mildly individualistic indifference. And the house names: KYOTO, PARADISE CORNER, HARLEQUIN. Then it changes as the incline steepens – car graveyard, a garage labelled MAN CAVE – the houses are smaller, less display, grey pebble-dashing, until the gardens disappear altogether, to be replaced by concrete car-pads. A youth delivers bright red menus for a Chinese buffet.

A bumper sticker: 23RD JUNE. INDEPENDENCE DAY. Another: JUSTICE FOR SGT BLACKMAN.

From the top of a steep road, the waters of the bay are spread out, half deep blue, half sky blue. The giant buildings on the Torquay heights stand out. Monolith Monsters. A scream from a house nearby. Then silence.

The long road is so steep and the street arrangement so uniformly bound to units of dwelling that there appears to be no 'street life' possible. No marks of public presence, no place to sit or meet, a giant ribbon development of small houses, terraces and bungalows. A Reliant Robin struggles up the hill. A van signed MARK THE SPARK ELECTRICIAN. A house called CORTINA.

There's an empty bungalow with a SOLD sign outside. I squeeze through the overgrown front garden and under the vast web of a giant Garden Spider, its huge body poised centrally. Inside, the furnishings have been removed, but from the creamy paintwork and the bronzy ceramics of the fireplace, and the original metal window frames at odds with neighbours' PVC, it looks like this home has never been redecorated since it was first occupied; a particular type of hermitage.

And then it all changes, in a kind of cosmic gear shift I turn off near the bottom and up a hill enclosed by tall red sandstone walls, past a house called LODGE and through a gap in the wall and over a metal stile. I clamber up what looks like a possible track under the sweeping cloak of leaves, and enter a world of dens, of overhanging tree roots, of improvised grates and chimneys, a canyon in miniature, a fantasyland for growing up in, the red earth and the roots making this place fleshy and internal, shadowy and illicit, socialised and naughty. I notice that what I thought was a bank of earth is an old sandstone wall and I clamber back down the crumbling slope, around this wall, up a set of steps and through an archway, up another set and onto a ledge beneath a long wall that stretches away to my left. I climb up yet another set of steps and emerge in a low key public area with an incongruous purple and orange seat, and then into a small car park beside a large chapel.

I know, from Salmon, what this is. A Father Pinmore had come here secretly in the 1880s to view the property of a virulently anti-Catholic landowner. While a local accomplice distracted the bigot, Father Pinmore, the procurator for Marist Fathers who were fleeing a ban against religious orders in the French Republic, sneaked about the gardens, becoming stuck in a hedge, his braces snapping and his trousers falling down.

By 1883 a monastery had been established and the tall gothic building here was opened as its chapel; the figure of Mary – known to the locals as 'The White Lady' – made in cast iron, towering six metres above the roof, looks back to France. The Fathers were joined by Marist Sisters and a Marist Convent was established in Paignton; then one for Sacred Heart Sisters in Goodrington. These institutions have all gone now; the monastery closing in 1970. Reading Salmon, and later, when I find a very old plaque to Belgian refugees, here over a century ago, I was becoming aware of these temporary diversities, that come and go, and rarely leave such a trace as this grand chapel. In 1940, Breton fishermen and their families (32 in all) sailed into Paignton to escape the Nazi occupation; when they returned in 1945 they took even their dead back with them aboard their trawlers.

The church had wanted to remove 'The White Lady' to their new building in town, but gave in to local pressure to leave it where it is; though what jumble of devotion and superstition lay behind these appeals might be rich to investigate; what Gravesian condensing of divinity?

Today the building houses a charity that runs a food bank and furniture provision in the town and provides counselling services. Later I experience a similar feeling at Oldway Mansion; a power around loss and spectral return, except that here it is of God and not a sewing machine. This is evidenced in the wreckages of old things: that where secularism, persecution and the decline of manufactures had all failed to destroy them, neo-liberalism with its indifference to the integrity of gods or machines, has triumphed in its destruction of varieties of public space. Yet it cannot quite dominate their ruins. I don't think to try the door of the chapel. I would not have hesitated if this was an Anglican country church; and I wonder later how much, apart from time, separates me from the culture of that bigot landowner.

At the bottom of Monastery Road, where it runs into Winner Hill Road, I feel as if I am coming into the Saxon part of the town. These are the tiny streets deplored by the planner Thomas Sharp, who was inspired by Haussmann's demolitions in Paris; I had never heard of him, until I read of him thanks to Salmon. Part of that same contempt for working class life, a 'for their own good' that likes to present itself as liberal, and that is, as I walk, taking such a kicking through the medium of Brexit.

Totnes Road, Waterleat Road, Waterleat Avenue, Clifton Road, Winner Hill Road, through gateway and up steps to car park of monastery building, Berry Drive, through path to Monastery Road, left onto Winner Hill Road, right onto Winner Street.

The road brings me directly out, shockingly and abruptly, on the recent murder scene on Winner Street. I immediately recognise it from the pictures in the local paper. Flowers are beginning to wilt in small bouquets. A Polish woman, Agnieszka Szymura, a shop worker, was knifed and died in the street. A man, Toryino Williams, has been charged with her killing. (The case will never come to trial; before my journey is over, I read online that Williams has been found dead in his Exeter cell.)

A house named THE OLD LABOUR CLUB – a 1990s' relic of the Blairite turn in the Labour Party. Blair is making noises about "a return" to British politics, and about the absence of a political force "at the centre". Real or otherwise, the 'council estate' vote for withdrawal from the EU has terrified a political establishment that included rather more people than even they imagined; prudishly admonishing the ill-informed and fearful, then fleeing wildly to embrace, trick or, once again, ostracise them. But the winds are not getting back in the box.

Off Winner Street, I turn into Palace Avenue and in a charity shop buy a copy of *Sir Constant: Knight of the Great King* by W.E. Cule and a sweet-looking 1930s' box of travel draughts. Later, when I open the box I find that there is no board, only counters. I am delighted! I have bought a game without limits, each square borderless and conceptual. A board made of frisky Labradors. I begin to leave the draughts in niches and on narrow ledges, wondering if I might one day return to move them on to another concept. Hadn't Yoko Ono or one of those Fluxus types played chess with only pieces of one colour? Without a board, the game of war becomes a dance.

Back onto Winner Street, between strange swimming sperm gates and through Sign Walk, into a car park ringed in breccias in Crown and Anchor Way, named after the pub where Torbay Lodge no. 427 was founded in 1772 and thrived until a dispute over ritual in 1824 climaxed with the Senior Warden gathering up every apron he could seize and throwing them onto the open fire. Along another breccia wall in Tower Road, I pass a red, mediaeval tower, wrongly attributed as the site for a Bible translation that never happened here; like the writing of 'The Waste Land' in a Torquay bus shelter or the filming in Occombe Woods. So many towers in this town, unexpectedly, and many of them, not just here, but at intervals along my entire walk, are Italianate; thieved parts of modernity stolen from the Renaissance to claim 'civilisation' for industries driven by imports of ideas and goods.

Into Gerston Place; I feel I might be overshooting something, as if I am one of those pebbles of limestone, smoothing too much in the flood of waters and polishing in sand; sliding over things. I halt at the mildly staid body of an old Institute turned 'Enterprise Centre', the words "SCHOOL OF ART AND SCIENCE" carved in its best custard stone. Down its side it spills its guts, four metres up, in an extraordinary mural, gross in its Pre-Raphaelite sentimentality and vicious in the irony of its erosion: the badge of Painting is now worn completely empty! Long lost is whatever image it had used to represent itself to itself.

I feel bad walking away, re-tracing my steps, like I am being painted-by-numbers; I am exhausted, though the day has hardly begun, and this neglected and constricted place needs a whole conference to itself. Few gems of nothingness as beautiful as this ever were. Such images beat my prose with a wooden spoon, hard against the edge of the mixing bowl. I run away slowly. Back to the tower made up of fruitcake rocks layered by flash floods, and turn up Church Path. It must once have been far less metalled than now. I check out the hall that has invaded the red walls, errant gravestones and mediaeval stone ornaments leaned up alongside its rubbish bins. A nervous elderly woman comes out to check on my noseying around the church hall bins; as politely as I can, I reject her offer of a coffee – perhaps because I think she thinks that I may be *in need* – and retreat to the neighbouring graveyard, with its gorgeous gas lamps, so long unused that even their adaptation to electricity is now redundant; a glass bulb fallen from its rusted socket and wedged in the frame.

The Star of David on the guttering of St James Church is a mark left by Isaac Singer, the sewing machine magnate, who came here with his Parisian wife, having been refused property by the anti-Semitic elite in Torquay; he paid for the renovation of this mediaeval church, with a vestry added by his grandson. A white slab at the foot of the church wall argues: "Those we love don't go away, they walk beside us every day". Its sentimentality gets me in the guilt bone.

A man emerges from a door to know nothing of the things that intrigue me about this building, but he does inform me that the suspiciously modern looking representation of the martyr was carved before the convention of showing James (of the Camino) with "sea shells". Shipwreck pilgrimage: James's corpse washed overboard in a storm, it emerges unharmed on the coast, covered in and protected by scallop shells. For one kind of pilgrim the many ribs of the scallop lead to a single point; for another the ribs begin at a single point and move outwards.

The tower of this church, one tower among so many, is red and fleshy. Even a cursory glance along the side of the outer wall gathers up some odd patterns: diamonds carved in limestone erratics and swirls in patches of concrete. Around the porch is something possibly Moorish. Inside it is far more brutal; a great empty space where folk would have gathered, standing, while priests gibbered behind rood screens, the mediaeval font like a fat hammer hollowed out. Gashed into the side of the nave is a darkness, and within it the representation of a shrunken and desiccated corpse, its skin sucked right back onto the bones. The face is drawn tight over the skull. The chest flesh stretched over rack-like ribs; the one leg left alone by Reformation vandals is thin, like a walking stick. A curtain stretched shallowly over a model made out of matchsticks. The only thing untouched is the monkish head of hair, shaped in the fashion of a 1970s' glamour girl, a Purdey. Its eyes are like the holes on a 'crazy golf' course. I take photos but can't get the sense of meaningless skin over a stiff structure of order, of wetness disciplined by wires. I try to get it on my grotty digital, but the light is too low; my final attempt is solid blackness.

I give up and wander off as a man enters the church and resolutely strides down the centre aisle, leaning slightly backwards. He is like a structure in baggy trainers and hoodie. His eyes are over-alive; I already warn myself against him. He throws himself, out of control, into a seat on the front row of the pews, pulls himself up straight, then takes his hands to his face and begins to sob until his whole body rocks back and forth. I find myself walking towards him; a man is disintegrating before my eyes, his limbs shake violently. I know he has noticed me, but... From his mouth come odd gulps; a dog stitched to a bird. I offer to leave the church, to vacate it for this man and his desperate sorrow.

"Would you rather I left you alone", I hear myself saying, as if I am speaking of someone else, "or would you rather talk about what is troubling you?"

"Can I talk?"

"Of course. Please."

"I've had bad news. Bad, bad. Terrible news."

I cannot read him. His hood falls back to reveal a head too big for the frame of sticks and metal stands that poke around in his trainers. His eyes are loganberry red.

"My sister killed herself with drugs, just like an overdose. Yesterday. I just heard."

That accent comes from somewhere around Birmingham.

I assure him that this is something terrible. I want to soak up his pain. But after that, I have no idea how this is supposed to go. I am speaking from a fake-efficacious script, of which I have only ever seen a tiny part, but I am doing my best.

"You are right to feel as you do. A terrible thing has happened and what you are feeling is a right thing to feel."

The man speaks of demons and I think of movies rather than real ones; he says he is starving and I think he means metaphorically; but he has neither eaten nor slept for three days. I don't notice the significance of anything beyond wondering how I should not offer him the tenner I have; that he is in need of a kind of sustenance that money cannot buy. I hold my hands, as gently as I can, behind my back; steeling myself against any kind of performance. I do not offer the tenner.

He says that he is thinking "mad things"; he skates carefully around the words, but, without saying as much, I know he is thinking of joining his sister unless someone can come up with a better idea. I once again affirm the reasonableness of his response to such a shattering event.

He doesn't quite say "at peace" but that is the spirit of what he seeks. He is alone, he says. I ask him what brought him to the town. I am hoping to trigger some other narrative for him to hang onto.

"I was abused by our father. She was too. But no one ever believed us and they drived us away, and now it's he, that bastard, sitting at the Christmas table. She had demons. I've been hearing the same voices as her. I've been thinking mad terrible things."

"No. There is nothing mad or wrong in what you are feeling. Given the things you have experienced, it's really completely right and normal for you to feel and think mad things. To get that terrible news, you are right to be feeling in a mad way. That's a human thing to feel like that."

"I've been so cold. No hot food and that. I've got no one here. No friends, nothing."

"Then you are being incredibly strong to take this kind of news on your own. You are quite right for it to hit you so hard. You're a sensitive person. You feel it."

I am trying to buy time. But I cannot keep repeating myself. I have kept to the script as I imagine it; but I am aware of reaching the bottom of the only page I have.

The man is here, in a church, it is a final resort.

"I haven't been in a church since I was christened."

A last chance chancel. This is no game. But I can be a mirror; reinforce his feelings, hoping to intuit some other way to keep him alive for a few minutes. Keep him where he is for the moment. I dare not leave him and fetch someone; where would he go? What might he do? But at the same time – what am I willing to commit to him? What is he going to ask of me?

I'd known how things would work up to this point, but now I am running out of ways to affirm this suffering man. He talks of demons again.

"If I was to go and fetch a priest? There's a coffee morning in the church hall I passed it on my way, they'd be able to get in touch with the minister. Is that something that would be helpful?"

To my surprise, he nods enthusiastically. But I am not too sure and I am not going to leave him yet. A woman in black comes creaking though the door. She is young and old; elegant, but clumsy, somewhere between beautiful and drawn, a hint of the stretched stone corpse about her grace; I think she might be a friend or even a partner of this man – I am running multiple scenarios – but she chooses a pew near the back and begins to pray.

I break her prayers.

She immediately embraces the man; once she has listened to me. Gets his name and gives hers. Why did I not think of that, do that? She praises me – "you are a good woman" – and sends me to the vicarage. But I am not, I have had to strip away most of me, to get rid of the fear and embarrassment. Just to be able to listen. Outside, the light is bright and unreal; the vicarage reached through a door in the old wall. I ring an unpromising bell but, after a while and then a creak, a rigorously washed and rotund woman answers, listens to my faltering narrative as if suicidal folk gather at the church regularly (maybe they do) and then thanks me peremptorily, hearing me for the performer I am, and shuts the door.

Moments later, on the street outside the wall, the priest or minister overtakes me on her way to the church. I lean on the graveyard wall, breathing hard, beside what Salmon says are the latrines of the old Bishop's Palace; in a yew tree a pair of jays are being bullied by magpies. The romanticist walkers write of their inner lives bouncing off the independent world just beyond the boundary of their skin, but I feel no distance. I feel totally compromised.

I walk on. Ashamed and in a kind of trance. I stumble along the road beside the church, cross the road and help myself down the steep stairs, trying to leave the encounter behind me; too real to be any part of my playful journey. It would be evil to incorporate it. I am writing about this with real misgivings and I have changed almost everything about it. I want to abandon it, like a stone or a building I can no longer afford to upkeep, or something amputated in an operation, something no longer part of me that is required to be handed over; rent to a landlord. I feel horror at the thought that Hazlitt was right and that 'the walk' is always and eventually about 'the self', when "long-forgotten things, like 'sunken wrack and sunless treasuries', burst upon my eager sight, and I begin to feel, think, and be myself again". I look around for some side-of-the-pool to put my hand on.

Up on the wall of the former brewery of Starkey, Knight and Ford are mouldings of three barrels, the three tuns of the badge of the Worshipful Company of Brewers, a livery company of the City of London, and a larger badge higher up, with a white silhouette of a knight's head on a green background. I imagine it is Sir Constant whose book weighs heavy in my backpack. I look for somewhere to sit for a while. Behind the flats is a beguiling set of successive arches, dark and pink and recent, but if I sit there I am in someone's garden. By the Clink, a mediaeval lockup, there is a circular flower bed and I sit on the red sandstone edge of that.

In an hour I have read Cule's book. It is wonderful. I had expected a clumsy evangelical text, but this (if stripped of its allegorical container) turns out to be an elegant symbolist drama. Later, I will read much of the Victorian and Edwardian literature produced (or adapted to film) in the areas of South Devon that I walk, works cited by Salmon – Mills, Mallock, Froude, Trevena – and it is always tainted, somewhere, by a sickly biological supremacy. There is always a flag or a race or a class. But 'Sir Constant' is unlike them all.

I'm not a fool. I can see that Cule's book excludes plenty, but I am impressed by its confidence in its narrow field to expand out to absolutes without losing touch with its objective correlatives, without requiring physical rather than philosophical or ethical enemies. A conceit around John Bunyan's *The Pilgrim's Progress from This World to That Which Is to Come*, the book takes its Christian allegory for granted and then finesses around its ornaments, like a mystic briefly disorientated in a theatre of memory. As a student of Symbolist art and performance, I recognise where I am with Cule; on an August Strindberg highway with a Maeterlinck sensibility.

I hope I will meet some of the book's landscapes and characters – the narrow valley, the empty suit of armour, the way channelled through a single doorway, the Black Knight who rises secretly in the night and changes personal maps; I think maybe I already did. But will I "fall under the spell of the city" and "see pleasant visions and rejoice in them, not being aware that they are visions only: and... lose all measure of Time and Duty"? Is Cule predicting that road of sloganised T-shirts and one-armed bandits, cafés and chip shops and tattoo parlours, pigeon wire around the classical pillars, and ancient Egyptian gods guarding its casino?

I love the book's chapel of voices that suddenly unfolds: "and lo! The walls of the great cross parted, leaving a wide doorway with a fair and open path beyond". I had already felt small moments like that; when everything seemed closed off and then, suddenly, a way had opened up.

I am re-reading the passage that caught me hardest; when Sir Constant, the questing pilgrim-knight, stays at the castle of Sir Joyous and at night discovers that his host's portrait changes from "bright and smiling in countenance" to one of "wild laughter, the brows grown heavy and leaden" and the label on the painting changes too, first to "Sir Pleasure" and then to "the name of that mighty enemy of the Great King whom men call Sir Self".

In my head I re-run the story; so the fear of pleasure is what is painted over with the whitewash of "joy" and "fun" and it is Sir Self who is the enemy and Great King of everyone.

I don't know... I am still puzzling over my partial inversion, when my self-indulgence is interrupted by a call to my phone. One of the conference organisers ringing from Plymouth: am I still in Paignton? Can one of her students, who lives in the town, come to speak with me about her research? Half an hour later, the wait spent re-reading my favourite parts of *Sir Constant*, Eileen arrives – a mature student, like me. She asks if perhaps she can show me around?

I never did quite understand what her research was, or why it would help her to walk with me. But walk we do and she commentates on whatever I show an interest in. Like the houses raised up on supporting walls, because there is nothing but sand under us, even this far inland we are on salt marshes, moisture rising with the tides and filling the cellars. I am not sure if she means right now. Nothing is fixed here. There is a 'Blue Velvet' feel; of lines not to cross. It feels very suburban, even in the middle of the old Saxon town, provincial and reassuring, yet it is also manufactured against doom; the storms at sea, the tides of working class holidaymakers, the lack of a clear identity of its own. Are towns supposed to have that any more?

I lead Eileen into backstreets and down an alley with a ballet school in a peeling warehouse: "for children aged 2½ to 21 yrs"; a gravestone tucked in a cubbyhole; "the best and most beautiful things cannot be seen or even touched": garden ornament Gnosticism – this in an elaborate car port that includes a former public drinking fountain, a spitting lion head painted royal blue; a ladder with most of its rungs missing; the almost illegible sign for a E VIC MEN'S CL B. I miss the ancient monument; its sign has been bent so far back into the hedgerow by a passing vehicle, but not a wildly tiled backyard with ceramic trees and birds and patterns that look like aliens from old 1950s' movies, and a plaster Pan. Then we explore up an old lane.

Eileen begins to narrate the journey in a way I could not: the haunted cottage, with the 'for sale' sign, that is always changing hands, NIGHT WORKER SLEEPING PLEASE DO NOT DISTURB, thick mud oozing up from under a manhole cover, orange trees, the remnants of an older monastic presence and stories of the more recent one I had already stumbled on, a billboard torn in half to reveal a cartoon removals worker with a terrifying grin brandishing a tiny house; it is hard to tell the Protestant chapels from the warehouses, both sport absurd facades.

Eileen points out the first Catholic Church; now housing. It had been a Baptist Chapel and when the builders were filling in the baptismal bath, another Peggy's Pool, Father Mulkern had joked: "There goes the last of Original Sin!"

All the time there are odd lengths of out-of-place wall, some grand, some stumpy and painted thickly; all speaking to an old arrangement, Saxon maybe, ill at ease with the recent town. It isn't a sinister thing; but a kind of irritated magic.

On the corner of Southfield Street and Cecil Road, by the zebra crossing are rubedo steps of breccias up to an elevated sliver of orchard. The old red apple warehouse, up for sale, seems positioned in the ruins of something much, much older; that is how the Marist chapel felt too, and the coffee morning church hall in the Palace ruins, anonymous modernity in old shells, while the houses here are palimpsests. Even the stuffy Conservation Plan attributes an "otherness" to them, Salmon says.

I am only a few feet above the pedestrians passing by, but the elevation has made me invisible; the afternoon walkers with buggies and preoccupations do not look up. On Southfield Street, we climb some steps to a semi-private garden that looks out over the town. The mediaeval and Italianate towers of the two churches pin the town to the sky. This is a welcoming private space, an assemblage of different subjective pruning and plantings, displays and deferences. The piping of the handrails, a wooden rail added to the metal one and then rotted away, the friendly jumble of privet and rhododendron, a deformed plaster pixie twisting his sightless eyes, scallop shells dropped from the concrete wall and leaving behind juvenile fossils. Looking out across the town, I think of the 36 slaves recorded here in the Domesday Book. Who were they? What mark of them is here? Those amputated walls?

Eileen takes me into the Catholic Church, The Church of the Sacred Heart and the Little Flower, where she is a worshipper. Inside, I am drawn to the statue of the Protomartyr of Oceania, Peter Chanel, founder of those Marist fathers whose chapel I had blundered upon; endowed with "marvellous meekness", his robes are of the same resonant blue as the lion fountain. There is a certain Dali-esque realism to Chanel's statue, a sur-reality, an above real, that has been lost in the victory of Parliament and text and in the dust of all those smashed statues and rood screens.

French priests and nuns, Irish fathers, Breton fishermen and their families, the Belgian refugees in the First World War. Salmon says that Agatha Christie's model for Hercule Poirot was a Belgian refugee. There is this heritage of asylum in these small towns, and yet no one seems to celebrate it much. Maybe no one knows it.

I say goodbye to Eileen, who has for a few loops within a tiny part of the town been a guide.

The giant milk bottle on the corner is not the wooden original but a concrete replacement, and was not always white. 'Itch Itchington', a local 'artist', once re-painted it in Coca Cola colours as an incoherent protest against sugar and invisibility, after first leaving a severed pig's head at the town's branch of McDonalds. The milk bottle, once advertising a dairy, has long floated free of function and become a simple, meaningful beauty, a Pater aestheticism, a symbol of bottle for symbol of bottle's sake. It is my favourite thing I have seen in Devon so far. The dairy itself, is not. It has become 'Women of Worth', an arm of World Christian Ministries: "liberating women and children". From the numerous pictures of white women handing over medicines to women of colour it is very clear who is doing the liberating. Christ is very white here. The seagulls keep up the screaming. On an advertisement hoarding 'The Black Farmer' is waving a union flag over his head, his arms lifted as if in surrender.

In Cecil Mews a garage-top sculpture of drift wood writhes wildly. I slide between the breccia walls like a limestone pebble polished in the cold flash flood sizzling across hot Permian sands. In Higher Polsham Road a single Georgian villa is a painful reminder of an elegance that once prevailed here.

FOR THAT MODEL RAILWAY EXPERIENCE. Closed down and boarded up.

Passing empty shops on Torquay Road, approaching the Mansion, I am thinking of how the rich have so clearly fled deeper into the countryside and behind their gates. How the big houses – Oldway, Redcliffe, Cockington, Torre Abbey – are all now in the hands of trusts, councils or hoteliers. The super rich have abandoned any physical accountability; their remaining visibility is the spectre of their former homes.

Coming at Oldway Mansion, climbing up the rocks, over exposed terracotta pipes and around scruffy palm trees about its fenced-off Grotto, dank water and cheap building-site Heras panel fencing, bantering warily with a group of young larrikins. Even though the sign on the steps up says "Mansion", I am caught unprepared, coming through the trees, for what I see. The scale, the detail, the theft, the de-composture. This is fabulous, this is Axël's Castle!

And this is being left to rot?

I follow a line of goats' masks, cast by Voltaire's of Paris, and then take the steps up to the southern side of the building, with its giant croquet lawn, emerald in the midday sun, a green rectangle commanding the fractal suburbs on the opposing hills. There are two Sphinxes here with the same, very human, female face; the model for the Statue of Liberty, Isabelle Eugenie Boyer, the wife of Isaac Singer. In this stone version of her, she looks away, not in disdain I think, but as if much more interested in something that is not quite here. Up above, under the gable, are symbols of warmth, wisdom and reason, abstraction and growth.

Just after I pass through, the house and grounds become the set for The Chuckle Brothers to play the live action version of the Hitman game; Paul and Barry guide a local man playing Agent 47 to 'take out' a Serbian arms dealer.

In the gardens there are figurative representations of Pan, hooves crossed, and a baby Bacchus with a tail (like a freakshow on Facebook), an imp carrying the mind to higher things, sur-irreality – these were 1950s' replacements for a broken muse and some putti representing secular passions. Two more giant and abstract Sphinxes guard the car park, wearing ram's heads for headdresses; one is treacherous, the other merciless; more purloinings from antiquity. Strangulators, squeezing the entrance. The association of learning and bad luck; that after the ordeal of education everything still remains to be done. They wait and wait; the riddles that would allow them to end their slaughters and ascend to heaven are unanswered.

The Pans are slow, great and still stone cold dead. Inside – or maybe it has been removed by now? – a copy of David's huge painting of Napoleon's crowning of Josephine. Women are worshipped here, but always on terms decided by men.

The great structure is suspended above a nothingness, disconnected from a monastic timetable of belief and tidal crafts of fruitcake palaces, losing its noses, eroded here and there, beginning to be rubbed by a lack of repairs, becoming formal and structural and more of an idea than a place. I think it is beautiful and unreal in its wreck, renovation would end its ruination. But in this interregnum it can float, unfunctioning, its excess of symbolism elevated by the administrative mess left by its entanglement with the economic downturn.

An elderly man – "been here 40 years, still an outsider, of course" – tells me that rain pours in through the collapsing ceilings. The council has "let it go".

Under some unruly tree cover beyond the circular Riding School there are extensive remnants of something ornately carved: a collapsed archway, possibly. A crash of columns, cornices, capitals and corbels. All coated in emerald moss. A definition of inside and outside is no longer required.

A ram-horned, dolphin-headed, feather-armed, trumpet-handed mutant at the foot of a tree.

The whole place is a diffraction of neo-classical theft and post-2008 composture; I love it. Never mend it, never give in to the outrage.

At the junction of Oldway and Upper Manor Road is a heterotopia, a cluster of spaces marinated with the ooze of vinegar and batter. Outside the Oak Tree Forge, rammed into the pavement, its roots crammed with cement, is a large oak tree. Opposite is a driveway with stumpy pebble-dashed pillars and in a garage forecourt is an odd, triple-layered concrete cake that has slid apart; different varieties of found art. Why have I not noticed before that there is so much free entertainment to hand?

> "When once we have begun to look with curiosity on the strange things that ordinary people pass over without notice, our wonder is continually excited by the variety of phase, and often by the uncouthness of form.... We can scarcely poke or pry for an hour among the rocks, at low-water mark, or walk, with an observant downcast eye, along the beach after a gale, without finding some oddly-fashioned, suspicious-looking being, unlike any form of life that we have seen before."
>
> Charles Kingsley, *Glaucus, the Wonders of the Shore* (1855)

The junction is busy with cars and pedestrians. Cider Press, Yarn Barn, thatched cottages and a pub with oddly-shaped windows: diamonds, triangles and thin rectangles. I take a simple pleasure in the line of cream and chocolate concrete bollards. At the Spiritualist Church on the corner an advertising hoarding promises a training for "deepening your evidence [for] the intelligence behind the communication; understanding the use of clairsentience in blending with the communicator... and being able to emanate from oneself the essence of the spirit communicator". It spells "contracts" instead of "contacts", as if everything is a 'trade deal' now. This week's medium is Jonathan Brown FROM LEAMINGSTON SPA. Beyond a show room, full of 1960s' Rovers covered in dust, I stop for lunch.

Church Path, through churchyard, the church of St John the Baptist with St Andrew and St Boniface, Princes St, along footpath by The Clink, though concrete arches, Littlegate Street, Milbrook Road, then Kirkham Street following it to the right and then left at the T-junction, right onto Cecil Road, right down Mill Lane, past Kirkham House, onto Littlegate Street and left down alley past dance studios, left into Churchward Road, right into Cecil Road to the end and the milk bottle, go back 20 metres and into Cecil Mews going north, cross Cadwell Road and straight on along back alley to Higher Polsham Road, Torquay Road going north, doorway into Oldway Mansions gardens, through gardens and round Mansion to the left, Oldway Road, at junction with Oak Tree Forge, right into Upper Manor Road, left onto Torquay Road and cross over to Brambles for good homemade food, restaurant quality at café prices (Braised beef and fresh vegetable including swede for £6.95).

Across from Brambles and the smashed windows of Fosse Healthcare ("Here to help"), past the ghost advert on the side of the Conservative Club, I climb up a handful of red stone steps and into Preston Gardens where something exotic has died. Its bark foamed up into a whale head bluntness. A thatched cat chases a thatched rat across a rooftop. There is no sun to read the sundial.

Turning up Preston Down Road, a sign says: "live happy! With Slimming World!" – John Trevena would not have been pleased; this is the kind of hedonism that would ruin the English stock. There are the faintest hints in the shaping of an exterior chimney, an arch and in a portal of that 'taste' that had once been a 'culture', even if it was someone else's. A garage, its cream door buckled, oozes bed bases and a mountain of leaves: the miscegenation of interior decor with the oak groves has burst the boarded cave.

I get caught up in a hunt for a cat around here. Passing a set of garages, a black cat with white markings crosses my path. I only notice it because of the superstition. A few streets on, taped to a lamp post, is a poster for a 'missing cat', Domino, and a photo of a cat very like the one I have just seen. I ask a passer-by for directions to the address on the poster and race off to it. Why this strikes me as going off on a tangent when I only have tangents to go on I can't explain, but it feels like an irritating diversion from my walk; a chore I could have done without. The owner, who is both graceful and grateful, says that Domino has been missing for five weeks, but that there have been numerous sightings and she saw him herself once, but was unable to catch him. She thanks me and goes for her car keys.

I rejoin my original route at a care home, where the road kinks round to the right. Two Filipino careworkers are taking a break on a bench. Eavesdropping, I nearly miss an almost overgrown turning onto some kind of track opposite. It begins dispiritingly at a utilities junction box. Then the path gets trapped at the ends of back gardens. Feeling that I am half-trespassing, I tread quietly. I hear the snuffling of a suspicious dog behind a fence and tip-toe gently. A concrete Romanesque archway has been breezeblocked, a wooden door has rotted solid into its frame; a gaping hole where a huge length of fence has blown down onto a plane of decking reminds me of the BNP graffito. Then it changes. It all changes. The psychogeography of a frightened siege town, of meaninglessness and hoaxery offered as normality, of the rows of closed shops punctuated by financial services with satirical names – Concise Wealth, Accounting 4 Everything – becomes an emotional landscape of relief and surprise. The abject track at the backs of the houses enters deep into the treeline and a world unimaginable so close to suburban roads.

These woods disrupt the nuclear logic of the suburbs. Raised roots and red earth, a thickening of feeling. Silent dogs creep up to sniff at my groin. The apologetic owners, two similar looking women – sisters? – know not to disturb the train of my thought. I follow them down the long red path tunnelled in trees. According to the information board this is Occombe Woods, the valley of the oaks, "Ancient Semi-Natural Woodland" free of human intervention (and garden escapes) since at least 1600. I like "semi-natural"; that's how I feel; conditional, contingent. When the path opens out onto a field, there is a view back to where I have walked today and yesterday: the churches, the pier, Redcliffe, Oldway. I can hear the whistle of a steam locomotive. The seagulls are gone; now there are crows, robins, leaves in the wind, and silence. The shade beneath the trees becomes darker; I notice that there are little paths off from the main track, up to a fall of creepers, a spring that has seen a huge collapse of branches; climbing into the chaos I can make out the sharp edge of a stone structure in there. These smaller and fainter tracks off from the main path are markers of the locals' attachment to the groves, the springs, the everyday magic of their long dead ancestors. This was all something important once.

Coming down I hold onto a branch as thick as my arm which breaks like a joke prop and I slide and tumble down onto the main track.

One of the twin-like women has paused where the stream from the spring crosses the path, crouching down to wash her hands; she looks up, as if she is waiting for me; as if she has something to say. I hang back until she is gone. I don't know why I ignore her.

Before exiting this wonderful space through a large rusty iron gating, I hunker in the grass for a long pee. The bank of dark trees rises like a wall. I hear women's voices in a back garden nearby.

On Sandringham Drive, its scimitar curve like a ripple of blast, I find three concrete frogs painted white on a thick front gate pillar; I find it strangely cheering that one has almost eroded out of all recognition. Outside a house called WHISPERS a van from Oak Tree Forge is parked. Walking knits everything together. I cross a busy road to look at the transmitter pylon there. Its sign warns "IF YOU HAVE A CARDIAC PACEMAKER OR BONES REPAIRED BY METAL/PLASTIC BONE IMPLANTS YOU MUST SEEK MEDICAL ADVICE BEFORE ACCESSING THIS SITE". The spectacle is corrosive.

Dame Sylvia Crowe, the pioneer landscape designer for nuclear power stations and hydroelectric dams in the mid-twentieth century saw these installations, even a single mast or a pylon, as "the outlier of human influence. Its prototype is the obelisk used by the 18th-century gardener to bring all the intervening land between the mansion and the distant monument firmly within the influence of civilisation... to banish untamed nature from the view". There are messages hidden within the signals.

At Occombe Farm I visit the deli and wander through the outdoor tables of the café; just as the neat lawns of Sandringham Drive have been something very different from the dire car crash of meaning down by the coast, so now I find a layer of something else; subsidised right-on-ness. Here there is a different way to meaning, defined by the stratigraphy of inclusion and exclusion. The best intentions poisoned by the grinding and infuriating refusal of the lowest to be righteous, to grasp what is best for them. Their persistence in rebellious self-harm and suicide. I construct Swiftian suggestions in my head.

I make my way down the narrow and heartless lane to Cockington. There is a brief respite on the John Musgrave Heritage Trail, named after and funded by a former British Intelligence Officer active in the Middle East; his body damaged by polio, he had walked with the mending flesh of subsequent surgeries.

Occombe Farm is growing flowers; just a small patch in a large field, but I hope they might soon fill it to its edges with bright colours.

Back on the nasty little lane, I wave to an approaching young driver, who does not kill his speed, but rashly misses my body by millimetres, pressed hard into the nettles of the hedge. I had felt in my chest an awful inevitability in the moment before he missed me.

I pass under three massive trees with pinnately lobed leaves. There are long stretches of straight road and my mind begins to relax to the tall walls of hedge that hem in my anxiety and turn it yellow and green.

Then coming up the lane, on their way to look for Gallows Gate and a field reputed to be 'hollow', are a group of ramblers who, gamely, had attended the conference; or attempted to. I had seen them at the conference venue, and later one or two of them had turned up for the papers. I hadn't heard any of them ask a question or make a point, but they had looked a little different from others at the conference. They say they all felt a little daunted, even snubbed. Though they had hardly arrived before the conference was over, it has made a big impression on them. They are puzzled to discover that there is more than one way of walking.

"Isn't walking all the same? That's what brings us together?"

They all agree with each other.

I try to explain how a "universalist" idea of walking might actually exclude those who feel marginalised.

"It brings you five together and that's fabulous, but what if I was wearing a burqa, would walking bring us together then? There might be different kinds of walking that would be necessary; different people may have different ideas about what they are free to do or where to go. Not everyone would see the countryside as a benign place..."

The women worry about how this imaginary companion might get over the stiles in her burqa.

"It's not a garment designed for public footpaths."

I shift the grounds. "Or imagine if they were a wheelchair user?"

The women had liked Will Self's talk and found him clever, charming and funny; they didn't seem to mind his kind of divisiveness. They had come to the conference because it was local "and something different".

"Different from what?"

Different from the other ramblers they had met, who, they say, tend to be snobby and exclusive, walking too far and too fast and certainly never ever getting lost.

"We're a bit mad!"

We say goodbye and for a while I watch them make their happy way up the dangerous lane. They do not look back, but I can see they are already in deep conversation about something. I wonder why they are so attracted to something like the site of a gallows and pit (hanging for men, drowning for women); or the massive subterranean passages discovered in the mid 1960s, running for "hundreds of metres and 12 metres below the surface". What could that be? The passages ran through a field called Daddy Croft – 'Daddy' sometimes interpreted as 'dead', sometimes as 'Devil'. Were these passages a kind of massive necropolis? Certainly much, much bigger than necessary for what the gallows would supply; its victims probably brought up this lane. Had people turned out to gawp at them? Did they gawp at Athelstan's anti-British crusade? Or at William of Orange's morbid procession, landing at Brixham and riding this way at the head of "200 Blacks brought from the plantations of the Netherlands in America" all wearing "Imbroyder'd Caps lin'd with white fur, and Plumes of white Feathers, to attend the Horfe"?

Despite its traffic, I am not glad to get off the lane and onto a gravelled Geopark Cyclepath; it all feels very bossed and managed and I take the first turn onto a red earth path I come to, sidling up beside fields and down steps to what I later learn is a 'haha' in the grounds of Cockington Court. I have wandered into a stately home!

In the field beyond the haha a young deer is being chased by ravens.

As I walk down 'Yonder Lawn' I think I am descending into a gentle park. An hour later, when I put together the gonzo information boards, chats with a possible priest and other visitors, the helpful man at the Court, bar staff and consulting Salmon, it all tells me that I am not.

I am deer, and this place is ravens.

Preston Gardens, Old Torquay Road, Preston Downs Road, at care home cross left onto footpath behind backgardens, same path through woods, at the old metal barrier turn right and walk uphill, at T-junction of paths, go right and into field, following path to the left into bushes on the other side of field, ignore the immediate right hand turn up to gate and carry on through the trees, follow signpost to 'Occombe Woods' across field and into trees, and out into field, past phone mast into woods with signboard 'Occombe Woods', turn right immediately down crumbled concrete path and turn left at the bottom past the information board, carry straight along for a few hundred yards until the path splits, take left lower or right higher, where the paths meet bear to the right, when the path forks take the right, through metal gate next to long wooden bench, Lindsay Road, left into Sandringham Drive, left into Preston Down Road, Occombe Farm, Cockington Road, John Musgrave Trail, Cockington Road/Totnes Road, left just before Warren Barn through gates and onto gravelled cyclepath, take right hand turn onto first red earthen footpath, take the first footpath turning to the right and then swing left through the stone portal, and immediately take the right hand set of steps down to the grass...

Chapter Five: Cockington Court to Corbyn Head

Up on the right of 'Yonder Lawn' is the first of the invisible wonders here; things that didn't happen or haven't happened yet, like the modernist village at Churston. This one is the National Hickory Collection; an ark of hickory trees (including pecans) planted in readiness for wholesale genetic wipeout in the US; after apocalypse, the new American Eden will start again from here. Making my way down the lawn, I enter, softly but rapidly, an intense weave of ideology; in a space where most people seem to feel that they are "getting away from it all".

I walk along a path towards the Court, a modest, but stately residence, pausing at three small gravestones; one is for Finn the gamekeeper's dog, shot by his master, George Giles, when in 1933 the local council bought the house and grounds from the Mallock family and dispensed with both their services. The hardy Giles, who took his baths in one the Court's lakes, lost his home on the estate as part of the deal and had convinced himself that a working dog could never adapt to a Torquay flat.

Outside the church are two plateaux; I cannot work out what their ecclesiastical function could be. Turns out they are tennis courts! And a possible solution to the mystery of Cockington's dead. For there is no graveyard here and no records of Cockington people buried in neighbouring parishes. Where did they all go? Did a squire of Cockington remove them into a field to build his tennis courts? Or have they always been taken to Daddy Croft field? Or maybe further away; the path from the church door a corpse road for carrying the dead over the hills?

Just inside the old West door, nestled away in a deep crevice, is a very long sanctuary bar; I doubt if many visitors ever mind it. There's no sign or information about it; unless you look closely it's just a hole. Somehow the bar has survived there, despite its redundancy, since the law of sanctuary was changed – and fugitives from secular law could no longer seek the protection of a church – in 1623.

> so rap on the knocker
> pull across the bar
> step out of modernity...
> and into sanctuary
> from the pressures
> and distresses
> you're not alone
> in a world in a world of its own

The church, its crenelated fortifications real rather than decorative, is dedicated to St George and St Mary. An odd designation, possibly something to do with the residence at nearby Torre Abbey of Premonstratensian canons proper, who had a special affection for Mary. The church was their chapel. In times before the sea defences, when storm waters ran almost to the edge of the village, the church doubled as a watch tower. I think of the White Lady on her lookout, and how a White Canon on the tower reflects her.

A 'monk's squint' in the tower – for a canon to check on enemies lurking in the nave – is a mark of long lasting fears. Notes in the Church Accounts speak of payments for "alteration of prayer for American war" (1780), "for form of prayer for Admiral Duncan's Victory over the Dutch" (1797), "for a form of prayer for Admiral Nelson's victory over the French" (1798). The church in the 18th century is a key national communicator and the emphasis on an international threat is a longstanding one.

The Church Accounts are surprisingly easy to get a look at; they record a woman named, rather wonderfully, 'Charity Ball'. While an entry in the *Overseers of the Poor Accounts* for Cockington records the three shillings spent on the burial of "Joan Smardon the pagon" in 1757. Was she part of a lost tradition, a non-attendee, or just a victim of gossip?

I find a bathetic text in the nave: "This electric blower was installed to the glory of God."

I stare long at the stained-glass window variously supposed to show Robert Cary, local squire, or St James of Compostela; the confusion arises perhaps from Cary's pilgrimage in 1518 to James' shrine at Santiago de Compostela in Northern Spain. The figure in the window wears the badge of pilgrimage – a scallop shell (or pecten), purloined for the logo of The Royal Dutch Shell Oil Company, which had started out trading in rare seashells.

A scallop has approximately sixty eyes; I may need a similar number to track all the world views contesting this quaint slice of a scones-and-clotted-cream county.

The rood screen depicts birds – or multiple versions of the same bird: each representing one of the sixteen qualities of the Christ upon which the human soul feeds. "Or sixteen different human moods", the ambiguous man quickly qualifies. This man, who might be a churchwarden or maybe a collarless vicar, is keen to explain the ongoing link between water and local power: in 1293, he says, on the Feast of St Catherine the Virgin, her symbol a wheel like a Beekite (he likes to digress), the squire Roger de Cockington traded the rights to the water of the Sherwell stream to the canons at Torre Abbey in exchange for which a Requiem Mass was to be said weekly for his soul. This had been discontinued at the time of the Reformation (dour face), but in 1988 (happy face) the Mass was reinstated in the guise of Wednesday communion. Warming to his fluid theme (later as I pass along the side of the modest Sherwell, its course hemmed into an unnatural channel along the side of the road, I think of running water as both sacred and up for grabs), he says the font was of unusual significance to the Premonstratensians who had their own special communion rite, and kept it for a while even after the Pope of the time (I think he said Paul V, but I may be wrong) suppressed other similar innovations; their rite was characterised by a solemnity that was out of synch with the new emphasis on the greater participation of the lay community in liturgical life. The Premonstratensians put the accent on mystery.

During the Easter octave (I have no idea what he is talking about now, but I enjoy bathing in these minutiae) vespers (now I am pleasingly imagining a scooter driven by a handsome young Italian through Rome) were concluded with a procession to the baptismal font. When Squire Cary gave the present font – perhaps to mark his 1518 pilgrimage? – the choice of Caen stone might have been intended as a flattering nod to the Premonstratensians' origins in Northern France.

The pulpit supposedly began life as a crow's nest on one of the lost ships of the Spanish Armada... er, well... I say that this reminds me of Melville's 'Moby Dick' where the whalers' chapel has a pulpit built like the prow of a ship. He has seen the film, with Gregory Peck as Ahab, his body pinned to the body of the great white nothingness, a screen between the appearance of the world and what is deep down beyond. The Cockington pulpit is covered in symbols; faces hidden behind later sculpted additions, figures to which have been added wings and sheep's horns. It is suggested, he says, that one of these heads originally bore a large pair of ears, "elephant's ears", a satirical swipe at Protestants who listened to too much preaching for their own good; the ears became angel wings when the Protestants won.

The ambiguous man is trying to sound as dry as possible, but the more arcane he becomes the more oddly erotic are the feelings of decadence that creep over and under me; as if I were secretly reading Là-Bas on a train or immersing in something by Théophile Gautier in a doctor's waiting room. There is not much difference, affectively, between the churchwarden's kind of local history, once you get immersed deep in the dark detail, and the noumena of the most abstruse symbolist theatre. A church becomes something thinner than the dogma preached there and the artefacts accumulated; maybe this is true of any place?

The most exciting things, to me, are some golden, twig-like shapes that decorate a few of the panels of the pulpit. They resist all explanation. They are not symmetrical ornaments and they are not decorative. If they are intended to represent trees... no. They couldn't be abstract, could they? Three hundred years before their time. The 'churchwarden' suggests that "they cover up rosary pictures"; but I am impatient of rationalisations and abandon my ecclesiastical lover to his sanctuary.

I barely visit the Court itself. It has little charm, but it is fun to imagine it as an ice cream factory in the 1940s.

Salmon describes the Court from the Conquest period, when there was already a Saxon homestead here, occupied by a Norman family, through the 'nation-forming' adjustments during the Middle Ages and the religious turmoil around the Reformation. The residents of the Court were directly plugged into national politics (raising troops, choosing sides, making defiant and loyal gestures) and this was always very dangerous for them – residents of Cockington were regularly beheaded or sent into exile: in 1388 Sir John Cary was attainted for treason and banished for life to Waterford, in 1465 Sir William Cary was attainted for loyalty to Margaret of Anjou and his estate confiscated, in 1471 he was taken prisoner at the Battle of Tewkesbury and beheaded. In 1646 the Royalist Sir Henry Cary surrendered to the New Model Army's General Fairfax; the fine imposed was so heavy he was forced to sell the Cockington estate to the Mallock family. The old bell on display in the church is decorated with Charles the First coins; supposedly they were placed there in defiance of the rule of Parliament, but I wonder whether – like the 'pagan' standing stone used as a doormat at West Ogwell church – this is a device for secretly beating the king's ringing head?

According to Salmon's tendentious history, the relative *internal* stability of the 18th and 19th centuries, following the arrival of William of Orange, greeted on the quay at Brixham by Rawlyn Mallock, Whig MP, signalled a great change for Cockington. Rather than invasion – by Saxons, Normans and ideas from Geneva and Wittenberg – now the invasion moves the other way, not by occupation but colonisation, by theft and the composture (this is Mentz's idea not Salmon's, but they weave together nicely) of the resources of other lands and their export back here. So another kind of invasion *does* take place, an invasion of alien materials, of money, of surplus, of labour in its fruits not its skins. Salmon suggests that it is a mistake to see pre-Glorious Revolution, pre-Industrial Revolution Cockington through the eyes of the Victorians, as a backwater bumbling along as it always had. But instead, to understand it back then as a node of political trajectory and power in a pre-industrial society; hence the Monday market and the fair granted in 1352, hence the fines and executions, hence the Abbey, the Armada prisoners, the leadership at the Battle of Tewkesbury, the defiance of the Parliamentarians in 1653, and the staging of the Glorious Revolution parade. But after William of Orange comes, things change. The local families of wealth, rather than battling *against* each other, contain and privilege their connections *among* each other – Froudes, Champernownes, Carys, Courtenays, Mallocks – and, while this provincialism reflects a greater national *internal* stability, something else new happens; because modernity is based now on navies, on careful long-term trans-oceanic looting, on tides, on shipwreck (Mentz again) and the coming influence of international 'instability', and the greater instability of all 'things'. Now 'things' are made in a different way, they are not what they appear, they do not grow in nearby fields, nor are they ground in local mills, nor burnt down to lime in nearby kilns, nor woven in the cottage down the lane, nor are they the fruits of trade with equivalent producers elsewhere; instead, they are driven by a surplus riven from its source, an alienation born of thousands of miles of splitting and rending. So, year on year, composture, breaking down, chaos and decay, increasingly predominates even over theft. This colours everything colonial, by merciless administration over there it sets everything here, for two or three hundred years, at the mercy of a madness of the sea.

Torbay becomes an international schizophrenic node.

Firstly, it becomes the haven and port of the Royal Navy, it is fortified with numerous watchouts and artillery positions, and then with the metamorphosis of the 'Grand Tour' into tourism, Torquay becomes a metropolitan-styled resort, a "gay watering place, with its London shops and London equipages" (Charles Kingsley, 1855), with an international visitor group, and imperial technology-tourists, like the Russian Admiral Popov representing the Tsar, come to see Froude's tank-experiments at Chelston. What happens at Cockington village is a hallucination directly related to this development: it becomes the domestic equivalent of an exotic location on the Grand Tour before the European revolutions closed it down. Where once the village was the agri-production motor of the big house's authority, barely worthy of comment in its own right, it is now subjected to an intense "tourist gaze", its forge is "one of the most photographed buildings in the world"; part of the same colonial transformation as India's or Burma's, the melting into air of what seems most solid: cattle, physical labour, bread, anvil. It all hinges around that moment when those 200 slaves pass through, their "Imbroyder'd Caps lin'd with white fur"; that is the marker, the tell, the moment when the most violent break possible is made between a people and their world.

Or just maybe it had been signalled a little earlier? Because Salmon says that eighty years before, George Weymouth of Cockington (a member of the Cary family), became the first ever European to land on what is now Maine; his companion James Rosier writing of the land as "woody, growen with Firre, Birch, Oke and Beech, as farre as we saw along the shore; and so likely to be within. On the verge grow Gooseberries, Strawberries, Wild pease, and Wilde rose bushes." Not so very different from what the Saxon invaders found when landing at Corbyn Head at the mouth of the Cockington Valley. When Weymouth returns to England he brings back with him five Native Americans, members of the Patuxet people: Manida, Skettawarroes, Dehanada, Assacumet and Tisquantum. These men, ostensibly 'recruited' for training as scouts, were put on show in Plymouth; maybe they came to Cockington too?

Whichever year it was, 1605 or 1685, the contract with things was broken, by taking people as their objects these men changed everything; from then on they, and we, live on the cusp between fluidity and nightmares, unsure of things, except by their representations.

Nothing, not even fantasies and fictions, (and writing is the one thing that holds best) is free of this vaporisation.

Salmon's example of this undermining of reality is a novel of 1877 written by Charlotte Dempster, called *Blue Roses*, a phrase which, like "black swans" (though Dawlish has a few), is synonymous with impossible dreams. The novel is set partly around "Portquay" (Torquay), "Rington" (Paignton) and "Ifflehaye" (Cockington Court) in "South Dampshire" (South Devon). Married unhappily to the squire of Ifflehaye, Helen Malinofska, a Polish aristocrat, never finds acceptance either at the

Court or in the village; at the climax of the book, she is reunited with her estranged husband in Paris and asks him to take her back to Ifflehaye, the "last of her Blue Roses". She asks her husband to help her to make him happy at Ifflehaye, but he clumsily replies: "you will get no help from me", really meaning, Dempster explains, that, incapable of communication or empathy, his humanity evaporated, he does not know how, to help her. Helen dies from the shock of rejection and the loss of her impossible dream: Cockington Court.

Backing away from the big house, I am struck by its combination of dullness and hopeless fantasy.

I think of the murdered Polish woman, lying dead in Winner Street, and wonder what blue roses had been trampled there.

I think of what is happening to me: I came here, an expert in symbolist aesthetics and now I am interpreting a lawn, under an avalanche of information pouring into my head and body; and I am somehow making a kind of sense of it. Which makes me highly suspicious of either my own conclusions or of how I am being manipulated by someone else. Because sense never arrives spontaneously. It is always, like places, under construction; never not there and never complete. So, have these boards and handbooks and 'spontaneous' conversations all been put in place for me? Of course, not. So – I do what I always do, when research hits a "no" – I turn it all around: how is what I am becoming right now drawing all these things to me?

According to Salmon, Basil Duke Henning in *The House of Commons, 1660-1690, Volume One* records that the Mallock who bought Cockington Court made his money by marrying the "daughter of a shady Jewish lawyer" with offices by Gandy Street in Exeter. This would mean, if the Jewish lawyer's daughter was also Jewish, that the first two generations of Mallocks at Cockington were Jewish by birth, even if not by belief. This is a part of the story here that is missing from the family history written by the anti-semitic W.H. Mallock:

> ...between the reigns of Henry VII and Elizabeth they provided successive Parliaments with members for Lyme and Poole. One of them, Roger, during the reign of the latter sovereign, found his way to Exeter, where, as a banker or 'goldsmith', he laid the foundations of what was then a very great fortune, and built himself a large town house, of which one room is still intact, with the Queen's arms and his own juxtaposed on the panelling. The fortune accumulated by him was, during the next two reigns, notably increased by a second Roger, his son, in partnership with Sir Ferdinando Gorges [the patron of Cockington's George Weymouth, coloniser of Maine], the military governor of Plymouth, who had somehow become possessed of immense territories in Maine, and was a prominent figure in the history of English trade with America.

Somehow....

The grandson of Roger, who dies as a minor in 1699, is reported by Mallock as having "distinguished himself by an accomplishment extremely rare among the young country gentlemen of his own day – indeed, we may add of our own – that is to say, a precocious knowledge of Hebrew"; so it is possible that something of the Mallocks' cultural inheritance was being preserved, though unrecognised, or hidden, by W.H.

The figure of the 'shady' Jew lurks in many of Mallock's novels, including *A Human Document* (not to speak of Dempster's *Blue Roses*, where 'shady Jews' serve as a useful plot device; a group of cunning capitalists who protect the heroine from 'Les Rouges').

All this twisted research bends my head in two as I stare down the Front Lawn with its picturesque massing of tree canopy, green sward and sky. The cultural diversity of both the owners, and the shifting and metamorphosing populations of passers-by: Saxons, expelled Celts, Normans, French canons proper, Jews, Turkish sailors drowned and buried by the church, black slaves from the Plantations of the Dutch, 7 shillings and sixpence in the 1797 church accounts for "expenses of burying a Man that was wash'd on shore (exclusive of the Coffin)", in the same year a mutiny was suppressed among the Navy in the bay (two leaders hung from the yardarm in sight of shore), and so on. While the pace was not as swift as now, perhaps, today's globalisation is not the first time that diverse immigrations and visits have occurred at Cockington; in his lecture at Chelston Coffee Tavern in 1895, Richard Mallock MP sets off the legend of Phoenician visitors and their importation of a rich delicacy: clotted cream.

Disorientating, but liberating: this has nothing to do with me! A Yorkshire girl, Devon is alien. I have barely spoken to anyone Devonian. I eavesdrop on conversations in French and Polish among the visitors here. I am not an organic intellectual. I am a sprain on the landscape. Just bruising through; there is no art to what I am doing! I am going with its flow. Crudely looping, and the space is looping, the texts are looping; it has everything to do with me. It has its sting in me.

William Hurrell Mallock was born at Cockington Court in 1849 and went on to become a well-known writer on political and theological subjects. He was a serious theorist of conservatism in politics and a dogmatist in theology, which makes him sound as dull as ditchwater, but Mallock was a very accessible and engaging writer and he pushed his non-fiction work to a mass audience. He wrote satires and novels that were very popular at the time, though long ago faded from fashion.

Mallock describes his childhood as "a long succession of Christmases, when holly berries enlivened their frames and peeped over the walls of the pew where my elders drowsed, and my coevals were sustained during the sermon by visions of the plum pudding and crackers which would reward them in a near hereafter. I can still remember how, before these joys began, we would group ourselves in the dining-room windows, peering at distant woods, in which keepers still set man traps, or watching the village schoolchildren on their way from church homeward, making with their crimson cloaks a streak of colour as they followed one another across slopes of snow". A fabulous contrast to the procession of the Premonstratensians in their clotted cream robes making their way from abbey to chapel across the red fallen autumn leaves. Yet, here was a world that Mallock perceived as fixed and deferential: "when a member of 'the family' passed, women and children would curtsy and men touch their forelocks... the differences between the two classes were commonly assumed to be static, one supporting and one protecting the other, as though they resembled two geological strata".

However, in Mallock's anti-utopian satire *The New Republic*, set right here, one of its characters, speaking for his author, says "we live in an age of change. And in all such ages there must be many things that, if we let them, will pain and puzzle us". This is quite a change of outlook from that of Mallock's childhood at Cockington, which he acknowledges as manufactured: "Our impressions... were sedulously confirmed and developed by carefully chosen governesses. One of these, young as she was, was a really remarkable woman, for whom English history had hatched itself into something like a philosophy. Her philosophy had two bases, one being the postulate of the divine right of kings, the other being her interpretation of the victory of the Normans over the Anglo-Saxons... she seriously taught us that the population of modern England was still divided, so far as race is concerned, precisely as it was at the time of the completion of the Domesday Book; that the peers and the landed gentry were more or less pure-blooded Normans, and the mass of the people Saxons; that the principal pleasure of the latter was to eat to repletion; that their duty was to work for, that their privilege was to be patronized by, Norman overlords and distinguished Norman Churchmen; and finally, that of this Norman minority we ourselves were distinguished specimens."

Such geology is not just in the mind. At times here, everyday life was just as controlled as in a totalitarian state. The grandfather of Richard Mallock (who died in 1900) sent a 12-year-old boy for transportation to Australia for stealing a rabbit from Cockington Warren. In 1588 14 men were fined for laughing at a joke – the joke, a pun ("ad Globus") was some play upon the name, and physique no doubt, of a neighbour, one Mister Ball (perhaps a relative of Charity's?). Justice, including sentences of capital punishment, was administered by the squire.

In a world where the rapidity of discoveries and the turnover of ideas had generated what he believed was a kind of intellectual "drift" among even the more philosophically inclined and had made "wise men" as unprepared and anchorless as "fools", W.H. Mallock strained to produce a politically conservative and theologically orthodox oasis in a world increasingly defined by positivist-wrecking modernity. Yet, though Mallock and like-minded contemporaries perceived the threat of modernity, they could neither inhibit nor administer it. Instead it administered them. The undertow of radical instability and fashionable controversy characteristic of their works, packed with doubt and scandalous narrative, pre-empted their own modernist failure. Mallock and his kind might seek after fixity, but no construct could provide it to them; only a race to the bottom of qualities.

Here was the re-emergence of the Cockington knack for backing the wrong side.

One of Mallock's successes, a novel, bears the strange title "A Human Document". Published in 1892 it is a romance of sorts, in which an upper-class 'cracker-barrel' philosopher falls in love with a sexy, 'prospective widow' from Hampstead; Mallock's characteristic blend of scandal and ideas. The book was successful enough to quickly go through several editions. As suggested in the title, the novel deploys a pseudo-documentary framing; and at least one subsequent critic has ascribed this to the author's attempt to give shape to slippery social, philosophical and emotional materials that he found troubling.

This self-reflexive tension becomes more significant given what then happens to the novel itself. In the second half of the 20th century it has an unexpected second life.

In 1965 the London artist Tom Phillips walks out of his home on a quest to buy a book at random. His only rule: that it should cost him threepence. A second-hand copy of *A Human Document* is the book he finds, buys and takes home. Over the next six years Phillips transformed Mallock's book into a completely new thing. Using various strategies he would select a few words from each page of the novel to make something like a short poem – once this was done Phillips then obliterated/ decorated the rest of the page in humorous, satirical, cartoon-like, erotic, ornamental, psychedelic confections, responding to whatever sense had emerged from or survived his shipwreck creativity.

A Human Document was transformed into *A Humument* and on its publication its novelty and subversion gained it much publicity and popularity; far wider than most artists' 'book works'; it was a kind of *détournement* of Victorian materials that were already dead; a kind of parody of *détournement*; *détournement* aestheticised, then. It remains in print, in a fourth, substantially revised, edition.

I am so pleased that this vaporisation is acknowledged in the Court, on information boards in a suitably liminal room at the back of the building.

Out front, on the lawn, a friend of the Mallock family, a young woman, a frequent visitor to the Court, took part in many family theatricals here. While this is generally characterised as her learning to overcome her shyness, just as significantly for her later working life, Agatha Christie was learning to grasp the art of theatricality. It is no accident that her works have transferred so readily to stage and screen; the dramaturgy is already written in. The pictorial sweep of the Front Lawn is suggestive of the so-called 'empty space' of theatre, theatre's universalising fantasy that there is a neutral, virgin, non-space, a launch pad, a mere airport lounge in which great performers do greatness, unhindered.

Such is a place like this, but without greatness; just the ache for something special.

William Mallock tells a great story about a meeting of the Primrose League (a social organisation of the Conservative Party) on the lawn in the 1870s. He despaired of the lack of deep philosophical support for Conservatism in Torbay (comparable, perhaps, to today's despair among some senior US Republicans at what their voting base has become), but was excited to hear loud cheers coming from around one of the numerous stages about the lawn on which local Conservative dignitaries were speaking to the crowds. Rushing over to find out what political idea was so inspiring the locals, he discovered competitors behind a stage attempting to climb up a greased pole and win the leg of mutton strapped to its top.

A 19th-century FUNLAND.

> Conservatism even with them was no more than a vague sentiment... I tried again and again... to call their attention to the sources from which our national wealth generally, and most of their own food, was derived, and particularly to the economic significance of a town such as Torquay, much of the wealth of which had its origin in foreign countries. In dealing, however, with these matters, I met with no response more encouraging than puzzled smiles; but whenever, for want of something better to say, I alluded to 'this great Empire on which the sun never sets', I was greeted with volume of cheers.
>
> (*Memoirs of Life and Literature*, 1920)

BREXIT!!

Salmon is very damning of the information boards at the Court, because one of them wrongly identifies Occombe Woods, the woods that had saved me from the suburbs, as the location of the "just a flesh wound" scene from 'Monty Python and The Holy Grail' in which a Black Knight is slowly dismembered, and yet, even when just a torso, fights on. According to Salmon, and everyone else online, this is a local myth that has somehow got into the 'anectdotasphere' and refuses to come out again. I think I understand why. For it matches with the other narratives of dark and unformed shapes, of half bodies, blank faces and the silhouettes of wrecks, and it entertainingly blasphemes the myth of resilience in the face of storms and bombs and floods and crashes and bear markets; it is the place admitting to itself that Teignmouth was burned down, that SIMLA was exploded, that the beach huts were smashed to splinters and the Pirates Chest, after surviving the storms, was first disenfranchised and then incinerated; that the reason the Giraffe Café is barely marked is down to good fortune and an enemy with learning difficulties.

I am getting a little tired of Salmon and his debunking of hoaxes and myth. He seems to think that the dissection of a myth somehow releases it, that rationalisation is liberation; he, like others, doesn't seem to understand the force of a myth's self-deception and intoxication and then work from there. I sympathise with the Reverend Hilderic Friend who, at the end of the 19th century, confessed that "a heavy charge must be laid upon the scholars and antiquaries, who, during the last quarter of a century, have done much to drive the poetry out of our Devonshire place-names, by bringing them to the touch-stone of linguistic facts and laws, by denying us the right to call in the Druids and fairies, the old Teutonic gods, and the heroes of chivalry to account for the rhythmic and poetic names with which our tors, streams, vales and villages abound".

I follow the scythe of limes along the edge of the lawn; 42 lime trees (40 for the nations, one for the GATT secretariat, one for the British Foreign Office), all planted in celebration of the 1951 conference of the General Agreement on Tariffs and Trade in Torquay; the early spadework for deregulation, globalisation and neo-liberalism. Shipwreck modernity, via the collapse of European monarchies, had brought the world, after the storm, washing up in Torbay. In 1951 those who had replaced the monarchies in power had gathered here to organise the backwash. Then, after GATT came the Bilderberg Group, assembling in Torquay in 1977; among their participants were Henry Kissinger, Giovanni Agnelli (the Fiat boss), Ralf Dahrendorf, Sir Charles Forte and Sir Keith Joseph. Of the three items up for discussion that week, the second was: "the future of the mixed economies in the Western democracies". I wonder in what detail the Thatcher/Reagan nexus was put into place in Torbay.

A woman is sat on a bench by the path, under the heart-shaped leaves of a lime, watching the cricket from a distance. Writing in a notepad. A rucksack beside her. She calls over.

"From the conference?"

"Yes."

"What did you make of it?"

"Were you there?"

"I saw you arriving as I was leaving."

"So, do you know why it all split up?"

"Did it? Or are we more together now than when we were all cooped up in one place?"

"Are you a walking artist?"

"That's two things really, isn't it? I write. I walk. Should one be any business of the other?"

I thought she bristled.

"I didn't see you at any of the fringe meetings?"

I explain that I am an academic engaged to write a report of the main conference.

"That's the mistake you all made. There is no "main", no "proper". Do you read poetry?"

I admit that it has been a while; PhD and all that. For three years most of what I read was directly linked to my study: Blok, Bely, Baudelaire, Mallarmé, de Nerval, Desbordes-Valmore. Mostly theatre, not much verse.

"No."

"Good. There is a crisis that you need not worry yourself about. When the poets have sorted themselves out then you should start reading them again. Here."

She hands me her notebook.

"I can't take this."

She is amazed.

"I thought you said you were writing a report?"

"I am."

"What's the point of a report without poetry? And *you* can't write poetry, obviously. How could you, when you don't read it?"

It was my turn to bristle.

"The others might not laugh in your face if you published your own poetry in a paper, but you would suspect that they were doing so behind your back? No? Or that they wanted to and were just being polite? See, you can quote me and I can take that worry off your shoulders. Quotation gives a paper a certain authority, doesn't it? The few academic books I've read are full of quotations. They plagiarise each other openly, and put the victim's name at the bottom; in poetry it's a much more subtle racket. Our great problem, Cecile, is that we are all in the same conspiracy, we have no secrets yet we still conspire to pretend that we are keeping something special from each other; maybe that is also our salvation. Enjoy your walk."

She gets up and begins to lope towards the house.

On the cricket field, a strange game is being played. The pitch slopes so precipitously down one side and up the other that a mighty clobber of the ball goes for nothing on one side and a feather touch on the other clears the boundary.

She fades from view around Finn's gravestone. I sit down and read the poems (I have interspersed them through the text.)

Cream-trousered fielders labour up the hill after the creeping ball; then speed helter-skelter hopelessly after accelerating fours. Everything has tipped. The light falls awkwardly through the trees in sheets. Salmon says that there's a kind of observable shelf above the pitch, a very old road, Saxon at the very latest, Castle Lane, a route to the 'British Camp' iron age hill fort at Chelston.

I can see a shift in the shadows where it should be; what should be light is dark, and what should be dark is light.

With all the 'theatre' of the strangely shaped ground, the sheets of light, the dappled canopy, white sidescreens, and zooming balls and arcing bats, it's all a bit reminiscent of the lab experiments of the great Hungarian Gestaltist Lajos Kardos, who first demonstrated how a person's perception of things, their brightness and their colour, is determined by array and the positioning of illuminations as well as direct light or the pigment of objects themselves; that there is always an "illegitimate" disturbance factor at the micro-level of noticing that depends, each and every time, on particular "temporary conditions and constellations".

The ball leaps off the pitch and bends by the batter's ear.

In other words, that what we see is not just an effect of the local thing, or of the light on it, but always also of the 'foreign' field adjacent to it; "no surface belongs exclusively to a single framework of illumination... Frameworks emerge and recede as we move about the environment."

No single framework... ever... frameworks emerge and recede as we move about the environment... I know this stuff from study of the gestalt tendencies in symbolism, but it has never struck me like this before – a sliced shot wrongfoots the fielder and goes curving to the boundary – that it might be real, that to actually realise a non-objectivist perception of shifting things in the real world you don't need to theorise, you need to *actually move*. That walking, if you know how to look, is a higher knowing, because to it is revealed the foreign fields, not just the local things (most mechanical transport would be too fast – no sooner would the eye identify a field than it would disappear, but a conscious walker would be able to see the emergence and recession of each successive one); that kind of walking and looking rescues reflection from opportunistic, atomistic, neo-liberal fragmentation and gives it to interleaving fields. No wonder the Gestaltists were suppressed; first by the Nazis and then by US behaviourists!

Even with deregulation no single objective field need be lost to fragmentation, because instead this kind of looking restores meaning as multiplicity of fields, not a fracturing and separation of everything! I think this is a pilgrimage. Something has brought me – with this knowledge – to the wonky cricket ground...

And I'd thought those experiments were just cultural background...

A gentle defensive prod sends the ball scuttling for another improbable boundary.

I watch for half an hour, walking around the undulating boundary rope, testing the theory. Back at the bench I open the notebook.

The poems are clearly written for and about (and possibly written in) specific and particular sites; but they have been cleaned out, bleached of details that would make them traceable. Much like the book of photographs of a Newton Abbot flâneur on sale at the conference: one of the few retail opportunities I turned down. This is as if her poetry were a secret operation, a covert undermining of place in favour of space: that the two concepts were separate continents engaged in a cold war, rather than shifting fields.

I watch the old road moving about in the shadows.

The ball comes spiralling upwards from the shoulder of the bat and five fielders set off to catch it, tripping in turn and rolling like cream-coloured logs down the incline and across the boundary rope. The cherry ball is caught by a dog and carried into the small trees high up on my side of the small valley, pursued by a complacent owner.

Two pilots fight for a joystick, architects dig feet from foundations
A tunnel is a handshake between false starts and demeanours
And on the table in the mill
They are laying glasses flat as maps
Until the planes find a kind of balance
In what each one leaves unfilled.

Something about deferral, I think. Possibly.

I wander away from the house, under the GATT limes. Past the dead tree to the left, its roots in a plague pit, where park gardener Charlie Fey was hospitalised after digging up bones and then ordered by "the authorities" not to speak of what he had seen. This is where a black silhouette had been sighted one dusk, dressed like the stereotypical anarchist in flowing black cloak and broad-brimmed hat, a 'bogeyman', caught in the beam of the bicycle headlamp of another of the gardeners, Jack Steer, in 1958.

I cross the grass, along the boardwalk and through the gate. There's a huge pub there, designed by Sir Edwin Lutyens. Not the obvious choice of architect for a village pub; but this one was a part of a larger plan of Lutyens's for a model modern village here. Like the modernist survivals at Churston, the pub is another false start for Devon. This could have been a pattern for a new kind of village; desirable residences, small trades, proper amenities, a pub to draw people to the place. The plans were pretty advanced. Lutyens got as far as designing the shop signs: for the mechanics, a car pulled by a horse; another sign had two spouting whales, but I don't know what that was for. This was a model which kept labour and amenities in the village and that might have transformed the countryside; instead of which the villages retained their appearances, mostly, but inside were increasingly hollowed out of people; growing tumorous dormitories and little used holiday homes.

Wedded to the innovations in farming that Salmon says were in experimental development on the nearby Dartington Estate (as much about factory farming as they were about the priorities of The Soil Association), was there a new kind of Devon emerging in the 1930s? One which for nostalgic and conservational reasons was nipped before it could bud? But which might have continued the narrative, which has now been severed and made 'historic', of cutting edge science and design, often with a military or colonial application – radio, gold refining, cybernetics, battleship design, relativity, algebra for quantum mechanics, underwater exploration.

I am back in love with A.J. Salmon.

I order half a roast dinner at the bar and sit outside, under the cenotaph shape of the giant chimney, to eat it. The Drum is an eerie place, humanised by its visitors; the proportions do not feel quite right, its bricks are too small and its frame too large. A cottage suffering from gigantism.

Across from the pub is a huge car park where the new village should now be, designed by Lutyens in a 'tree of life' pattern. I assume that Lutyens's nod to memorial in the pub chimney's shape has something to do with the 43 names on the First World War memorial in the church; at a rough guess that was maybe as much as a third of the male working population of the village at the time. No wonder it "has never recovered, destined to become the chocolate box cover village of the tourist". A cause of resentment that occasionally surfaced in tales of cattle driven at tourists, drivers mis-directed and the antics of a fake beekeeper who would make great play with a smoke 'gun', collecting coins for a children's apiary that somehow never materialised.

Across from the pub is a giant mill wheel, which Salmon claims is broken, adding a photo of it covered in emerald moss, apparently past the point of no repair. Well, it is certainly 'working' now. Driven by water from a large pool above the path, though I cannot make out what, if anything, it is driving. The pond is eerily still. In the time of George III ("it is said", Salmon again) the lady of the Court liked to be driven about the estate in a gilded coach. When she died, the coach was left out to rot, eventually collapsing into the pond,

> *Ever after, passers-by may catch a stirring,*
> *In the waters dark and deep, and a*
> *Splinter will surface, partly gilded, partly green,*
> *As if waking briefly from the clutch of sleep.*

Down past a linhay, I reach that part of Cockington "where time has stood still" – hahaha! – this is the crossroads around 'The Old Forge'; today it is still turning out tiny horseshoes. It is as mutable as anywhere else in the complex. Its ersatz qualities sit neatly in a discourse of fixity and identity: the 'Weavers' Cottage' here was actually a farmhouse; the 'Old School House', only briefly a school, is really a Devon longhouse where folk lived with their animals under the same roof, built on a slope so the animals could be kept in the lower part from where their effluent ran directly into the street. It's a shop now. I briefly look in; an examination of the back of a packet of sweets labelled "Cockington" reveals that they were made in Market Harborough. In 1929 it was rumoured that 'The Old Forge' was to be dismantled and taken to the US; questions were asked at Westminster.

My roast at 'The Drum' was good, but I'm sorry not to have eaten at the tables outside Rose Cottage (though the menu is nothing to write home about); I overhear the place described by a visitor as "like The Prisoner's Portmeirion" and that's about right. A pianist under an awning is playing the theme from 'Jurassic Park'.

I follow the main route through the village proper, its houses built on the same ground plans as the original Saxon settlement. Salmon cites *Devon Notes and Queries* from 1910 in which a Mrs Eliza Hingston has written about the people who lived in these farms and cottages, including her father George Madge (born 1807) who, at ten years of age, was apprenticed for ten years to a Mr. Shapley, a farmer at Chelston, establishing a lifelong relationship and friendship. Describing a time when Madge would have been coming to the end of his working life, the Reverend Hawkes read a paper to the Devonshire Association in which he outlined the conditions of Devonshire labourers; their basic wage was supplemented by corn, cider, straw and other things that came direct from the employer. At harvest time, extra hours were rewarded with an "abundance of meat… and to give cider without stint".

The direct 'presence' of the productive land and the longstanding relationships, of control for sure, between farmer and labourer, but also its standing outside of the usual commercial nexus, is the material basis for a degree of nostalgia about this "more stable" society, "as if all the village was one family with the Court at its head". That stability was yoked to a direct connection through things, often unmediated by markets, tied to the caprices of the seasons and the capacities and adaptations of organisms rather than buyers and sellers. One can see inside the rosy-tinted nostalgia a grain of something like the improvised economies that emerge out of devastation, such as the informal mushroom harvests that have developed in the ruins of the great US forests, where logging has moved out and a heterogenous group of loners, outlaws and migrant pickers with traditional skills has developed an economy which bypasses the market-setting of prices. I had read about this in Anna Lowenhaupt Tsing's *The Mushroom at the End of the World* and I wonder if this kind of 'to the side of' the market, yet within the bounds of a market-based economy, is in any way both sustainable and exponential, and if so, if the crucial driver is the thing itself, released from being product; was there some defiance of alienation there in the thing released from commodity?

Salmon spoils his hopeful narrative with some folkloric nonsense from an 1877 account of Sleuth Hounds in Cockington: "I have ascertained from an old woman, a native of Cockington, that she has many times heard the sleuth hounds at night. They will go over the roof of the house, but never enter the door, and never do any harm unless you meet them." These hounds are common in Devon, common all over; but what were they *here* exactly? A very distant and guilty Anglo-Saxon memory of the 10th-century expulsion of their Celtic/British neighbours by Saint/King Athelstan who reputedly regularly used the route to Dartmouth that passed Gallows Gate to launch his raids of ethnic cleansing? The hounds are a violent threatening force, and yet only to those who see them; that is, only to those upon whom they call; Saxon neighbours who stayed quietly in their homes in 926 while their Wealas neighbours were being expelled may have come through without a scratch, but were they henceforth haunted by an irreconcilable pack of myths that visited in the night? Or were such stories a Victorian folkloric invention of a 'superstitious peasantry', a convenient fantasy for those seeking to turn a fungal relation into a geological one?

I take the lane out of Cockington, rather than the footpath through the trees.

A little way down, on the right, is a wooden gate, jammed ajar. A sign warns against tipping, but not against trespass. I dip in. Beyond the gate is a second barrier: a fallen tree draped in ivy. It looks like an insect monster. I dodge under that too. Not so easy. Now a special space unpeels. An old quarry, at the base of which are growing huge, thin trees that search up for light, all their green at the top of enormous narrow poles. The face of the quarry has crumbled since it was last worked; in one part there is a spoil pile of fragments, worked by rains, in another part a giant overhanging ledge of reddened Devon slate, the size of a tank, juts from the face. A thing powerful, a thing immense. Just the thingness of it! I should have used the loos in the pub. I squat under the ledge, daring it to fall on me at this one moment in two hundred million years.

Zipping up, I stand under the tall thin sentinels and let the silence fall down on me. I begin to detach from the carnival of the Court and Rose Cottage, from the military-trivial complex of Torbay. I feel an isolated peace descending, a hermit-quietude inside all this carousing; all this thundering mass whirled around me – not just the history, but the shipwreck, jellies and foreign fields – and then just me.

It is as I am about to test the one remaining part of the quarry that I see the tent, and then the extensive regalia of homelessness. I tread carefully and quietly back across the hybrid floor of slate bits, semi-submerged cans and spongy moss.

Thomas Moran drew here. Thomas Moran, the great painter of the US geological landscape. And he could make no more of this place than me. Something between grandeur, dumb stupidity and rank injustice; his drawings here are like child's scribbles, more like the surface of storming water than rock. When he got back to New York he painted Cockington Lane, with a bend that is not there; though he might have been painting the turning into Old Paignton Road and mis-labelled it? The painting has that green cave thing I will be repeatedly entering; that luring green maw I will come to love, oblique turnings into a potential for just about anything, places where anything might be waiting.

But Thomas Moran! Here. It is as if I had bumped into the subject of the Mona Lisa, alive and living in poverty in Cockington... but then she was, wasn't she? The mostly forgotten Eugenie, model for Lady Liberty, had she haunted the lawns, or was never invited, as the third wife of the "flamboyant" (read "Jewish") Isaac Singer?

There is no plaque in the quarry, no recognition of a visit by genius; only the sign against tipping and a neglect of the space that has made a kind of safety for someone vulnerable.

On the road I meet the spectres of extras shooting the silent movie 'Nelson'; chasing the King's soldiers, only be turned on and chased themselves.

At the junction with the Old Mill Road, at a giant Beekite-like turning circle, I take the left. Going straight to the sea seems dull now. At the top of the short sharp hill I find myself at what must have been a very grand residence once, now multiple flats and 'cottages'. The former home of William Froude. I knew from Salmon it was in some part of this property that Froude had constructed tanks, including one under his attic, in which he tested battleship designs in miniature. Froude was the first to make such experiments; and engineer-pilgrims still travel here from Japan to show their appreciation, Salmon says, though I see none.

Opposite Froude's place, weirdly, is the Hungarian Consulate! I am in the middle of nowhere, I am in a village zone between two quiet seaside towns and I am being avalanched by sensations and narratives and displaced powers. Behind the walls and the hedges there are HUGE houses here. Turns out that the Honorary Hungarian Consul is a local councillor; helping Hungarian nationals in the South West with their problems and queries. Their Consulate building is a self-catering holiday property, with two imposing eagles on its gateway, it is called PROTEA: according to Wikipedia "the genus Protea was named in 1735 by Carolus Linnaeus after the Greek god Proteus, who could change his form at will, because proteas have such different forms".

CAMELOT, SHANGRI-LA, MEDINA; house names here. Utopias, individualised and gated.

> ...the motto of the future is freedom – holy, awful individual freedom. We shall each be free to choose or evolve the religion most profoundly suited to us.
>
> W.H. Mallock, *The New Republic*

I wonder if I should stop looking at Salmon's guide.

Not many engineers have a law named after them, but Froude's Law of Comparison has been influential in engineering and zoology. His Law states that the speed attainable by either a creature or a ship, where there is some geometrical symmetry, is proportional to the square root of their length, that the relation between a ship and its model (and, in theory between a squid and its model) can be calculated from its displacement and length where speed is the same; that flow divided by the square route of the sum of external field and length produces a Froude Number by which different designs, different warships, different squids can all be compared.

I don't really get it, I'm repeating what I found online, but what seems exceptional is that this Froude Number can be used in respect of real seas, of real choppy waters, not just on a theoretical plane.

Froude's Law determines that the energy generated by a steam engine is proportional to the square of the scale of its boilers, that the amount of heat energy transferred by a ship's boiler is limited by its surface area rather than by its volume, and that a similar limiting factor applies to creatures, that the work they can do is proportional to the surface area of their lungs.

It feels strange to be thinking of the design and manufacture of immense and immensely destructive ships, while walking up the tiniest of lanes, confined by tall Devon hedges; I could be in the middle of rolling hills and green pastures, a mile or more from the nearest farmhouse, but I am approaching a morbid laboratory.

I turn down the beautifully named Seaway Lane. Salmon mentions a plaque. A man is bringing out rubbish from his house. He asks me how much I know; I know a little. "I'm very lucky, I have a lovely flat garden," he says, and gestures over his shoulder, "because Froude levelled the ground here to build his first experimental tanks. The first tanks were built here, so I have a lovely flat garden". He marches me a few metres down the lane to the large stone plaque and goes back to attending to his rubbish. A 4x4 pulls up; a woman leans over: "did he say the experimental tanks were on his lawn?" Yes, he did. "I'm in the marine trade." And with that she guns the engine and drives away.

Two of the ceramic tiles from the street name have been lost: S WAY LANE.

On first looking on the bay from S(ea)way Lane, it could be a different sea from the one at Paignton. I have no idea why I feel this. A Bow-born author I will have cause to rage over later in my walk once remarked upon "a favourite thesis at Oxford in my day, that there was no proof that Napoleon had ever existed, because nobody had ever seen him" (Reginald Blomfield). Which might explain why Devonians had poured into small boats and out on the waves – thousands at a time – to view the progressive-dictator display himself, under arrest aboard the 'Billy Ruffian' (HMS Bellerophon) in the bay. Perhaps, they had come to see if he actually existed; or, if not, if they could bring him into existence. Napoleon was another of those manifestations of the Devil who regularly appear in story form in Devon, luring erring parsons into the sea or dragging their hooves in snow or purloining the names of things. It is said, repeatedly – on the understanding that if you say a thing enough times you bring it into being (I hadn't seen a negligee yet) – that the Devil's most powerful weapon is the idea that he doesn't exist. Rather like "charity begins at home" – well, that's not charity, then, that's self-interest – this is one of those sayings that do not describe but rather create meaning; the Devil has no separate existence from such phrases, but that is an existence. He's a primitive and protean form of ideology, or 'Spectacle' as the psychogeographers like to call its contemporary form.

Today our demons do not hide their existence, complaining that they cannot help how they are. For sure, they say, we are constructed – by all your eyes – and that is all there is, and all that there is is is. Like those tedious plaques for the Trafalgar Way – Salmon has a picture of one disappearing into a shrub by Exeter's council offices – machines in the same process; the delivering of representations of victory. Each one crafted at the expense of the blood on the deck of the Bellerophon. Lieutenant Lapenotière's journey by coach is a scribble in alloy, a first dribble from the lip of a young Spectacle; but that is what it always was. A strategic reality made by the tactic of eyes, now made large.

The traffic on the road that separates the hotel from the beach is so intense I have to walk a hundred metres or so to find a place to cross. Finally there's a gap in the stream of cars and I can look over the thick red walls. Off to my right I can clearly make out, in the waters, the sickle shape of the stone pier built for William de Falaise, the second Norman resident at Cockington Court, for his travels to France and back. It doesn't look much like an international port any more. But it's a reminder of just how connected we have been; the ports along this coast once licensed to carry thousands of pilgrims every year.

I find it incredible to think, up on the top of thirty metres of rock and concrete, that all this was brought down in 1859 by huge waves, that the road was scooped out by the storm right up to the walls of the hotels behind me; and that greater storms are coming. Before I can make my way to the beach, thinking maybe I can find some of the walkers there, I recognise, from Salmon's description, what had been Livermead House. Built in 1820 for the Reverend Roger Mallock, it had been a seaside guesthouse for visitors to Cockington Court, among them the Christian Socialist Charles Kingsley, a friend of James Anthony Froude, and famously author of *The Water Babies*. Rather later, when the house had been commercialised, a 13-

year-old Gracie Fields, who would go on to make a fortune singing songs like 'Red Sails in The Sunset', a reference to the ochre sails of the Brixham fishing fleet she would have seen in the bay, stayed here. There are still five of the once four hundred Brixham trawlers afloat, and I think I see the red sails of one out there now. I want to, anyway; maybe that is enough.

Kingsley stayed here for some months in 1854, while his wife convalesced, and during that time he scoured the beaches at Corbyn Head, Livermead and Preston and wrote *Glaucus or The Wonders of the Shore*, inspired by the zoological writings of the 'Last Thursdayist' Philip Henry Gosse, the populariser of the home aquarium, who lived in Torquay. "You make God tell a lie," Kingsley would say to Gosse of his theory that God had included a deception, millions of years of fabricated fossils, when he produced the cosmos in a single moment around 6pm on the 22nd of October, 4004 BC. Kingsley's book is filled with precise descriptions and exquisite illustrations of the rock pool universes of tiny animals, most of them long since fished out and poked into obscurity by the very interest that Kingsley sought to inspire. The rock pools here are as stripped as the crystal cave at Saltern Cove.

Glaucus was a fisherman who took to the sea and became a submarine shepherd, tending to sea life in the meadows under the waves; like the sward of sea grass on Torre Abbey Sands, where, long before low tide, I can make out the meadows of Zostera.

I had read Salmon's theory (Salmon is a bit like a Devon version of the character on 'Goodness Gracious Me', Mr-Everything-Comes-From-India) about a chain of 19th-century technologists – Babbage, Clifford, Julian, Peacock, Froude, Heaviside, Lethbridge – all living or working along the coast from Starcross to Paignton. In his *Glaucus'* Kingsley adds 'life scientists' to the chain: "No wonder that such a spot as Torquay, with its delicious Italian climate, and endless variety of rich woodland, flowery lawn, fantastic rock-cavern, and broad bright tide-sand, sheltered from every wind of heaven except the soft south-east, should have become a favourite haunt, not only for invalids, but for naturalists... the original home of marine zoology and botany in England... For here worked Montagu, Turton, and Mrs. Griffith... Here, too, the scientific succession is still maintained by Mr. Pengelly and Mr. Gosse... the soft sandstones and hard conglomerates of the new red series slope down into the tepid and shallow waves, afford an abundance and variety of animal and vegetable life, unequalled, perhaps, in any other part of Great Britain".

Not any more.

Among the creatures Kingsley finds on the Institute Beach, beside de Falaise's pier, is a model of self-transformation:

> ...look at the mouth of the shell; a long grey worm protrudes from it, which is not the rightful inhabitant. He is dead long since, and his place has been occupied by one Sipunculus Bernhardi... finding the mouth of the Turritella too big for him, he has plastered it up with

sand and mud... and has left only a round hole, out of which he can poke his proboscis. A curious thing is this proboscis, when seen through the magnifier. You perceive a ring of tentacles round the mouth, for picking up I know not what; and you will perceive, too, if you watch it, that when he draws it in, he turns mouth, tentacles and all, inwards, and so down into his stomach, just as if you were to turn the finger of a glove inward from the tip till it passed into the hand; and so performs, every time he eats, the clown's as yet ideal feat, of jumping down his own throat.

Wow. *That's* what I call seaside entertainment! But Kingsley is interested in more than a freakshow. Contemplating the oceans in which the grey limestone cliffs – I can see them now, under the pinky grey evening sky, in a sweep from Berry Head to Daddyhole Plain – were formed from the silt of billions and billions of animal deaths over tens of millions of years, he describes a 'tree of life':

all tiny things, the lingering and, as it were, expiring remnants of that great coral-world which, through the abysmal depths of past ages, formed here in Britain our limestone hills, storing up for generations yet unborn the materials of agriculture and architecture... To think that the whole human race... has been rushing out of eternity and into eternity again, as Arjoon in the Bhagavad Gita beheld the race of men issuing from Kreeshna's flaming mouth, and swallowed up in it again... and all that while, and ages before that mystery began, that humble coral, unnoticed on the dark sea-floor, has been 'continuing as it was at the beginning'... while races and dynasties and generations have been: '*Playing such fantastic tricks before high heaven, As make the angels weep*'. Yes; it is this vision of the awful permanence and perfection of the natural world... which would at moments crush the naturalist's heart, and make his brain swim with terror, were it not that he can see by faith, through all the abysses and the ages, not merely '*Hands, from out the darkness, shaping man*'.

Well, I have no such faith. Don't want it and don't seek it. I do *want*, however, to reach out with my hands to take and shake the hands in the darkness shaping me; but I am nervous. It is a darkness to which a young and precocious William Mallock, on the publication in 1876 of his *succès de scandale*, *The New Republic* – set at a thinly disguised Livermead House, "a cool villa by the sea" – reached out and touched.

Cockington Lane, Old Mill Road, Seaway Lane, Torbay Road.

After three years' immersion in Symbolism's lateral and allusive strategies of meaning, a *roman-à-clef* is familiar territory. I find a copy for sale on Amazon Marketplace, order it for the Grand Hotel (there are 'No Vacancies' at the Livermead House Hotel), next-day delivery. It comes in time for breakfast, and I enjoy the musty, slightly sexual smell of its yellowed pages and cracked binding. Over breakfast and coffee, sat in the big window overlooking the bay (I'd got an early alarm call to secure a good table), I skip the theological dialogues and consume the rest.

I taught myself to speed read in my twenties and it is coming in useful now.

The book tells of a lightly disguised gathering of the intellectual celebrities of the day: John Ruskin, Matthew Arnold, Thomas Carlisle and others. The few female characters are either anonymous or trivialised ("Miss Prattle"); the most rounded, Lady Ambrose, is a simulacrum, a copy of no one real, while the avatar for the poetess Violet Fane is described in the introduction, by Sir John Squire, as "a communal Egeria". What the hell does he mean? That strange thing, a woman who can write? A sex-pilgrim for the collective exploitation? It is not the only reference to Egeria – author of an account of a 4th-century pilgrimage to Jerusalem – I have come across. The travel writer S.P.B. Mais opens his book *We Wander in The West* (1950) with a rich conflation of colonialism, serial monogamy, *genius loci*, sexual conquest and pilgrimage, describing how he always travels "in the company of Egeria, not always the same Egeria. I have gone through life in search of Egeria and Egeria and I together have gone through life in search of the West Country. Both are elusive."

In this male construct, walking the landscape is both an exploration and an appropriation of an eternally renewable territory with "always something fresh to discover". This is a familiar lie about 'virgin territory' in which the female adventurer is flattened into a metaphor for territory possessed by men; a woman walker expected to represent the route itself and play the subsidiary role of exchangeable companion.

The young host of Mallock's seaside party prepares menus with different courses of conversation and then struggles to keep the guests on message. John Ruskin wants to blow up anatomical museums and Wolverhampton. While some of the intellectual preoccupations of the time have long passed into obscurity, there are details that still startle: a melancholy monument to loveless and skewed relationships straight out of Wilde, a pair of salt-cellars that are "models of a peculiar kind of retort invented for burning human bodies and turning them into gas".

The biggest excitement around the book's publication was the effect it had on the career of Walter Pater, represented in the book as 'Mister Rose'. Mallock's homophobic depiction of Pater started a bilious stream of anti-gay characterisations by du Maurier and others. It drove Pater to withdraw from applying for the Oxford Professorship of Poetry. Yet, Rose is the most interesting of all the characters, a monster and an exemplar. If it were not for the putrescent context – Lady Ambrose says of him "he always seems to talk of everybody as if they had no clothes on" – Rose might now be a household name, pre-empting postmodernism with his call for an architecture "of no style in particular, but a *renaissance* of all styles". His apocalyptic description of the city of London pre-empts T.S. Eliot's by 48 years; he recounts "a delicious walk I took… by the river side, between Charing Cross and Westminster…

there went streaming on the wide wild waters with long vistas of reflected lights wavering and quivering in them; and I roamed about for hours, hoping I might see some unfortunate cast herself from the Bridge of Sighs. It was a night I thought well in harmony with despair."

Rose pre-empts the symbolist serial killer so beloved by misogynistic literary psychogeographers.

In the Conclusion to Rose/Pater's *The Renaissance*, a work of theft and composture if ever there was one, I found a pre-emptive paean to Phil Smith's 'mythogeography', with its primary sources in mobility "our life is a perpetual motion", and multiplicity, "a flood of external objects" burying experience benignly. Sustaining the rush of things, Pater decries "that thick wall of personality through which no real voice has ever pierced". He disconnects the cold hand of identity from the fundamental elements (including experiences) which burst the body; celebrating instead "the action of these forces that extend beyond us: it rusts iron and ripens corn", and dissipating the anthropocentric focus: "birth and gesture and the spring of violets from the grave are but a few out of ten thousand resultant combinations.... face and limb is but an image of ours, under which we group them – a design in a web, the actual threads of which pass out beyond it".

Field thinking! An ally for the quantum walkers!

All this sets the scene for the entrance of Dr. Jenkinson, the avatar of Mallock's real-life personal hero, Benjamin Jowett, theologian and influential Oxford tutor, who gives a sermon from the stage of the guest house's little theatre. Jenkinson/Jowett poses before a backdrop, preaching "in the middle of a gorge in the Indian Caucasus – the remains of a presentation of 'Prometheus Bound'". He describes a spirituality which evolves, like ape to human, from a fear of God to a love of God. Christianity, he argues, is emerging from and outgrowing its "deeper unity" with principles found in all religions; somehow the present status quo comes miraculously crawling out from the "imperfection" of its past and is transfigured. What has been evil is becoming good, slavery and colonial rapine are superseded and forgiven as the building blocks of a divinely commissioned modernity. A servant lowers the front curtain "and Faust and the young witch again covered the preacher from the eyes of his congregation".

The ridiculous staging is a ploy on Mallock's part to distract from the sermon's, and his own, synthesis of religious belief with a newly savage materialism: "in their last analysis a pig and a martyr, a prayer and a beefsteak, are just the same... note the truly celestial light that science throws". The preaching ends with the apocryphal words of Jesus Christ, reported by Clement of Alexandria: "The Lord being asked when His Kingdom should come, said, when two shall be one, and that which is without is as that which is within, and the male with the female – neither male nor female". In Mallock and Jowett's universe all was uniform and is becoming uniform again and it's not turtles but reductionism all the way down...

The New Republic: culture, faith, and philosophy in an English Country House is a remarkable book. Even after almost 150 years, it's a rattling good read. It is funny, witty, surprising, even shocking, and prescient: it condemns the worn-out aristocracy, the "marriage market", mass production and industrialised cremation; it proposes a very modern kind of historiography: "History, in its true sense, is travelling in the past… your histories of dates and battles are at best but the Bradshaws and the railway-maps. Our past must be an extension of the present". It pre-empts globalisation and a mobilities-paradigm: "being, as we else should be, merely *temporal* people, who are just as narrow-minded and dull as those merely *local* people – the natives of a neighbourhood – who wear gorgeous ribbons at flower-shows in the country" and salutes the hegemony of science's alliance with materialism, which "once came into the world like a small street boy throwing mud…. and the indignant world very soon drove it away. But it has now come back again, dirtier than ever, bringing a big brother with it, and Heaven knows when we shall get rid of it now".

Culture is a YBA freakshow: "our generation would rather look at a foetus in a bottle, than at a statue of the god Apollo". (Cue Hirst and his cow and calf halved in the Spanish Barn at Torre Abbey).

When I took the train to Paignton I expected to join a small group of ambulant intellectuals trying to generate a critical vortex in a quiet tourism backwater. But I found a backwater that is remarkably unquiet, its ghosts rattling and its intellectual narratives ending in inflamed stumps. Behind the faded grandeur of declining seaside resorts and an older revenant of fishing villages, woods, farms and country courts, there is an angrier and cleverer conservatism, a legacy of modernising reactionaries irritated by 'geological' relationships, slowness, thingness, mushroom economy and jelly longevity. Mostly, this revolutionary conservatism – like Lutyens's village – never happens, except now by default in shabby cuts to social spending and the progressive mouldering of public space. But there is an impregnation of disgruntlement, a bilious irritation that the opportunities for a brilliant and modern reaction have been squandered. That everything has been scaled to disappointment and humiliation; rather than real navies in the bay, the area is reduced to models in the attic. The thousand trees ripped up for Nelson from Manscombe Woods ("the evil valley") have returned as a farcical reciprocation in Torquay Rotary Club's gifting of "A Thousand Trees" for verges in 1966. The wars with France and the US that bathed this coastline with insecurity and vulnerability have long cooled, but fear remains – the squire of Cockington Court set up his own artillery station in the late 19th century, in 1900 a tremor along the Sticklepath Fault mistaken for the rumble of French guns in the bay – and now such anxieties, digging themselves out of their graves, miserably scaled, fear not great navies but drowning refugees. The Brexit vote in Torbay was huge, unlike anywhere else in Devon: over 63% to 'leave Europe'.

Chapter Six: Corbyn Head to Babbacombe

I slip out of the Grand and down to the beach. The tide has receded a little and I spend a while climbing over the rocks and looking in the rockpools through Kingsley's words.

"Cast one wondering glance, too, at the forest of zoophytes and corals, Lepraliae and Flustrae, and those quaint blue stars, set in brown jelly, which are no zoophytes, but respectable molluscs, each with his well-formed mouth and intestines, but combined in a peculiar form of Communism, of which all one can say is, that one hopes they like it".

I cannot see much and I understand even less. But my scrambling and poking and peering reminds me of being a child. The last two days have felt childlike, as if I have actually followed through with my threat, aged six, to run away from home; as though I had not stopped at the corner but kept on going, irreversibly, my plastic bag of toys and drinks squeezed damply in my hand.

I stand on the rocks and look out to the limestone cliffs beyond Torquay; I look down, I look up to a shimmer of sunlight on the gently swelling bay, and I look down and I cannot believe what I see. The rocks I have been standing on, assuming them the most natural thing possible, a chunk of cliff eroded away by the waves, are a construct! There is a line in the water! And when I look more closely, what I thought were rough inlets to search in for crabs and small fish, are the gaps between huge plates of cut stone. Slabs, about four feet wide, and three or four feet sticking up out of the sand, lain one against another in a straight line, turning in at the end to make the curl at the edge of a harbour mouth. There is nothing in Salmon about this, but it is just as clearly a pier as anything on the Institute Beach at Livermead. I climb up onto Corbyn Head and sure enough the structure is as clear as anything from above. I imagined these beaches were playgrounds, but they are industrial ruins.

I had not intended to come up to the Head again. The Rotary Club plaque irritated me; am I supposed to care who these people of 1966 were, to recognise them by their trees, probably all brought down by now by Dutch Elm, Ash Dieback and Sudden Oak Death? But I am up here and look around. There is a sad memorial to a group of Home Guard civilians and an officer killed when their artillery gun blew up in their faces; and just beyond it, two policemen are guarding a section of the cliff edge metal fence that has been ripped aside. The officers do not want to speak, once they have ascertained that I am not a witness, but a man walking a dog tells me that a BMW went over last night, crashing through the barrier opposite Seaway Lane and then through the fence and now lies on the rocks below. A body has been recovered. Had the car run out of control on Seaway Lane? The man shakes his head: "sometimes life is too much for people, you know?"

I agree.

I am starting to feel like a rubber-necker and walk into Torquay; although I am not quite admitting it to myself, I can avoid woods there. I backtrack past the Grand and on to the town centre, along the prom, ready to be narrow-minded.

> "The drinks they get thrown up, in Torquay,
> These streets will help you get knocked up"
> (Lady V, 'Torbados', a parody of 'A New York State of Mind', 2010.)

> "Drunkenness and the other pathological consequences of the free use of stimulants... tend in their turn to become honorific... the superior status of those who are able to afford the indulgence."
> (Thorstein Veblen, *Conspicuous Consumption: unproductive consumption of goods is honourable*, 1899.)

Salmon writes:

> *Torbay is a fabrication. There was and is no material reason for it. It is a hallucination that became property and people are trying to carry on as if they are still unconscious. There were no natural resources here for new nineteenth century towns, except the stone; the whole bay is a bubble, villas built entirely from work elsewhere, belief in itself and the power of the gaze upon nature. Today, there is a thriving criminal arboriculture; the secret razing of trees in one garden to open up a vista for a neighbour; a thriving trade in gaze upon a terrain that few enter. The bay is an over-extended temple to the transition from holy days to holidays; secular in the sense of not believing in the nature in which it has faith, the malevolent colonial gaze turned on its own navel. In the phase before this present one, when working class 'Brits' were persuaded to valorise temperature over meaning, traditional English seaside resorts shrivelled until the Sea Change programme poured millions into piecemeal seafront regeneration. Axed by the incoming Conservative Government, the material elements are already eroding. Short-termism returns; the race to the bottom and the cheapest chips. The original precariat live here. Tourism and war have always been inextricably linked: the nineteenth century European ruling classes rehearsed their exile, the Dreadnought fleet was reviewed in the bay, the Red Arrows would sweep over the beaches and big army helicopters woomph woomph over sunburnt kids, airborne recruiting sergeants. They have*

been 'fighting them on the beaches' here long before World War Two.
The quiet of the Westcountry, far away from centres of radical working
class population, is ideal for non-centralised intelligence work, for
listening stations in Cornwall, currency manipulation in Ivybridge,
military technology in Newton Abbot, nuclear weaponry in Plymouth,
submarine spying and first-strike capability at Dartmouth. Since the
end of the Cold War these have all been in decline. The area is subject
to the politics of boredom, relieved by the prospect of once again playing
a part in apocalypse.

I pass a police-box-blue shelter where T.S. Eliot nearly wrote 'The Waste Land': intending to come to Torquay for his wife's convalescence (like Kingsley before him), the couple went to Margate instead. So he wrote it in a shelter there.

On the other side of the road is a sports ground where The Goodies filmed a sketch in which an MCC side play a violent form of cricket against an eleven from the 'Rollerball' movie (1975); as mayhem escalates the action switches from the sports ground to the lanes around Cockington, where a bewhiskered cricketer first bowls grenades and then an atomic bomb. There is the familiar blast and mushroom cloud and the narrator announces: "and so it came to pass that the MCC inherited the earth and retained the ashes".

So, a 'waste land' *was* made here.

Beyond the sports ground, water is jumbled and jittery in concrete channels. A limp ornamental pool compares poorly to the reedy, rushing stream at its side. The pool tails off into a shallow concrete channel; one of those odd functionalist concrete constructions that escape their reason for being. Salmon says there were big disputes here over water; the Cary family at the nearby Abbey built a weir in 1750 to ruin the Royal Naval watering hole – where the ornamental pool is now – from which the Mallocks were selling water to the ships of the line. This water had refreshed land grabs in Gibraltar, Minorca, Sardinia, Grenada, Bengal, parts of Vietnam and so on, hydrating wars that won Britain the 'rights' to supply slaves to the Spanish colonies in the Americas. Something so pure and transparent is a medium for a holocaust.

I somehow miss the big swan gates for Torre Abbey, distracted by the ceramic tiles of a now defunct drinking fountain (I saw so many that day!), and end up following a long, forbidding wall, then distracted by the multinational crowd in smart suits with dangling lanyards massing outside the International Riviera Centre. It is some ticketed event, but I walk around the back and find an entrance to a lower floor and join the queue on a stairwell being ushered upwards into a dark auditorium. I love this. I am not malevolent. I feel like those men on 'Person of Interest' who can get into anywhere. Maybe we should all do this more often, all infiltrate everywhere. I am in the upper gallery, close to the drop to the performance area; theatrical smoke gushes and disco-colour spotlights throb; are they going to unveil a new sports car?

A complimentary programme on my seat discloses that I have gatecrashed an international gathering of global geological park administrators! Even better, the opening ceremony will take the form of a geo-opera. I am scribbling notes madly; challenged by my friendly neighbour I pass myself off as a journalist blogger.

For an opera about rocks there are not many rocks in it. But then, as the libretto makes exaggeratedly clear to the delegates, this – is – the – Anthropocene. It is a strangely (I suppose, appropriately) archaeological performance; part 1920s' Max Reinhardt spectacle, part 1930s' Brechtian *lehrstück*. A last hurrah for a theatre that has somehow survived through the English community play and become a geological phenomenon.

A group of 'Human Beings' labour like seething rocks under a large tarpaulin. We really are deep in German Expressionist territory: this is Kaiser, this is Toller, Teutonic rip-offs of Strindberg's symbolist greats! Not what I expected first thing on a Torquay morning!

After lessons in molecular biology and the scalar relations of deep time, the 'Human Beings' emerge, earthy, grimy and dusty, their 'timeless' peasant/cave-dweller costumes filthy in an artistic way. I would have liked real mud.

These particular 'Human Beings' are very prone to tribalism, they chant "eat, survive, reproduce", choreography by Ayn Rand, and are fated to be lectured by a group of experts: the geologists. The 'connected by stone' theme is contrarily contemporary, given the divisiveness around the EU referendum. Onstage, 'the great unwashed' (I struggled all the way along Cary Parade and Fleet Street trying to remember this phrase!) discover their togetherness under the guidance of a wise elite – the opposite of what is happening outside, where the blood of Eastern European workers is adding an extra layer of mineral to English pavements.

I love the music. I want them to have stone singers, to set the spotlights on crystals, to roll great rocks around and let them resonate to the strings of the Bournemouth Symphony Orchestra. I hope the organisers will be screening, perhaps as a fringe event, the recently rediscovered 'Monolith Monsters', a 1950s' b&w monster movie in which the villain is a mineral. At the end of the mini-opera, I sneak out, by the backdoor again, congratulating the aerialist who is showing off a burn on her thigh.

Outside, I can more easily read the programme. I realise that I have been subject to the same synchronicity that other disrupted walkers report: for the music is written (and conducted) by Hugh Nankivell, who I knew, from preparatory reading and a reference in Salmon's documents, had been one of the three members of the GeoQuest, an intense week-long journey with daily 'mis-guided' walks, public feasts, performances, and workshops in schools, nurseries and nursing homes in 2010. His two collaborators were the seaside entertainer 'Uncle Tacko' and the Crab Man, who I hoped to meet up with; he was based not too far away, but had been ill. Something struck me during the opera, and I could not place it; a song that sounded familiar, a variation on the hymn 'Abide with Me' with the lines 'change and decay in all around

I see / o thou who changest not, abide with me' but sung with the second line as 'those limestone bones, abide with me'. Geology for theology. It is in the online film of the Geo-Quest I had watched for my preparation. I should have recognised Nankivell with his distinctive frizzy hair.

My walk has taken a distinctly rocky turn; the ensemble playing of the performers was strikingly good, and though 'rock' was present as a character only in wood and canvas representations of it, it still "appears as the mover and shaker, the active power, and the human beings, with their much-lauded capacity for self-directed action, appear as its product".

I find the Abbey, eventually. I need to decompress after the geo-operatics. I have read the walker and zombie runner Kris Darby's reflections about a white carpet that was set down between the sea grass beach at Torre Abbey Sands, across the links, and the Abbey's Spanish Barn, where Gormley, Hirst and Long were exhibited. The barn was named for some Spanish sailors who were imprisoned there after the Armada defeat. Although there are clear records that the prisoners were transferred to prisons in Exeter and Plymouth, a local rumour, often more reliable than they should be, holds that the prisoners disappeared. Murdered? Or hidden in the coastal villages, marrying into local families? The landscape writer W. G. Hoskins, born in Exeter, describes a "Spanish-looking people... found in some of the coastal districts of Devon", but attributes these qualities to "people who migrated by sea from Spain and Portugal nearly four thousand years ago".

Everything shifts. My body is challenged by deep time and the lack of anything that will ever be fixed. I cannot quite go with that, yet.

The remains of the Abbey, presumably the result of Henry VIII's dissolution of the monasteries before the Cary family arrived, have been sculpted back into cliffs. Huge chunks of thick wall standing on their ends at crazy angles, like faulted beds tipped out of the horizontal; glued together by a really old *nouveau riche*. The only thing that will make me feel like these ruins do is Triangle Point at Meadfoot Beach. I am suddenly falling apart and the ancient chunks of stairway, propped on pillars and disappearing into fake edifices, are not making me feel any more stable.

In the gift shop I buy a copy of a programme for the 'Sublime Symmetry' exhibition, but I cannot get myself to visit the ceramics themselves. I have been enjoying the ceramics I have found 'in the wild', in abandoned water fountains and cracked into the surface of footpaths, but the thought of an exhibition in an enclosed space is too claustrophobic for me at this moment; I flee and sit in the gardens. Rather as the rock opera has no rocks, so the pamphlet – 'The Mathematics Behind De Morgan's Ceramic Designs' – has no mathematics. I ponder whether the sporadic ceramics I see every day of my walking are all pieces of one global assemblage of symmetries and that, when finally put together, they will add up to one cataclysmic equation, spasming all things in one swift solution. My experience of such assemblages is that they end in banalities, some cliché like 'know thyself' or 'live more in the present'. What else does anybody know, where else does anybody live?

There is supposed to be some unique 14th-century 'tree of life' grave carving in the free-admission area, but I am not sure which one of the various patterns it is; there are some circles, and a shape with a large circle at the top and symmetrical necks branching to each side, and a weird stone figure in bits, but otherwise the shapes and symbols are foreign to me; and having failed I do not want to go back inside and try again. I know that pattern is important, I have seen it two or three times on my walk, and I cannot recognise it. My eyes have not adjusted yet.

I try the gardens, instead. This year is the 50th anniversary of the Aberfan disaster, when a slag heap liquefacted and engulfed a Welsh primary school. There is a flower bed dedicated to the memory, planted after the surviving children were brought here for a break. I shiver at it. It is just a heap of plain dark soil now, waiting for new bulbs; it looks distressingly like a model of a slag heap.

Two minutes in the Palm House and my body surface is a playground of perspiration; I feel instantly sweaty and oily. Under my shirt I am a hot dolphin. The plants have strange labels:

TOUCH ME AND SEE WHAT HAPPENS
SQUEEZE MY LEAVES

I am the only visitor in the Palm House, along with five young men, in green uniforms, tapping their hearing aids, mouthing words, physicalising the dictionary, muscling ideas, re-enacting prole, loose and focused on just about enough, squibbing the plants with their hoses, water running voluptuously down the green rubbery skins of succulents. Like sea water over sun-oiled bathers. I make my flustered excuses and leave.

I find The Chalkers in the Abbey's 'tea shoppe', poring over their plans – disappointed not to find them spontaneously chalking! – I tell them I have seen none of their signs. They are working on a large sheet of paper spread between the three tiers of hand-decorated cakes and an elephantine teapot. The paper is broadly gridded and The Chalkers are filling it with arcane symbols.

"Not arcane, just not representational; only meaningful in relation to each other..."

I question them on the authenticity of hobo and burglar signs, but they are indifferent.

"We're not looking for another f***ing genealogy."

A tourist at a neighbouring table flinches.

They are keen not to be the final arbitrators of their signifieds. Once the signs are in use on the pavements, the grid will be destroyed.

"In use?"

"The first time we see that someone else has chalked one of our marks: that's the signal to burn the grid."

One of the chalkers relents sufficiently to tell me how an elderly couple "down the road in Plymstock" had a new drive installed in 2009; unasked, the contractors had made a pattern of brickettes, four squares, each with another square within, and joined at the corners to make a central square. Since then the couple have been answering the door to a procession of rogues and cowboys; they were victims of the 'Da Pinchi Code'.

I tell her that I'd read of chalked and sprayed signs outside people's homes – an open book to mark a vulnerable female, different colours for different kinds of dogs, dangerous or not, circles like a spread of coins to denote wealthy occupants, and so on.

"That last is a sign for how many cables are in an underground duct. I've no idea about an open book. But I know what they are, generically; they're marks left by the utility firms to indicate what kinds of maintenance work need to be done there."

One of The Chalkers elbows a silver bowl full of sugar cubes onto the carpet, and the others disappear from the waist up, bent under the table hunting cubes, like the mystics in Blok's *Fairground Booth* who, scared, disappear, leaving only hollow costumes. I sneak a photo on my phone, confident, given the multiplicity of such codes, logged in books from Henry Dreyfuss's unfussy *Symbol Sourcebook* to the artiness of Michael Evamy's *World Without Words*, that this one is unlikely to attain even a moment of authority.

I am minded, from Evamy's book, that the motivation for some of the most impressively surreal imagery is a need to inform far-future beings, when all currently existing languages have died out, of the abiding dangers of the present's nuclear waste. I suggest to The Chalkers that all these grids are coloured with that sense of warning. They strongly reject any backwash from apocalypse, insisting that their grids are as celebratory as their cakes.

"Have you done any actual chalking yet?"

They look, pitying, at me. I look up. I can see for a hundred yards or so. The footpaths around the Abbey are crawling with chalk marks, like red crabs on Christmas Island before the crazy ants get them. Those yellow crazy ants are one of a number of 'tramp species' inadvertently spread around the world by human commerce; so perhaps walking artists should feel a special sympathy for them, and for all invasive plant species and visiting aliens?

I pay for my tea and walk away, careful not to tread on the crabs.

> If plays, prayers, manifestos, news reports, feedback, dissertations, confessions,
> Novels, wills, government bills, bank notes and directions
> Were drawn in chalk on walls
> Imagine how the rainfall would change everything.

Off the King's Drive is one of those miniature worlds that park designers in – when, the 1950s? – lovingly crafted. Thumping big rocks, maybe the designers' insurance against dismantlement? As a child under the shadow of their heady, dark trees-cum-shrubs, these were miniature jungles to me, a wormhole to the worlds of relatives in

Tasmania and South Africa I could only visit in framed photos; slithering places of a thrilling dread, and just the same now! In the oiliness of the Palm House, and in this dry rockery, there is grist to Edward Said's mill.

The obvious way to go now is along the back of the beach, but do I want to follow the way the terrain leads me? What if I walk over the top of the big rise rather than round the bottom of it? Go straight to the summit, in fact? See everything. Then maybe go home, summit reached?

I slog, uneasily, up the hill. The road bends steeply to the left, the traffic straining at my elbow; a huge yellow mansion looms above, ghastly like a septic ghost, a yellow sign. I persist by the derelict and boarded Shedden Hill Hotel, malevolently crouched half way up. On the side of the hotel are the simulacra of two tired male faces emerging from a chiaroscuro of grime on deep blue ornaments; one seems grumpy and resigned, the other terrified, chewing all ten of its fingers at once. I shiver and carry on and then don't, turning on my heels and racing back down the hill as quickly as I dare.

I watch the waves for a while. There is a convulsed bridge over the busy road that destroys the beachiness of the beach; its concrete foot in the sea. Beside and around it, the waves strike along the sea wall and against the foot, then veer off at an oblique angle, so that when they rebound against the next incoming wave, rather than one wall of water bouncing off the other, there is an interference, a diffraction which creates a kind of moving knot in the water, tightening and undoing itself, unravelling and retying, as it runs along the line of the incoming wave. It's like a bolus swallowed in a tube and then swallowing the tube itself; Kingsley's clown jumping down its own throat.

There are two kinds of pattern in the water. The reflection that transports a here to a there, reproduces itself, but also replaces somewhere else with itself. When that kind of *reflection* is the main metaphor for comparing and connecting things, it reinforces analogy, homogeneity and conformity...

Thumph, shuuuuurl, resssh. Another wave hits the wall, turns back, entangles with the oncoming wave and diffracts.

This is the second pattern: diffraction is a kind of dynamism in the matter of the world. It is what the theorist Donna Haraway calls a "metaphor for the effort to make a difference in the world". This works all the way down, so at a certain level, incredibly small things overlap, interfere, and make a difference *all on their own*. Below a certain superficiality, things are socialistic and entangled.

"One hopes they like it."

The neo-liberals can keep their selfish gene, we have quantum waves!

In the 19th century, Symbolist poetry went beyond the conventional metaphor – this over here is like that over there – to the idea that only *everything* else over there defines this tiny thing here. Similarly, diffraction makes a fool of any science that only looks at stuff in order to separate it from everything else. It indicts any system that separates materials without a thought for how that changes everything else.

I am not a mirror.

I've been reflecting on things as I've walked, yes. But I've also noticed how some of the things I've reflected on reached out of their own accord – people, sea slugs, sharp limestone rocks, gusts of wind, whatever – and entangled with me. Reading all those blogs and papers at home and on the train down, there *was* a dividing line, a big difference between the writers who only reflected on their walking and those who were caught up, snared, tangled up in it.

I was asked to Devon as a researcher. I'm 'Doctor Oak', almost. I wonder if I have ever properly understood what research is. That only if I put myself at the mercy of my subject, only when I am caught up and becoming part of my subject and only when that subject is caught up and disrupted and diffracted by me – leaving a footprint, climbing a fence to trespass – am I really researching.

I look at the diffracting waves; and they make me feel intellectually energised and emotionally trashed.

I displace to the place. I back off from the waves.

There are several obscure plaques at the bottom of Rock Walk, some of them so bleached as to be unreadable. One, about sea grass, almost illegible under the growth of lichen. Ha ha. Those I can read are perverse disruptions of this bay's malevolent gaze: "The peasant oft, so glory's service charms... Joins the bold crews and dares the strife of arms". (Rev. Charles Short)

There is a life-sized model of a rhino on the pavement, caged behind metal crush barriers, for H&S reasons.

Anger surges through my body; it's wonderful!

I cross the thick stream of traffic back to the promenade – the ultimate de-romanticiser – and hang over the railings. The means to bring people to the place destroyed the place the people were travelling for. Everyone has transport now, but no longer any 'where' to arrive at.

In 1910, not so long before the First World War, there was a review of the Fleet here; the haven for the Royal Navy had moved from Torbay to Plymouth once a breakwater had been built there, but the Fleet had returned to the stamping ground of Nelson and his captains, all very patriotic and nationalistic. There was the king, there were the Dreadnoughts, what could possibly go wrong?

Then an enterprising and independent flier, Claude Graham-White took off in his small plane from the green below the Abbey, bisecting the white carpet of the Office of Subversive Architecture, and circled above the battleships. Insulted by Graham-White's impertinence the battleships began to raise their guns in mock belligerence, and then they stuck, unable to raise them to the angle at which they could threaten Graham-White's plane. There, for all the thousands on the shore to see, was all future naval power entirely at the mercy of the air. For once, a spectacle had rendered up a truth.

Following Graham-White's flight, cities would burn and oceans boil; it began here. The transference of imperial dread from sea to air; vaporisation. And is still under way.

He claims to be the caretaker. Theatres don't have caretakers any more, do they? I don't think so. We seem to walk through doors just as the corridors beyond them become empty, as if he knows the timings, the shifts of personnel. As if he has memorised worksheets and punchings in. The stage is dark. There is just a little green from the emergency exits. Hordes of minor characters pursued by fleets of green bears. He sits down in the middle of the darkness. I am not particularly enjoying this. I do not like dark. I think he senses it. Not that he wants to unnerve me, but he wants to move me, and he has no right.

"Where are you?"

"Where am I?"

"That's the question."

"On a stage. In the darkness."

"That's two places. Where *exactly* are you?"

"I see your point..."

"I don't think you do. Let's just suppose that you and I are characters in a play. What play would you like that to be? 'Private Lives'? 'Oedipus Rex'?"

"A Dream Play."

"Very well. You are Agnes, the daughter of a goddess. Let me be one of the deans. It really doesn't matter which. Where are we? Come on... dung heap, castle? What? You see, you can't give me an immediate answer. If I were to give you any longer you would fabricate something. You're intelligent, you have a reasonable memory. But more telling is your spontaneous uncertainty..."

"If you give me a moment..."

"I won't. A moment will lead us back into the dung heap. And we have a castle to get to. You will dismiss that as hopelessly phallic, no doubt. It is not. It is the lack that is significant; above any soaring towers. This is not middle-Ibsen rubbish, this is real Swedish symbolism; not the Norwegian mess. This is the real Villiers De L'Isle Adam thing."

"We're in Devon. How do you know all this?"

He laughs and his genuine chuckle explores all the rows of the most privileged seats.

All the time along the coast I would come across thieved-orientalism – SIMLA, the ancient Egyptian statues in the casino doorway on Torbay Road, the adobe calf, the missing minarets, Pan – but what came next, the modernist naturalism, the TV behaviourism, the melancholic Corries and Eastenders and Benefits Streets for whom everything is continually collapsing and nothing ever changes; victimhood becoming a badge of bitterness for separatists who did not choose their separation. Life imitates art because art has become imitation and imitation is now a thing not a representation, and Mimesis is now a god in the pantheon of ideological machines.

No wonder the local small businesses had kicked up a fuss when the Office of Subversive Architecture put a £10,000 white carpet across the Torre Abbey lawns. Absurdity has no place in the face of moribund realism, just as it had none in

Jenkinson/Jowett's scientific theology; because it is already there. Just as fascism is already there in libertarianism; freedom to do what the hell you like, whether justified by anger or desire, is a machine for making victims.

The most obvious way to characterise the victim-anger – "waste!", "rubbish!", "profanity!" – of the hoteliers, traders and shopkeepers is as something conservative. But Kris Darby hints at something more volatile; for while he emphasises the warmth and transformation of the space for positive visitors – the same applies to those already hot with fury at their own impotence, almost ready to wound themselves in order to harm the things intended to do them good. That hot and angry conservatism is the face of a coin that has victimhood on the reverse. And that coin is naturalism (scientific, theological and theatrical); the currency of the stage on which we are sat.

Salmon describes a performance on this stage by the late Sir Norman Wisdom, the last Dauphin of Albania, bouncing child-like about the stage, well into his eighties, performing all his pratfalls, rolls and flips. The only thing he couldn't do was his hunting horn blast: the act had taken too much of his breath away. As a young lad, Wisdom had escaped an exploitative, dead-end job, joining a fellow-worker and walking all the way from London to Cardiff, sleeping in barns and drinking from streams; his friend had promised him that when they got to Cardiff his family would help them both, but once within the city, Norman's 'friend' ran off.

Further east of here, Wisdom made a movie – 'Press for Time' (1966) – at Teignmouth; hanging out the front window of his hotel every evening to sign autographs and chat with the fans. All his life, he dared not be deserted again; he had turned his victimhood into a powerful, if needy, conviviality.

Fans who hung around Norman's Teignmouth hotel for nights on end turned out, with other curious locals, for a special screening of 'Press for Time'. At one point in the movie, Norman commandeers a bus to chase after a thief who has stolen his bicycle; everything became very odd for the town audience as the bus careened down the bridge to the station, then turned a corner and was instantly on the other side of the river, turned onto the promenade and was back up by the station. The town was being shattered and reassembled in front of its residents... a lesson in a *détournement* that cares only for the abstraction of its act.

"That's the loveliest thing... there is no boundary, no centre, no arterial road, no suburb, there is nothing where we are right now. We are held in the magic of the stage; but it has no place. Athens, Arden, New York... it's irrelevant where our play is set, it is always going on in the same place – nowhere. So, when a character says they are in 'Athens' or 'Elsinore' or 'Wapping'.... these are not real places to which they refer. The action of a play moves backwards and forward in time, but always in the same nowhere. Now, what are the consequences of this for the stories that the punters come to see? Pretty big. I am sure that you are aware that there are actually only a handful of plots; the quest, the investigation..."

A door at the back of the stalls opens a fraction. A silhouette of someone slight is framed. The door shuts again.

"Yes", I interrupted. "I'm aware of that idea."

"...they can all be boiled down to this one thing: transformation. No transformation, no theatre. I'm sure this is true of other things – forms seem to travel – but when you've found your alchemy, why keep looking? And how does this transformation occur? By a shift of level. The character, the community, the whole milieu must go down and then come up again, must die and then rise again. So, a double shift of level? Down and then up. And when the character or whatever returns from that other place, the place that has always held up this one, its basement, its foundation..."

"You said that there was no place..."

"Try to keep up. Whatever sinks, whatever or whoever falls through the nowhere into whatever holds it up, brings something back up with it when it rises; something it did not have before. That is how *the whole thing* works. It is not the characters that die in a theatre, it is space itself. The moment places are named, their fate is sealed and the action moves on. The set is changed. Palaces turn into painted flats; only a feeling of something real persists. Atmosphere. That is the lesson the theatre has for you, Cecile. Every stage direction is a sudden Pompeii or Aberfan."

"I saw the flower bed... just soil..."

"...heroes, lovers, pilgrims; they do not die and fall beneath the world; instead, the world dies and falls on them; and what is left in memory is ambience. Build your castle on that."

And, for some reason, I think of SIMLA and its jelly spaceship.

"Tragedy is about dirt, about rock, about plastics, about gas. It is their death and not ours that makes us civilised and high cultured. So what does that tell you about things as they are, right now?"

"Do you mean the Anthropocene?"

"Well, I don't mean the Counter-Reformation do I, dearie?"

"You mean... there is some... special role for the theatre?"

"Not the theatre, but the stage. Stage occurs arbitrarily, accidentally. Theatres have to be built, but stages are everywhere, and they will be crucial to the working out of the myth of the next few years. Did you ever see one of those awful kitchen-sink, naturalist nonsenses? 'All My Sons'? 'Chicken Soup with Barley'? And wondered why the picket fence suddenly peters out at the edge of the stage? Why the kitchen does not go on forever? Well, that is no longer a necessary question. We have a deadline now, drawn in the sand. A foreseeable end to reality. On any accidental stage, anywhere now, we can portray the tragedy of the end of space, of time, of human consciousness, all buried beneath the death of the Earth and its theatrical transformation into something genuinely other; into whatever consciousness is when it is not human, or unhuman or dishuman. We will be the first humans to really live, Cecile, because we are the first to really die. We can pass nothing on. Like Rutger Hauer, the robot who 'saw *such things*', it is 'time to die'. Find the stages, Cecile, find the stages..."

Suddenly, all the lights go up. FOH. Spots. Wash. The lot. Just a lightning blizzard of brightness. Pain zig-zags across my forehead. Stars dribble about off the end of my nose. By the time I have composed myself I am alone on stage and being harshly addressed by cut-outs in the orchestra pit. I don't care any more.

"Tell me," I say to the shades "if the world dies, what would be the last thing you would want to put on your stage?"

Silence. A kind, middle-aged woman in an unkind suit enters stage left, flanked by a bruiser in a dinner jacket. "Please come with me. Members of the public are not allowed on the stage." I feel myself slow marched through the waves of light. Exit stage right. Down a short flight of curling steps; going down in order to come up again. Is this my ritual? Along this skanky tunnel? Another one that The Beatles were smuggled down, no doubt... and into the sunlight, exceeding anything ever delivered by the National Grid. I white out again. By the time I can see again, they have gone, but I can still hear the bruiser's voice, whispering hopefully in my ear, "I'd see 'The Rocky Horror Show'".

I stagger across two lanes of traffic, light cannoning off the rear bumper of a camper van. I end up on my arse, my back to a wall and the back of my head pleasantly grazing the rough stones. In front of me is a plinth. I push myself up on my palms and stagger head first into it. I smother the thing. A drip of blood plops onto the metal plaque; maybe bronze or copper or something even more synthetic. The plaque says: "How many eyes do you dare to look through?"

What the hell is this?

And who the hell was *that*?

I run up and up and up the stairs to the top of the cliff, but there is text after text; lactic acid begins to burn through to my shins, nagging texts keep edging into my vision. At the top is a viewing platform. Gasping for breath, I take in the view across the bay to Brixham and consider catching a ferry there.

I climb back down the steps and follow the prom, wondering which Princess the Theatre is named after. Salmon does not say. A stone and plaque marks 'Speakers' Corner' – 'opened' in 2005, but apparently no one ever speaks or listens there. How real is a right if it is never used? Nearby there is another ironic monument (I would later find an exact copy on Exeter High Street), made in a composite-concrete, polished to look like granite, a family group, their legs lost in a goo of abstraction, odd for something celebrating the 'Year of the Pedestrian'. It is rusty with lichen; two males restrain a central female figure. More like the arrest of a protestor than a family stroll. The faces blank and hollow. The Crediton-born sculptor had grown up in a building business and as a child had made her own pre-cast concrete shapes. Unknowingly perhaps, she was inducted into the same craft as Eleanor Coade, the businesswoman from the Exeter wool industry who had refined clay recipes and double-firing processes for her own composite-concrete, Coade Stone, the super-weathering material that was still keeping many of the neo-classical figures and ornaments I passed defined.

I turn away from Cary Parade, and its ghosts of mountain lions.

In the town, headlines on boards outside the newsagents speak of a DEADLY WONDERING SPIDER. It turns out to be a find in a bunch of supermarket bananas of the eggs of a Brazilian Wandering Spider, its venom capable of giving a male victim a four-hour erection; a globalist conspiracy of priapics is evidently at work. Torquay has form where spiders are concerned; it was here in the late 19th century that False Widows (*Steatoda nobilis*) from Madeira first disembarked, part of reverse-colonialism, they have established their own colonies in the county and across the south coast and are now making their way north in the rising temperatures.

I turn up Fleet Street, the bottom of the old valley.

It is hard to believe that the ruling classes and royal families of Europe had once chosen to come here, as revolutionary Europe got too hot for them. They set the models for what happened here, and then as these spaces were popularised after the First World War, they were never made democratic; the original models were simply hollowed out and then their shells were hollowed out again.

Symphony orchestras became bands became electronic jingles; the sentimentality and nationalism remained, but now refracted through Gary Gilmore's Eyes (a proto-version of The Adverts started here). Holiday was a time when a railway clerk could pose for a week as a station manager, a labourer as a ganger, a maid as a lady-in-waiting. Imagination and mobility maintained the continuum of aspiration; no new sense organs were evolved, no one had two new ideas to rub together, after the wholesomeness of rationing and meat and two veg, sugar and fat colonised everything, the fish inside the batter had first to be driven to London, frozen, and then driven back. What had been exceptional – a holy day broken from the working week – was made a part of the homogenous system, and, globalised. After the first few pioneers, the ruling classes, the royalty and aristocracy of Europe had come to wane here, suppurating in the pinched splendour of Torquay, among villas occupied by industrialists. Its parody of democratisation in the shape of reactionary modernism was fully realised when the prurient colonial gaze was turned on itself and then by rail the working classes came pouring in along the GWR, Midlanders spending a week on the beach and promenade watching each other watch each other.

No wonder Michael Winner made 'The System' here.

No wonder the nightmare makers lived here.

That yellow spectral rotting wound, up there above Rock Walk, the amber signal, turns out to be the former home of Edward Bulwer-Lytton of "dark and stormy night" fame, while the blue ruin crouched beneath it was a hotel owned until 2007 by Brian Lumley, author of *Necroscope,* a novel about those who are able to communicate, on peaceful and equal terms, with the Great Majority, the dead. Indeed, Lumley's hero not only communicates, but teaches the dead to communicate among their expanding community.

If you put fury in a gentle rocket
Where do you think it would land?
If you fished for hands with crab nets
What washes up on your beach?
And if one of you was the boat and the other the sky
What sail would tie you together?

Something about gaps as connections, maybe.

Cathy Turner, one of the speakers at the conference, writes in her *Dramaturgy and Architecture* book about gaps, material ones and those between function and poetry in the same material thing (in her case, Tatlin's tower): "the possibility that it exists not simply as a functional container, nor as a representation of heroic men, but as the performance of an idea which, despite this is 'put to good use.'"

As I walk, deliriously, up Fleet Street I try to imagine the mountain lions that once lived here. Padding through Sports Direct or the Licence 2 Fill Sandwich Bar. Numbers, quantities, scalability. The valley has been overwhelmed. It is easy to see where the elitists became disgruntled with democracy. I imagine Bulwer-Lytton, imagining himself as a mountain lion perched in Warren Road looking down on the middle-class pygmies below and formulating his *The Coming Race*; it was he, I read in Salmon, who coined that phrase "the great unwashed" I had been struggling for earlier, right under his gaze on Shedden Hill.

I had briefly looked at Bulwer-Lytton's writings: there are mystical overlaps between his works and those of certain European Symbolists, but the similarities turned out to be deceptive; where the scenarios of even an arch-reactionary like Maurice Maeterlinck are dispersive and intangible, with Bulwer-Lytton they are clunky and monocular and empty. *The Coming Race* is responsible for the 'hollow earth' theory, taken to the final stupidity by a few Nazis who believed that not only is the earth hollow, but that they were living on the inside of it. Firing a few shells at Denmark guided by their theory soon cured them of this nonsense. The same novel popularised the idea of 'Vril', a liquid force controllable by mental training. It provided part of the name for the meat extract 'Bovril', and it is still cited by contemporary Neo-Nazis as the gooey essentialist yuck in which their race theories are forever stuck.

At the top of Fleet Street I try different ways out. Abbey Road feels desperate. I stop looking in people's eyes. There is an underlying feeling of violence barely suppressed. Women rip into a taxi driver, shouting instructions for some kind of animated search. A huge bouncer-like figure sighs in the shadowy doorway of a long closed-down business. I am looping back towards the Great Majority and The Coming Race. The pressure is incredible; as if the statistics – the 8 years less the poor live than the rich here, the suicides (twice the national average), the divorces (third highest in the country) – are all here in ambience. This is Unhappiness, walking like a lion in the streets. I retreat to Pimlico, where the locals had once acted the part of anti-monarchist

Neapolitan rioters for the cameras, routed by Nelson's lobsterbacks. This is where the old poor of Torquay, billeted on the exposed Fleet, running with effluent, had rioted with the help of navvies working on Brunel's new railway line, and tore into the bread shops on Fleet Street. Some years later, a body turned up in an unmarked grave near Torre Abbey; the bones were dated to this time. Had the same authorities who had been refusing for twenty years to provide a bathhouse for 'the great unwashed', covered up a killing? It would take a cholera epidemic, burying 66 poor folk in 6 weeks, before the sewer-stream was enclosed – bottling up the excess and the fury of a people I still feel roaring just below its emotional manhole covers.

Flood is the new social media, the new sex, the new sharing of fluids; the climate will be turning us all amphibian. When melancholy becomes militant, the drain covers will be lifted and the effluent will be free.

I retreat down Fleet Street, because I can still hear that horror. Still smell that stench. Fastfood grease is little different from people fat and I like both.

I skirt the harbour.

Although I know that I can get straight to Babbacombe, passing the Museum – where a finger and thumb print have been found recently on the glass of the locked display case of a mummified Egyptian boy, on the *inside* of the glass, that is – I take a digression up Beacon Hill instead, past a morosely netted flock of birds and penguins, everything screeching. I might have been less affected by the miserable calling of these snared organisms, if I hadn't known from Salmon that this, in a previous incarnation as the Marine Spa, had been the venue where Baron von Ribbentrop, on a Nazi charm offensive, was feted by Torquay Town Council in 1937. Nineteen – Thirty – Seven!!!!!! Four years *after* the opening of Dachau concentration camp.

A view to a beach where Agatha Christie nearly drowned. A graffito in big letters: WHEREVER YOU WILL GO. And the Grand Hotel, where the aforementioned surfer, archaeologist and thriller-writer honeymooned in 1914, stormed in 1918 by mobs of local extras for 'Nelson', and where the body of a Sri Lankan man was found in 1997 in Room 131, dead from cyanide poisoning. Scars on his shoulders and the vial of cyanide in a leather necklace linked him to the Tamil Tigers. His final note: "I'm very sorry for what I have done here, but this is the place I had to be to carry out the deed", alongside the money for his last meal, plus tip. What was so special about the Grand Hotel, or perhaps about Room 131; why such a site-specific political suicide?

I turn up Parkhill and, after admiring a now redundant lift shaft, turn right up a long and daunting set of steps, the first of many today. The strange thing about these long climbs, some inside grey three-sided tunnels, some stinking of vegetable waste, is what they do to mind and body. Lactic acid for the soul; grim and puritan. Devon is not flat.

Big walls, and a surprising path into St John's Woods, walking down the backs of gardens. Up on Daddyhole Plain, past what appears to be yet another redundant drinking fountain, this one shaped as a crenelated castle. I am now standing on top of the great pillars of limestone I saw in the distance from the turning into Clifton

Road at the top of Paignton. That seems a long way back now. A long way back. I am amazed at how far walking can quickly take you.

I choose a path at the far left of the plain and it leads me up and down, hugging the edge of the cliff, around a tree shaped like an upside-down squid, and then squeezes me between a wooden fence on one side and a metal one on the other, fringing the abyss; until I come out through a trampled hole in the metal fence and signs – "sheer cliff edge stay away" – warn me of the danger of the path *I have just taken*! Well, thank you for not saying so at the other end! Finding my way down with the help of a very old railing, I am almost back to where I started on Daddyhole Plain.

Trying again, this time I find a way down to a beach, Meadfoot, where I am transfixed by a giant triangular rock and, climbing up to it, lie face down on its huge slope. I can see how it is aligned with another great chunk of rock far out in the water, part of some massive broken bed of black rock that has tipped up like a sinking aircraft carrier. On its 'deck' there are the soft pudding shapes of stromatoporoid sponges, parts of "that humble coral, unnoticed on the dark sea-floor". I reach out and cup one of the 400-million-year-old animals in my palm.

Lying flat out on the rock – it's called Triangle Point – I can see right across the bowl of the bay; soft Permian sandstone carved out from between the jaws of the much harder Devonian limestone (though it should really be called New Jerseyian, because that's where the better examples are). I love this little outcrop of rock under cliffs where (according to a local I speak to) there was once a tiny and uneconomic gold mine in the breccias. I wonder how many visitors make it up to this end of the beach and clamber to a world that feels so alien and special to me. I am floating among stone sponges at a crazy angle, drowsing in the hallucinogenic colours of the rocks, each surface has stone stories of coral smashed in storms or the slow tipping of whole sea beds; and above are the remnants of something like today's Libyan deserts. I am travelling now.

Nothing appeals to me at the café, so I make my way along the sea road.

THE THROWING OF STONES IS PROHIBITED

A giant gabion under the cliffs has been bent by an unknown force into something like the shape of a stranded whale. I turn inland into the valley; light entertainment gathered on this road in the 1970s – Max Bygraves, Bruce Forsyth, Larry Grayson, The Crankies – and then up another calf-burning set of steps.

Where are all the other walkers?

At the end of a short road, there is a turning off the junction into 'The Bishop's Walk'. Why not?

I am all alone on The Bishop's Walk. At first flanked by a tall grey wall, and then by green; at times in a tube of branches and leaves. For thirty minutes or more of walking I meet no one. The path was made for a Bishop, Henry Phillpotts, the last of the clerical super-rich, a combative Tory autocrat who kept a grumbling and divided church together (mostly) with bullying and compromise. He was high-church by inclination, favouring ritual, yet opposed Catholic emancipation. He disliked the idea of 'being born again' at baptism (baptismal regeneration) and refused to allow one of its champions to take up a post in the parish of Brampford Speke. For Phillpotts, the walk was a space for repose, somewhere that things could be unified and resolved, indifferent to a geology that was holding him up and that would bring down his timetable of creation. It is and is not such a space for me.

I decide that I should contemplate as I walk, settling on solitude and property as my subjects.

This path is meant to be walked alone; I will ignore anyone I pass.

Phillpotts needed to own and control the land to be alone. This vicar of the ethereal (as profoundly religious as he was immensely powerful and obscenely rich) could manipulate the material world, even its vistas. Nowadays, the path, mostly enclosed by mature trees, has few views, contemplation and the interior gaze is somewhat enforced; at best there is an occasional glimpse of yellowy-orange cliffs through the boughs. Later there are views back to Hope's Nose with its end sliced off, like a vandalised mediaeval idol, by quarrying.

I try to own the path.

Can a woman ever really own anything?

The path is public land now (I assume), certainly a public right of way, but am I safe? Am I really within *my* rights and on *my* land?

What is the murder rate for strangers in leafy parts of Torbay? About the same as that for terrorist acts perpetrated by Syrian refugees in the US, I guess. Zero. Yet, as Alain Badiou claims, a zero trumps a mathematical set of ones, and an indiscernible thing, like the likelihood of one's murder in the safest of all places, produces an event of fear, an 'evental' anxiety.

A branch pokes across the path, like a stork's beak. Another like a cartoon snake.

"Trust in me. Just in me. Shut your eyes, and trust in me."

Passing no one from start to finish, I draw some comfort from an article someone had posted, collected by Phil Baker – an acerbic commentator on those who have passed off earth mysteries as psychogeography – and written by an amazing woman called Celia Fremlin.

She owned the London night.

Reporting in 1979, Fremlin had spent three years, one or two nights a week, "deliberately roaming the streets of London between 11pm and 3am and talking to the people I meet walking alone, particularly the women, about their experiences and their feelings".

She had been a late-night walker all her life, wondering what her fellow walkers might be doing, thinking, feeling: "the young man striding out of King's Cross station: is he feeling as confident as he looks? This old man weighed down by a mysterious bundle, what is he thinking, as he stands there with his back to me, staring into those empty windows? And here is a girl, young and lovely, in a long evening dress.... why has her escort set her down without a word in these insalubrious reaches of the Caledonian Road?"

Instead of wondering, she decided to ask. Inspired by all the scare stories she had heard at dinner parties about walking out at night. They did not match her experiences; she had begun to wonder if she had just been lucky: "was I due for a sharp and painful lesson?"

Time changes space. How differently would I feel now if this was night?

Of the 200 women Fremlin interviewed none had experienced sexual assault or actual physical injury while out at night, "most were inclined to pooh-pooh the alleged dangers of the night" – although perhaps her sample was skewed; how many of those who had been assaulted would continue to walk at night? – and she quotes women, young and old, who "go around all over the place", "just for the pleasure of it... I control it completely", "I love that feeling... the stars... the sky... that I have the world to myself".

Fremlin does get told about incidents that are frightening – an encounter with a naked man with a paper bag over his head, for example – though "all ended harmlessly" (at least in the sense of avoiding physical harm). What had frightened Fremlin on her walks, though, were a string of "sad or tragic" encounters; a suicidal woman, a mother unable to cope with her schizophrenic daughter, and then her encounter with "some huge dark object blocking up the pavement" which turns out to be a very large woman, who, on seeing Fremlin screams at her, quickly followed by an apologetic husband explaining "please forgive her, she cannot bear that a person should see her, the way she is now" and that her only exercise is to walk, unobserved, at night. Fremlin notes "here I was, taking away from her the one hour in all the 24 that she could call her own".

Then she broadens it out; and nails what takes away ownership of the hours, not just from this woman, but, literally from millions of women (the 40% who at the time did not walk out alone at night): "here in the midst of our glittering Permissive Society, with women's lib going from strength to strength, millions of women will sit imprisoned within their own four walls, unable to go out in the evenings unless their husbands choose to take them. They are exactly like their oppressed Victorian sisters of 100 years ago".

A whispering campaign of fear, fuelled by the creative industries, social commentators, media and politicians, the 'mugging' panic of the 1970s, not so very different from similar scares around drugs and crime and young black men in the US, was cultivated around the same time, with extremely profitable results for a privatised incarceration industry. The TV told you that outside was terrifying, so you stayed at home, and watched TV tell you how terrifying it was outside and what to buy to forget that outside was even there.

Was this connivance of commercial (and, shamefully, public) media, with all its advertising revenue (and licence fee) resting on ratings, in a conspiracy against women, to keep women (as the main household purchasers) watching, really very different, say, from the conspiracy of the big corporations in the American Legislative Exchange Council's lobbying for profitable higher sentencing policy, like the execrable Bill Clinton's triangulatory 'three strikes and you're out'?

Using fear to incarcerate black men 24/7 in privately owned prisons, using fear to incarcerate women 12/7 in front of TV sets.

Fremlin: "for responsible people – in newspapers, on television, and among feminists themselves – to be actually encouraging these life-destroying attitudes seems to me a development far more frightening than anything currently going on in our night-time streets".

For a while I pause at a shelter. TORBAY MAFIA. Even in my perturbed state I do not believe that one. FREE CANDY. And an arrow to here. That is more sinister.

Despite my anxiety, I hold myself still. I wait and wait for ideas to come. Or for a real quest to rise. I don't quite believe in my absurd setting off into obscure paths and suburbs in pursuit of walking artists. I know I am partly running away; I know that. The conference was always going to be a chance to think through some things about where life is taking me after my doctoral research. My 'perfect' French and Italian are assets, whatever the outcome of the Referendum; but I will have to think about schools for Sophia. I am only a very partly free agent. The more I sit and think, the more aware I am of the heavy armour I am walking in.

I sit a while longer until it begins to dawn on me what I have done. I am deep into this path. Unlike the paths on Clennon Hill and Primley Park I have not turned back in fear. I am deep in the green and lost in shadows now. To turn back might mean being on the path even longer than going forward, and perhaps to run into whatever it is I think might be chasing me. Am I with Celia Fremlin in the London night? Or am I still walking inside a paranoid TV world? I get up, and stop.

In the City of Dreams (in Cule's *Sir Constant*), Sir Fortis is living in a 40-year-old daydream, seated beside his discarded armour, the coat of arms on his shield washed away, sword rusty in its scabbard... and yet, he gets up, and sets off on the journey he has been dreaming of.

Sir Constant, the exemplary pilgrim, thinks of this as a waste of time, but it is a Bataille-like surplus, isn't it? Part of the accursed, unrecoverable and irredeemable excess that can only be spent luxuriously. I am only learning anything here, I am only determined and re-determined, because I have sat with absurd graffiti and my own 35 years of daydreams and fear and 'understood' their message to me. Yes, I will find the walkers, but only if I am chasing my own illusions along the materiality of the road.

I walk. Less afraid. More distracted.

The Bishop's Walk ends at an empty notice board, green and yellow with micro-colonies, and a road, across which is a car park, and in which two crowds are milling. I wonder if they are enacting a satirical version of the demise of our conference, but it turns out to be a dance of geologists modelling the clash of Gondwana and Laurasia to form Pangea. The giant continents are being marshalled by two of the 'Geo-Quest' walkers – Uncle Tacko and the composer Aeolian Hugh – whose 2010 walk had created (accidentally, by their own admission, things just piled up) an 'art of living' journey around Torbay's Geopark, each day consumed in workshops, walks, misguided tours, performances, parish notes and feasts. I had watched Siobhán Mckeown's film of how it became a rolling festival as repeat attenders multiplied and people began to join them for the non-formal parts of their journeys.

I whisper congratulations for the morning's opera and leave them milling and churning the planet across the car park, back in a time when Devon was in the Middle East. We would be bombing ourselves.

The break-up of Pangea made wet empires possible, sea power. What might have been a barrier to mobility was its opposite: a disaster for the world. Once mapping began – that blight – the sea looked like the negative of the land, susceptible to the same occupation and possession. As I walk away across playing fields, the two land masses are clicking small stones together in their hands, fifty or so of them; a strange sound like the rushing of water up a beach. Or the breathing of a bronchular idol.

Palæologia Chronica: a chronological account of ancient time was written by Robert Cary, of the Cockington Court Carys, and published in 1677, shortly after the family moved into a dis-established and partially demolished Torre Abbey. Cary's book is a very early attempt to calibrate "ancient time" (time as revealed by geological and palæontological study) with the Bible's chronology. This became a sharp and culture-changing debate in the early 19th century, partly due to discoveries in the caves at Brixham and Torquay – I knew I couldn't be far from Kent's Cavern, now: I had seen the name on signposts. Excavations here had undermined the place of 'The Flood', the first chink in a toppling textual edifice.

Passing a vandalised sign on a football changing room – "boots to be wo n" – I find the steps, more steps, up to Kent's Cavern. I drink a bottle of Luscombe's Sparkling Apple Crush in the café and smile at lanyard-wearing geo-delegates. The Apple Crush is better than good. It is a hot day. I like to find something local or regional if I'm somewhere I don't know. Not because local things are always produced under any qualitatively different economic or social relations, but for the selfish reason of keeping myself alive to novel tastes. I like the fizz with what tastes like actual apple. I set off again.

At the top of Ilsham Road are two more redundant drinking fountains, one elegant and proto-modernist, the other hyper-gothic: twin fish heads, maws full of teeth.

I decide to walk Middle Warberry Road. This was Palk land. Bleeding with tigers. Land that Palk (like the Carys and Mallocks) had refused to sell to the "flamboyant" sewing machine magnate. Buried in the middle of it was Eileen Nearne, long dead before her body was found, carrying the invisible burden. Expert at invisibilising herself, and plagued by The Invisibles. Once SOE, always SOE. There is a memorial beside the fishy fountain and it gives addresses.

At intervals three middle aged women, sharply dressed and brightly made up, perhaps the ghosts of Eileen Nearne, cast sparkling eyes on me. Each one speaks, over-friendly, solicitous. Extras from The Truman Show perhaps? I am a stranger in the kingdom of the absent. Huge walls. Bridges over gateways. Anonymous piles glimpsed through shrubs. Where those who once guarded secrets come to die with them. And that probably isn't true now, either. Otherwise they would not be doing their job. They will always turn up, when they do, in unexpected streets; 'who would have thought it! Her?' The 'little old lady' whose past is only revealed on her death; when the medals secretly presented are found in her flat by council workers. The psychological problems that followed torture, for half a century or more pulling her down. The hyenas of pain. The teeth juggled in dark caves. The work she could only talk about in disguise, in another language. As if the war were never going to end. Never did.

Peter Cook, the comedian, was born here. I cannot find the plaque, but there is a plethora of enigmatic doorways in giant walls revealing little. Will that do?

What I do exactly identify is MONTE ROSA, the house built on the site of CASTEL-A-MARE, where in the first two decades of the 20th century some portal to the Great Majority had opened up among the Tiny But Very Powerful Minority. The house had been empty for a while, and was starting to fall apart. Enter the spiritualists: séances were held, sounds of running were heard, doors opened and closed (more portals) of 'their own' accord, but things really took off when some choirboys decided to break in after Evensong, armed with candles and crucifix. One just happened to be a future novelist: that always helps, the ghosts perform, when they know it is worth their while. Once in the house, the aspirant wordsmith noted his thought processes slowing down, as if he had been given an anaesthetic. One of the boys became separated from the others, there were sounds of a struggle, and the victim/medium emerged with an account of a dark shadow moving quickly at him, a shape in the form of a man but without any features. Then the phrases begin to build up: "this entity was not alone", "as if everything had gone into slow motion", "the atmosphere had changed", "it was black, shaped like a man", "I could see no face, only blackness", "it made no noise as it raced at me over the rotting boards", "black, silent and man-shaped, it rushed from the room and knocked him to the floor".

What was this black absence? Was it composed of the same material as the shape at the bottom of the Front Lawn at Cockington Court? A furious power in the form of a man without light, without reflection? A man without depth, only outline and emptiness. A human surplus denied human-ness? Was this the energy of excesses, profits, thefts, come from the colonies, unable to contain their absenting of the human from human life forms, in the shape of a slave?

The house was demolished and MONTE ROSA built on the site. Google Street View shows it under a massive storm cloud, with the shape of a skull in the bottom right panel of the far right window. I find the force is still at work here; as I pass by, the wall opposite has been dragged down and its gatepost is lying smashed on the pavement. The house name is visible on the pieces in the gutter: EDWINSTOWE, a town in Nottinghamshire the Crab Man passes through on his journey for the *Mythogeography* book of 2010:

"Setting off through E----stowe, passing Maid Marian's Secrets lingerie store, the Crab thinks of the Ranger, telling him how the authorities will soon close the Visitor Centre in S---wood Forest in order to build a new one in a distant field. The present one attracts too much damage to the forest. The Crab, dreamily, imagines the present one, left to the forest's tender mercies, like that layby at New -----ton, adapting, managed by the forest for the benefit of 'forever'."

The levelled gatepost looks like the corpse of a 'Monolith Monster', a beast that destroys by toppling, threatening the world not in the world's Fall, but by a series of relentless raisings and crumblings, wave after wave; going down in order to bring back something new.

After a brief venture through an archway in a wall, to a plot so heavily overgrown it is clear no one has ventured in for months, I take an alley (downhill this time), marked by an amputated Victorian lamp post, to Lower Warberry Road, where a gorgeous yellow sandstone lion rests on a gatepost, its huge front paws casually crossed (as were Pan's hooves in the garden at Oldway, does that crossing symbolise something?), looking across to the valley where mountain lions had once sipped at the stream that still occasionally pushes up the manhole covers and floods the buses on Fleet Street.

I could just about see where the new flats were going up, on the site where Oliver Heaviside lived towards the end of his life; he had by then shifted from eccentric to sinister. Ostensibly the tenant of Mary Way, the unmarried sister of his sister-in-law, he imprisoned Mary in her own house, replacing her furniture with blocks of granite, refusing to allow her to go out without his permission and getting her to write to friends to tell them to stay away. He forced Mary to sign a contract in which she promised to wear "warm woollen underclothing" and "never to marry a nigger".

It was a next-door neighbour of theirs who had broken into CASTEL-A-MARE and seen the thick, dark entities: "black, silent and man-shaped".

It was eight years before Mary, rescued in a raid on the house by her nieces, was released from her servitude; by then she was in a semi-catatonic state, spending her waking hours staring into the flames of fires that Heaviside kept roaring to satisfy his thermophilia.

Salmon tries to set all this in the context of Heaviside's "genius"; his intuitive guess about a reflective ionised layer around the Earth, his facilitation of long-distance cable transmissions by installing periodic induction coils and his development of operational calculus. Wrong, unforgiveable; like Heaviside. Unforgiveable. The W.O.R.M.'s real "genius", or his genius loci, rather, was to take his work on electromagnetic waves, facilitating the crucial technology for expanding a geographically limited and contested empire of things into a globalised and incontestable empire of information, and to distil it down to a single house, and a single soul, staring into a screen of flame, irrelevant to comfort, all difference prohibited and all subjectivity vaporised. That was his "genius". Where Mallock, Bulwer-Lytton and Trevena were political, Heaviside pre-empts the post-political, the post-human. He intuits Nick Land's shift, from the Earth's molten core through horror to the digital Alt-Right.

Beyond a high wall, window cleaners are using sponges on giant poles to reach up to the highest floors of a block of retirement flats. At least I assume they are cleaners. I can only see their long poles reaching like the feelers of mechanical aliens from Wells's 'War of the Worlds'. I keep noticing stuff about water, evidence of piping and water management; what had been kept – in what was then Britain's wealthiest town – from the poor in the bottom of the valley.

Torre Abbey, the King's Drive, Torbay Road, Shedden Hill, Torbay Road, Princess Theatre, Cary Parade, Fleet Street, Abbey Road, Fleet Street, Strand, Victoria Parade, Beacon Hill, hard left turn up Parkhill, right up steep steps, Vanehill Road, path at the end into St John's Wood, Daddyhole Road, bear right at red telephone box onto Daddyhole Plain, if you go to the far left corner of the Plain and take the footpath, at the end of this path there are warning signs to have never taken it(!), and it ends, anyway, in the road from Daddyhole Plain so rather than follow this dangerous path, instead take Daddyhole Road, and look to the right for an archway in the wall, go through this, down the steps to Meadfoot Beach, Meadfoot Sea Road, Ilsham Road, take a set of steps to the right, Bishop's Close, at junction take the signed footpath to Bishop's Walk, Bishop's Walk for half a mile, cross Anstey's Cove Road, through playing field, turn right along Ilsham Road, up steps on left to Kent's Cavern, café, out of Kent's Cavern, bearing left through car park, left up Ilsham Road, right onto Babbacombe Road, left onto Middle Warberry Road, take footpath on left down to Lower Warberry Road and turn left along Lower Warberry Road to Babbacome Road and turn left.

Outside St Matthias' church there is a utilities box, a sub-sub-station, long disused, its corporation paint peeling in slim curling strips of murky green, exposing scars of swimming baths turquoise. It rusts away next to a rotting tree stump. I resist peeling away the dusty wood fibres for fear of disturbing stag beetles or other unlikely creatures I hope are digesting the base of the great being. I have seen so many amputated lamp post stumps, redundant public drinking fountains, chopped faucets at pavement level, and dud metal boxes in thick, dead paint with the relief of CORPORATION or DEPARTMENT, and, most impressively, TORQUAY ELECTRICITY UNDERTAKING. Testimonies to a time, now long gone, when the provision of utilities and the maintenance of fabric, were civic obligations rather than businesses.

I dither at the door of the church; what's so special about churches? Apart from their being often open and it being odd for anyone to object to you entering one. Untrue of most other non-residential buildings. Open churches are indictments of the policing of space that we put up with. I tentatively enter the porch; the 19th-century gothic is a poor, stiff and lifeless copy of a mediaeval church. Why am I bothering? I never get through the door, halted in my step by a poster on the porch notice board for a JOLLYWEEN PARTY CELEBRATING LIGHT. It takes me a moment to take it in, then I get it. This is an attempt to take back All Hallows' Eve from the readers of Harry Potter and the trick-or-treaters, to fight back against a Devil that none of their enemies believe in, let alone worship, a conspiracy in hell that the Church has created for its own purposes. On the face of it, what could be sinister about a JOLLY celebration? But the "No Fancy Dress Please" is chilling. These people are *scared* of fancy dress, *fearful* that the Devil (that they have invented) might pollute, even possess, their Jollyween Party. In what? The clown costume they have on the poster?

A few days later an epidemic breaks out across the country and I see people brandishing bottles as weapons, chasing a clown out of a supermarket car park.

A few doors along I come to a house named HALLOWDENE.

In a local newspaper, provided free at one of the hotels I stay in, a well-known and 'beloved' regional broadcaster worries at "the dark side of celebrating the equinox".

That afternoon I come repeatedly upon the undaunted commercial exploitation of the attractions of demons – HAUNTED HALLOWS: A MONSTER SELECTION WITHOUT THE SCARY PRICES and HALLOWEEN EVENINGS OF MINI HORRORS at the Model Village – but I didn't think *they* were JOLLYWEEN's target; it is not the representations of magic and spirits, it is the unorthodox intuitions of those who suspect there is more to the world than its appearances. I hope I am not offending anyone here, but I have very little time for the sentimental (and very, very occasionally sinister) nonsenses that pass for spirituality in many New Age and neo-Pagan groups. They seem to be passing round and round amongst themselves a few 20th-century tropes of ancientness. Where is the innovation and mad rigour of Strindberg's 'To Damascus' trilogy? Or the melancholic existential conspiracy-testing of 'Axël's Castle'?

The evangelicals were picking off easy targets for their own ends. I am worried where the dynamic of their witch hunt, begun with children's parties, will end.

Then a signpost I cannot believe. I must have passed under it and missed it on my previous loop. One of those brown heritage signs. The top half is for "Kents Cavern Prehistoric caves", but under that, painted over in brown but still visible by its raised surface: "Gleneagles Hotel Inspiration for Fawlty Towers". How can I not go and look at that?

At first I think they may have built a Watts Tower in place of Fawlty Towers, but it is a giant red crane. The hotel that inspired the TV farces has been levelled and a block of retirement flats is being built. I check with one of the building workers, hi-viz jacket, luminescent hard hat and disinterest; yes, yes, this was Fawlty Towers. I nose about, but there is not much left to see. However, an alley overlooks a surviving patch of the hotel's garden, including one palm tree.

Basil: Do they have palm trees in California?

Mr Hamilton: Burt Lancaster has one, they say, but I don't believe 'em.

The firm developing the property is Churchill Retirement Living.

Major: Black? Churchill wasn't black!

I'd always wanted to be Polly. Even as a child I'd hoped to have her vulnerable capability in the face of the chaos of the adults around me.

First Cook and now Cleese, giants of the single-sex public school comedy that had wrestled the media from the likes of Bernard Manning, Frank Carson and Charlie Williams. With their roots in the misgivings and miseries of Britain's upper middle class, they have held comedy in a grip so ferocious that, while I was walking, a researcher would reveal that since 1967, when Cook was at the height of his game, of the over 4,700 comedy panel shows broadcast only one – only one!!!! – had consisted solely of female comics.

I backtrack onto Babbacombe Road, twice passing beautiful modernist and art deco blocks of flats, and then the Palace Hotel; a leisure re-appropriation of the Palace built for the Bishop who had made the Walk. I call in to Reception to ask if maybe there is a chapel or some revenant of the Bishop that I can visit, but there is none; the concierge explains that only the central part of the building dates from the Bishop's time. The wings were added in the 1920s.

"There's some information over there," and he waves his hand, but I find only glass cases of trinkets for sale and details about the gym. I stand for a moment, blankly, so as not to appear rude, then leave, out past the art deco garage, with its tennis player weather vane, and into a part of the road openly cut from the limestone bed, stained a whitish blue on one side, and pink on the other.

Now the houses grow more suburban, then terraced. Then the remnants of quarries, even a working supplier of sand and gravel. An older stone cottage, set back behind a terrace, looks like it might have been a residence for stonemasons. A pub, The Masons Arms, with a pair of compasses, splayed wide, on its sign.

This change of architecture awakens me to just how many *enormous* houses I have been passing by all day; reminders that, while there is still money here, Torquay was once much, much richer. That it has maybe been a mistake on my part to see it through the faded glamour of the democratised 1940s, when ordinary folk, like my Nanna and Granfer would pour down from the North and the Midlands in trains, stop in guesthouses in Paignton and trespass into Torquay. The resort's origins have since been mediated to everybody by Basil's tortured aspirations at Fawlty Towers, despite the show's outdoor scenes being shot in North London: "Well, may I ask what you expected to see out of a Torquay hotel bedroom window? Sydney Opera House, perhaps?" But it was magnates, billionaires and plutocrats, not insecure hoteliers, who first built here; then, quickly, the besieged aristocracies and monarchies of Europe joined in. The town had its own symphony orchestra. Parts of the front were openly policed to keep all but the hyper-respectable away. Yet, it was always abject. Its disease was fakeness. Kingsley described the symptoms here:

"You are half-tired, half-ashamed, of making one more in the ignoble army of idlers who saunter about the cliffs and sands and quays, to whom every wharf is a 'wharf of Lethe', by which they rot "dull as the oozy weed"... and worst of all, at night a soulless réchauffé of third rate London frivolity; this is the life-in-death in which thousands spend the golden weeks of summer and in which you confess with a sigh that you are going to spend them."

Salmon finds these words a more radical assault on everyday life than anything written by the situationists:

> Kingsley had everyday life down for a life-in-death, while the situationists merely imagined it as survival meaninglessly repeated.

The big Mediterranean villas, the importation of dying monarchies from Europe, the attempt to make a southern European cultural resort in rural, coastal Devon had delivered a monument to the defeat of the very people for whom it was built, in a town where they were still scared of France in 1900. Each property had been built as a last redoubt against a confused Somewhere Else. Huge limestone walls are everywhere. In many streets there is the permanent feeling of being shut out. I feel exhausted and melancholic. I have discovered so much, but so little to raise my spirits. I feel as if I am being tested, an initiate rather than a researcher. I have hardly met anyone today. The Chalkers and some weirdo in the theatre – who was that? The Geo-Questors, of course, briefly, but they were working. I have set myself on a foolish pilgrim task and distracted myself from my commissioned work. I resolve to re-think and book myself into a B&B for the night on Babbacombe Downs. I am too tired to go out in search of other walkers and sleep a long deep sleep, remembering no dreams.

North up Babbacome Road, turn right into Asheldon Road (site of Gleneagles Hotel on the left), retrace steps and turn right onto Babbacombe Road, right down Babbacombe Downs Road.

Chapter Seven: Babbacombe to Newton Abbot

Out of bed, an OK breakfast and straight into it. I'm not looking at any map, so I don't know where I am going, but Beach Road is a pretty obvious clue and I take that. Past the Theatre advertising 'Ultimate Genesis by Los Endos', glad I'm missing that, and down the sharp incline to an edifice with another plaque. Oscar Wilde was here in the winter of 1892/3, consummating his romance with Bosie. "It's a lovely place," Wilde wrote to him, "it only lacks you".

Wilde retreated here after the banning of his play 'Salome', his Symbolist displacement, it was a natural genre for him; he was always shifting the surface away from the layers of what he was saying. How could Bosie touch him and know that he was really there? No wonder they rowed, and Bosie left in a tantrum.

The building hangs over me, the wall immense and the angle downwards steep. I am flopping down hard on my knees. Too early in the day for this!

Wilde was here at the time when he was writing that "Socialism would relieve us from that sordid necessity of living for others.... the majority of people spoil their lives by an unhealthy and exaggerated altruism"; he imagined a progressive egotism, by which, not at the expense of others, but to the profit of others, self-realisation would be freed from wage slavery and real slavery, and from the poisonous obligations of fear that accompany them both under the guise of faith and deference.

Wilde overplays his hand.

Just being shocking and 'perverse' (but not really) is as tiresome as Trump. But there is something inside the flaw especially for us now; the idea that pleasure comes from nowhere else than from within, that we refuse to have our desires created for us, but make and then satisfy them for ourselves; breaking the tentacles of the Spectacle in a slimy mess of desire. Wilde is revolutionary, he is anti-reformist ("it is immoral to use private property in order to alleviate the horrible evils that result from the institution of private property") and severs the tradition of radicalism from the pottage of Puritanism. But he is elitist; he is playing to the wrong gallery; for him there are no 'gods'. No West Quarter. No 'Romany Rye'. But he is anti-authoritarian: "if Socialism is Authoritarian... then the last state of man will be worse than the first". Too much of what he writes is clever-clever, but from the heart of the public gaze he grasps, with steel sharp clarity, the significance of this: "Through the streets of Jerusalem at the present day crawls one who is mad and carries the wooden cross on his shoulders. He is a symbol of the lives that are marred by imitation." There it is. Almost a century before René Girard; straight to what the Spectacle destroys; its imitators, those who think they flatter It.

The dry yet slippery road twists and the sea comes into view; greyish brown and unsettled. The chalkboard at the Cary Arms says that there are grey seals around the harbour wall, but I cannot see them. I walk following the prom, and enquire at the café about the house of Emma Keyse, the elderly woman murdered here in 1884 in the John 'Babbacombe' Lee case; victims are mostly forgotten and the cases, unless the victim is already famous, named after the assailant. A man sits at a table, he says that the house has gone, but that there are some ruins in the trees at the back of the beach. In fact, the house, The Glen, stood on the waterfront, where the car park is now...

So what is in the trees? Perhaps I should have climbed in there? I don't think so. What am I going to find out after 132 years of fable and uncertainty?

Why am I even bothering to engage with these histories?

Too much of the time I am relying on Salmon, notice boards and the web.

But later, at my guest house, when I read up on the case online, there is a reason there that I was drowning in these details, stories, analyses. And there is a certain 'something' that was never ever there, smothered by how much of the information-stuff there is. There is no 'place-sense', no 'space-logic', no understanding of these terrains that can give you any hint of what might come next; yes, there are anecdotes and documented events and tales, but there is nothing in the way of a sited narrative.

No wonder the man, sat at the café table, had no idea of where things had been; where is the incentive to attend to the details when there is no attending to meaningful space?

Lee, the convicted murderer, was taken to Exeter where, on the scaffold, the trap failed to open three times, and, although there is no law to say this, his sentence was commuted to life imprisonment by dint of superstition. The execution was intentionally bungled by a hangman who had no inhibitions about selling lengths of his noose or acquiring a murderess's dress for Madame Tussaud's. Lee was present at the murder, caught by Emma Keyse *in flagrante* with his girlfriend Kate Farmer, and another couple, Elizabeth Harris, a house servant (and Lee's half-sister) and her lover (by whom she was pregnant) Reginald Gwynne Templer, a married solicitor from Teignmouth. The impecunious Miss Keyse, who had once conducted Prince Albert around The Glen, in that moment, saw a lifetime of respectability ruined and demanded that the police be called. Perhaps with the assistance of Lee, she was murdered by Templer who then fled while the lesser orders manipulated the scene to give the impression of a burglary gone wrong and set fire to the house. Templer immediately offered his services to the police, but then became Lee's defence lawyer. He mentally collapsed and was replaced by a solicitor who would himself later hang for the murder of his wife. Templer died a couple of years after the trial, in Thomas Holloway's grandiose Sanatorium for the very rich at Virginia Water, from the effects of syphilis ("general paralysis of the insane").

The Templer family were immensely rich and powerful, owning much of the land immediately north of Torquay. James Templer, the patriarch, was responsible for the building of the Stover Canal, his son George (an 'am dram' enthusiast who had six children with his mistress before marrying into the Kennaway family of Escot House) is responsible for the granite railway at Haytor, its rails made from the same granite it exported for the building of the British Museum, the National Gallery and Rennie's rebuilding of London Bridge. In the 20th century the Templers were a significant force in the higher echelons of the British Army.

The successful prosecution of John Lee, on the basis of questionable, circumstantial and tainted material evidence, his subsequent deliverance, and the removal of his half-sister to Australia were organised by powerful men through the offices of the Freemasons. Lee and Elizabeth's mother (the family described by a contemporary MP as a well-known "witch family from Newton Abbot") was cousin to a Mary Jane Harris who in 1865 had been indicted along with Charlotte Winsor, twice the widow of men who died of industrial injuries who lived in an isolated cottage on the edge of Torquay, for the murder of Harris's baby. The "witch-like" Winsor was, supposedly, the final resort of women with a baby to dispose of; her practice, though nothing is said of this at the trial, being to hold the child by a hand and a foot and the mother likewise to enforce her silence and then together to lower the victim into a tub of water. Harris's child was, according to Harris, who turned Queen's evidence, smothered by Winsor alone, though Harris was present. The trial – for the death of a child found wrapped up in a copy of *The Western Times*, discovered close to Torre Abbey – followed revelations in Torquay about numerous murdered children; like Lee, Winsor escaped the drop, on a legal technicality.

Given that many of the young women likely to experience an unwanted pregnancy were working as servants in the big Torbay houses, a network begins to appear of rich and powerful male sexual privilege, an unreliable spectacle of respectability, informal networks of malleable laws and enforcements across which silence is traded as goods for sale, and a desperate poverty translated into the smoky language of Satanism.

Or not. Because there NEVER is a resolution like this into meaning. No sooner does one narrative emerge by which other narratives are made understandable, than all the parts unhitch and unhinge, and the whole thrashes into bits. No wonder Fredric Jameson suggested that conspiracy is "the poor person's cognitive mapping". Without access to some tool of analysis, the options are a radical separateness of tiny pixelated informations or a paranoid over-explanation.

I am not discovering anything. Except that in some cases there is no possible way to discover anything at all.

The waves are washing over the promenade ahead. I time my run and get to the wooden bridge, with the breakers gently crashing below, lifted out of any danger. In a tiny cove, the waves are fizzing under the walkway, the name of LEE traced in concrete on a step: FIZZ + LEE WAZ ERE. Up ahead and above I can see the massive rockfall of red sandstone and the ruined villas on the top, bent and threatened. At the point where my path sneaks around the giant sandstone pillar of the cliff railway, the narrowing path is pounded by tall waves. There are lulls when the path is briefly clear, but it will take good timing. A couple with walking sticks wave me ahead of them, warning me about the "seventh wave", the unpredictable giant that borrows energy from everything around it to climb up above the rest.

I am extra careful. Just after our baby was born, I had let my ex take her out onto a sea wall during big waves. I had got nervous and left them there with about six other people, strangers, and walked back to the harbour. There was suddenly a mighty thump and water pillared up through a blowhole right next to me. I turned to see a huge body of water spilling off the sea wall and, to my ecstatic amazement, everyone safe. Although I had said nothing, they had all, including my partner with our baby, taken their cue from me and retreated. It was crazy that we were ever on that wall. And I am getting a little flashback of that sick stomach of craziness right now.

I look for a wave with extra energy whose reflection I know will eat into the energy of the next incoming breaker. I wait and wait and then take my chance, skipping across the wet concrete and up the steps to the beach. Which is fine, but the couple with the walking sticks have also decided to chance it on my judgement and follow me, at their rather slower pace, and now a wave is chasing them. I shout and they are able to hurry, I run back to give them a hand up the concrete defences, with the water breaking at their ankles; I watch them blithely walk away.

In the Museum Room of the Cliff Railway, on the front where all the buildings had been destroyed in the storm of 2014, one of the volunteers waxes lyrical to me about the finances of their operation. He points to a picture of the beach in 1960, packed with people – "that's me!" – and yet, when I ask him to point himself out while I take a photo he is loathe to – "maybe it's a taller person".

"One hundred thousand people we used to get then, and they ran it at a loss! Council run, you see. Now it makes a hundred thousand pounds profit a year, since it was a private company, well, a public trust company, we've got our own Donald Trump!"

"Really?"

He changes his tune.

"Well, huh... God help us all if *he* gets in!"

I had been struck by his remark about civic provision. I think of all the public spending cuts that have been under way since... well, pretty much since I was born in the early 1980s. What a brilliant device this is; you so denude the spending on publicly owned or democratically elected institutions that they seem to be to blame for their own lack of action. And then you have these men, like the man in the Museum, these evangelists against the public, always present in apparently benign spaces, drip drip drip, slowly dragging us up the Cliffside of neo-liberalism.

A handprint in concrete, and then a name, maybe ZEE maybe LEE. And another redundant drinking fountain.

It sounds like the Tardis. Grinding up the cliff. The winds are driving the ferns crazy, where they'd found a knife a week after the murder, a weapon that Lee could not have disposed of, but most likely caused the wounds on Miss Keyse. The defence made little of it. I cannot see any remnants of a house.

At the top I consider stopping for some early lunch at the café, with its views over the Channel, but decide to go hungry for a while. I pass a car plastered with posters, a sign on the top reads NEW EVENT!

An oil tank in a garden has been decorated as Thomas the Tank Engine, and then another sign:

WALK THROUGH WORLD WAR 1 TRENCH *experience the sights, sounds and smells*

I buy a ticket for the Model Village. I want to test its representation of the world against my conversation with the Privatisation Man. I notice a few things about the Model Village: there are police everywhere. The population of the village is far more diverse than that of the radical walking movement. There is an emphasis on media, including a filming of The Tiny British Cake Off with a miniature Nadiya; at an unsigned Fawlty Towers a tiny Manuel is forever smacked over the head by an angry Basil; a Superheroes Mansion; Mulder and Scully at a mediaeval joust; an opening of a new Star Wars movie; and leisure, with zoo, football ground, and cricketers disappearing into long grass. This is a meta-model-village; so there is an entrance to Babbacombe Model Village in the Model Village and, once, a sign says, the house-on-fire had really burned down in the night. The Senior Citizens Social Centre is grimy, its paint peeling. Bankrupt firms – bankrupt in the real world – have been removed from the model High Street. The only signs of production I can find – as distinct from mining, quarrying or distribution – is a Broken Biscuits 'factory'; it is not clear from the models whether broken biscuits are made there or complete biscuits broken. A house is being squatted. Parked cars are wrapped in giant spider webs. The railway station is named after Dr Beeching who single-handedly smashed up the publicly-owned local railway system in the 1960s, or as it explains here "famous for sanctioning the closure of many of the UK's uneconomic railways". There is much ancient heritage – druids at Stonehenge, a white chalk horse, Morris dancers, Kent's Cavern – but the only hint of the colonial is in the racialisation of the models.

Cockington appears as Mockington, with a Dram Inn; though the model-makers have ignored Lutyens's design and plumped for a thatched Tudor building. It is a very potent silencing. Everything modern has come from elsewhere; Devon is allowed to retain possession of (and its resort to) the rural past.

I stay much longer than I mean to. I think it is the 'meta' feeling, the sense that in model form it is possible to think the whole thing, to loop back from any part into the whole. Even though the model, like the real Devon, resists place-meaning, there is at least a model for how a meaningful space might be made, arranged and rearranged, even if these are not the right pieces.

I have barely walked a hundred metres out of the Model Village when I am thunderstruck by Kelvin Court, a tiny cul-de-sac off Petitor Road, three sides of terrace around a central ornamental garden with its own ersatz standing stone. It is *exactly* like a giant version of part of the Model Village!

I weave a way through green-jacketed officials spilling out of the golf club, through a metal gate at the end of the road and set off vaguely northwards along the coast path. I feel no less anxious about these quiet spaces, but I am just *doing them* now.

The path is voluptuous. Glowing green caves. The roof is howling. The wind that had whipped up the white horses is raging in the canopy of trees. At times the path is almost hidden by freshly fallen leaves; as if my path were being sprinkled with petals.

The text on a bench spooks me something rotten:

> David and Lorraine
> Somewhere in Time

As the path contours inwards I can see how tall the cliffs are on the opposite side of an inlet ahead. Towering above me, even though I am high up on my side. There is a small concrete-like building way below and what looks like a short cut, branching rightwards from the path.

The cove is catching and channelling the wind. The trees scream and the tops bend. The main path is disappearing beneath the fallen leaves. The loneliness and inwardness that I felt on the Bishop's Walk is blown right out of me. I am scared, not by an imagined threat, but by the real power in the huge trunks creaking, their energy of position at any moment translatable into a crashing fall. All along the path I have passed through arches made by fallen boughs and trunks. Occasionally a twig or a small bough comes rustling through the canopy and settles in the growing piles of leaves. I am crawling along the side of a noisily snoring beast, fearful of waking its true force.

I tread carefully down the precipitous short cut. Away from the main path the wind begins to catch in my scarf and coat. I lean inwards, but under my feet the tiny path is disappearing and, disbelieving what I am looking at, I see my feet balanced on roots protruding out from the red cliff, nothing but a rosy crumble between me and the hundred foot drop into the combe. I dither.

What am I doing? I am not in my comfort zone. I am making rash, bad, rushed decisions. In Leeds, in Sheffield, in Huddersfield the paths I take I know already, I can't even remember when they might have been new to me. I have worn them smooth since I was a kid, but I have always walked the same ways. Even when my destinations changed, from office blocks to libraries, the routes were barely different. But here – and maybe in Leeds, Sheffield too – just a few minutes from the ordered suburb, you can be ill-advisedly creeping down a path that turns into roots above a precipice.

Scuttling back feels more like dodging a bullet than retreat.

Back on the main path, I erupt in a huge relief. Glad that I have been respectful of the power around me; even if tardily. The trees could not care less; they carry on yelling as if nothing has happened.

I get down to the broken road and the concrete building. I decide to have a quick look at the inlet that must lie at the bottom, but on taking a step downhill the wind rips off my scarf and flings it up the road. I take the hint and, recovering it, choose the path into the woods without a look back. This path rises and then contours again, drawing me under a huge, huge cliff. I feel as if I have stepped out of England; there are skull-shaped caves high up in the red face. This, then, is a 'Valley of the Rocks'; not the famous one in the north of the county by Lynton, all bleak and exposed, uncovering what Southey called "the very bones and skeletons of the earth", lionised by Coleridge and Wordsworth and their failed tale, 'The Wanderings of Cain', but green and cathedral-like, its roof of leaves and floor and walls of red crumble, a desert raised up in groping sheets. Salmon says that as Torquay became popular the new residents would gather here to listen to concerts of orchestral music. Today there is the stringy roar of the leaves and an occasional cymbal crash of a falling bough; a strange hollow in the sandstone that might have been a throne for a master of ceremonies.

I tail a couple walking their dog into a car park. They seem to be straining to not notice me. I climb up to one of the carved (I assume) shapes in the sandstone; maybe they are spooked by my looking down on them. They herd their spaniels away.

A young woman, mid-teens, is leaning on a wall, texting. I ask her what the nearby big building is. Mostly to confirm my prejudice that people never know what is immediately around them. She takes the skinny cigarette from her mouth and explains how the film industry had made movies right here about a century ago, but it all went away as quickly as it had come. She says I have been walking through its movies' locations.

There is nothing in Salmon's guide; maybe he did not expect the walkers to come all this way through the trees. Later I find on the web how quite a few movies were made here at what was then 'Cairns Torquay Film Studios', opened in 1919. The company transformed some of the spaces I had been in: Torquay for Naples, Corbyn Head into a magic cave for 'The Rocks of Valpré', while Rock Walk (where the plaques and texts were) stood in for a jungle in 'Unrest': "the paths are covered with artificial jungle grass, a human baboon clings to the branches of an old ash tree and sailors climb over the steep slopes as if they had landed on a tropical island". Nothing very famous was filmed here, but there was one hidden and forgotten transformation that struck me more than the others; filmed in the 'Valley of the Rocks', it was a prototype for the Narnia mythos and I was amused to find a Narnia lamp post in the car park of what had been part of the studios, now Watcombe Hall, a stone lion over its front door.

This movie is 'Where the Rainbow Ends'.

As a play, 'Where the Rainbow Ends' was massive in its time, the sister production to J.M. Barrie's 'Peter Pan'. Opening in 1911, it ran, every Christmas, for

47 of the next 49 years. Almost no one has heard of it now; I heard Leslie Joseph mention it on the radio recently; but she could remember almost nothing about it. I read the novelisation, written by the author of the play, Clifford Mills. Terrifying. *Mein Kampf* for kids. It kicks off with a shipwreck; the child characters' parents lost at sea when returning from colonial duties in India.

Steve Mentz cites "Northrop Frye's resonant joke that names maritime disaster as the 'standard means of transportation' in literary romance"; here it serves to provide the children with motivation to seek transportation by magic carpet: "If Faith thou hast... The carpet genie will inflate... thy slave he'll be". Faith, like Vril, is someone else's servitude. The children's evil guardians, Uncle Joseph and Aunt Matilda, trigger their journey, following a promise in 'The Rainbow Book' that "all lost ones were found in the land Where the Rainbow Ends".

I thought of all the benches, the endless memorial benches, I have passed. And, sitting, reading this sentimentality, realise I have never sat on one of them, never seen anyone sat on one.

In 'Where the Rainbow Ends', Uncle Joseph deprives Cubby, the children's pet lion cub (Aslan in training), of his Colonial Mixture – "the one thing that would keep a British lion strong and powerful... Equal parts of Canadian, Australian and New Zealand Iron mixed with Indian and South African Steel". For Uncle Joseph is a self-hating Englishman. He refers to the Cross of St George as "that pretty bit of bumptious bunting", so that even Bertrand, the French dealer – "he had missed a bargain and just imagine – his great-great-grandmother had been a Jewess" – is disgusted and breaks off their business deal.

The children call up St George, who manifests as a pilgrim in a dingy cloak and dusty cowl: "thus humbly clad, unnoticed and unsung, do I lie hidden in the hearts of men". This is the grand entrance of entitled-disgruntlement personified. And he is quickly whingeing on about how St Patrick and St Andrew have their days celebrated, but not his: "who ever wore a rose on his day"? After the swaggering nationalism, the self-pitying resentment of its more extremist forms; prelude to very bad things.

Uncle Joseph, armed with a piece of magic carpet torn off by the subaltern William, conjures up a Dragon King to recapture the children and the book, and the action shifts to the Dragon King's domain. Within it is an enclave, a tiny piece of empire, safe ground protected by the red and white flag of St George. Close by, though, are the big bad dark woods; and inevitably the children all end up in their dangerous shadows. I had been scared to enter them in Paignton, but not here on the Bishop's Walk or in the Valley of the Rocks. Something was changing in me.

At the conclusion of 'Where the Rainbow Ends', the children save themselves by cobbling together a makeshift flag of St George, and calling the knight to their rescue.

At the top of Watcombe Beach Road, I cross a busy main road, for a moment back on the John Musgrave Trail, and then follow a sign to Brunel Woods. Sounds interesting. I briefly touch the edge of suburbs. There is something suddenly like relief; stood beside two plaster winged lions and looking out of a relaxed homogeneity. After the sonic bashing of the storm, I understand, for once, the appeal of being as far as possible from wild.

At the top of a climb, I turn left and then up yet another set of steps, posted for Teignmouth Road. The steps bring me eye-level to a dangerously busy road with no pavements. I turn around and hammer my joints back down the concrete. Turn further down the road and find a better footpath directly into Brunel Woods, up to a small clearing full of sculptures. There are strange twisted shapes, beginning to rot from base upwards and a wooden Isambard Kingdom Brunel; the carving of his waistcoat and watch chain has produced a cadaverous effect like exposed ribs, like the tomb in Paignton church. Nettles reach up to Brunel's knees. It seems a little perverse to carve him in wood rather than cast him in metal.

The woods are full of fallen trees. One great trunk, fallen across the path, has to be crawled under.

I come to a wire fence; Brunel Manor is visible on the other side. The land was bought by Brunel for a house to retire to, but he died before the building was barely begun. It is now a Christian Holiday and Conference Centre. I follow its border and then worm up a boarded alleyway, where two knots in the wood, a little green mould and the shadows of the trees have made a spirit of The Grinch. Then down long suburban roads, punctuated by a plastic bag, bulged out by the wind to look very like a Dicynodon from the late Permian period. Coming out on to a very busy Great Hill Road. I follow it for a while uphill, worrying that the pavement will run out as the houses begin to drop away, but the road splits and I can take the narrow, quiet fork.

Over a hedge the whole valley, all the way to Dartmoor opens. From the bottom of the valley one huge hill, rounded and dumpling-like, rises up, dominating everything around it. In the very far distance, a twin-peaked tor sits on the skyline.

I wind along tiny lanes, worried about speeding traffic. But it soon feels as if I might be out in the wilds for a while. The sun shines hard, the wind drops and the gaps in the tall hedges reveal the occasional startled rabbit. Yet no sooner have I settled into this tentative pleasure than, unexpectedly, the tiny lanes loop back to a junction with the busy road, and neither direction seems to offer anything in the way of a verge, but plenty in the way of racing vehicles, vans and lorries driven hard at each other. I do not want to get squeezed by one of them. Tight corners, very fast traffic; no one driving on this road expects to meet a pedestrian.

I don't seem to have much of an option but to give in, turn round and retrace my steps back to the suburbs, try some other way out of the town. There is a gate a few metres up the road on the other side, maybe I can cross a field there and get to another lane? Or at least see my way to where there might be a safer route? It seems odd that my tiny lane has so suddenly run out.

I dash across, but I never reach the gate. Instead, before I get there, I find something extraordinary. A small gap in the hedge and the tiniest stretch of path bending into shadow; but once I step into that darkness, I enter the rich red and green funnel of an old hollow way. I am Alice falling down the rabbit hole. This place is not now. Who would ever come here? It is almost impossible to walk; regular streams of water have left large stones dotted along parts of its floor. It is hard to mind much else than these ankle-breakers. And I do not want to fall here; I might wait a month before someone came along to pick me up. Or meet a horse; there are some droppings, maybe a week or so old; I pretend to myself I can tell. The red base of the path is defined by another channel that has been cut into it by rainwater, sharp enough to have been cut with a spade. Every now and then, a sizeable part of a bough lies across the hollow. I am not surprised, when I sneak a look at an A-Z in the next town, that this is called 'Fluder Lane', though why it is marked as if a car could get down it I have no idea. It is difficult enough to walk.

Fluder Lane not only came to my rescue, but claims my soul for its quarter mile of red and green darkness, its boulders biting at my ankles, cupping my head in its green palms. Up until now I have been walking through towns, occasionally in a green space alongside their suburbs, but now, for the first time, I am stumbling down an old hollow way into something quite different. I know from the signs I have passed that there are no towns this way. I think of my daughter. Why am I being so melodramatic? OK, I am a city girl, at home in the Northern conurbations, in Naples and Paris, but I know the moors, I have been out for a hundred afternoon strolls and a drink in the pub afterwards. But this is somehow different. I have no map. There are no pubs. There is no moor.

I do not know where I am.

It is a green world, hot now and dry, stinky and loamy despite the winds, the bane and spoil of fertilising new life in the rotting heap; the unnatural heat of clamminess, too close to be polite. Twigs poke and nettles sting. What do I imagine lives here that can threaten me? And yet the green is alien. I am uncomfortable. And yet, it is also wonderful. I can feel beneath my fear a kind of joy. To be just an hour or two's walk from a model village and 'ye olde filme studioes' and yet already to be entering the Shire down a quarter mile of initiation.

Eventually Fluder Lane spills me out onto a tiny metalled road, watched by horses from their field, and I follow its incline. Across the road a tall sapling has been brought down by the winds; and no one has come this way in a while and shifted it. I feel very alone. In good and bad ways. I become angry that I feel like this. Then I become absurdly grateful; for not having to feel fear unambiguously and unrelentingly. I am starting to imagine myself exemplary and my walk meaningful.

A junction with cottages. One with a thatched gate! I take the route signed Coffinswell as a kind of gothic rebuke to the twee gate. The lanes are elongated. It is hot. I am very thirsty, and hungry. I begin to love this too. The greenness, the effort, my knees beginning to complain, but I have no blisters! I slide through the land; no one knows my quest. I pass unseen by farms and cottages, only the birds remark on me.

I remark, once more, to myself: Devon is not flat.

Treacle Barn; rusted farm equipment on display. I do not pretend to myself that this is any kind of real place. At Coffinswell, I finally find the pub I have been dreaming of for the last three miles. Breakfast at Babbacombe seems an awfully long way away. It is shut. The Linny, mediaeval, historic. But shut.

I am still stood sadly at the door when a woman in a black waitress's uniform appears behind the glass. We shout to each other.

"What?"

"Closed?"

"What?"

"Closed?"

"Yes. Sorry."

"I couldn't bother you for a glass of water, could I?"

A second woman appears with a key and lets me in, while the first woman reappears from the kitchens with a long thin glass of iced water. I drink it in one gulp, thank them and leave. They say they have not noticed any other 'walkers' recently. Maybe I had lost them all now.

I feel I should have stayed and chatted longer; once I had finished the water they had offered me "something else, now you're here?" but I didn't want the alcohol to take the edge off my anxiety. It was helping me to feel the colours more distinctly, to get the ironies and poetries more sharply. The road is intoxicant enough. I had never walked like this before, not knowing where I was going or how to get there, or if I would get there. At times my walk seems to hang by a thread. At other times to be walking in different times simultaneously, and at different ages; I feel very young, then suddenly, frail and vulnerable and rather brave. The exhilaration at the simplest of discoveries is my reward. I am on a treasure hunt.

I had not realised until I check Salmon later, how appropriate it is that I am given water here. The village has a "welle", hence the name – of course! – mentioned in the Domesday Book; and it has its own anti-apocalyptic timetable: an unburied woman who every year takes one cock's stride towards the churchyard; one of those investments that will never be cashed in.

I don't understand the countryside. I don't understand unhuman animals. I don't trust them. I am much happier in the worlds of a symbolist Strindberg or a melancholy Maeterlinck. I am happy in the most morbid of the castles of Villiers De L'Isle-Adam. I am not comfortable in these old lanes with their high hedges, but I am excited. Scared and thrilled. By the rabbits scampering and the sudden views across huge distances. The twin summits of the tor and the single voluptuous rise of the hill, almost hovering there above the valley floor, a green cloud.

I turn off before Doda's 'holy well', stopping a car at the junction. The driver cannot tell me the name of the lane, nor exactly where it goes – "I've just driven all the way from Worcestershire!" – but he urges me to take care: "it gets pretty narrow". It should get me to the main road in about a mile and a half, he says. I am starting to wonder where I will be sleeping tonight. I am not sure about barns and fields, Norman Wisdom notwithstanding.

I am skilled now at distinguishing the sounds of carburettors from the roar in the leaves. I pass a building site for a huge villa. The very rich are still building here, but more privately now; they will have a massive vista of hill and moor. A huge pile of white ash smoulders with resentment.

At the top of the lane, safely negotiated, I can see the busy main road. I have yet again connected to the very vergeless road I am avoiding. I can see a turning off up ahead but it may be too far to safely run on the road. I am not an athlete. And I fear the cars far more than I do the waves.

Many people have faced this same fear. And it is shared in the landscape. Pacing back and forward in indecision, I notice a small gate with a rotted signpost, just before the junction with the main road, and a footpath running inside the edge of the field, parallel with the busy thoroughfare. I enter.

Red. Redness.

This is so Devon. So old. I have never seen soil like this before. It is lipstick red. So bright in the late afternoon sun. This is the golden hour now and it burnishes the upturned clods of recently ploughed dirt.

I tread carefully, particularly where the farmer, carelessly or maliciously, has ploughed the path into ankle-twisting traps. This is how treasure hoards are found, the sun catching the edge of a golden plate turned up by the tractor.

There is someone else thinking the same. She is crouched over the edge of the ploughed ridges, balanced on a sliver of remaining path. I recognise her from the official conference site. She was showing a group of paintings in the lobby, but painted *with* the landscape. Rocks, red soil, white chalk. Things tied together with red string, children's rhymes, the kind of simplicity that hides unspeakable things. It had put me in mind of escaping from the house onto waste land where the trace of an old steelmakers had been.

"You're Helen B?"

She is. Collecting red soil from the field. She slips on her flip flops – "do you walk in those?" "yes" "wow, I couldn't, I have to have boots, you must really feel the road under you" – and I help her carry the soil to her car, parked in the lane on the other side of the field. There is red dust on her white shirt. I ask her about "process" and she laughs.

"I'm exploring how walking affects painting, in gathering ideas and materials and content, but also the walking in the painting itself, how painters walk in the studio..."

"Your work reminded me of trespassing into old factories as a kid..."

"A lot of people say that."

"What's the red and white about?"

"Ah..." she laughs again, "When I started my walking for this set of paintings, it was during the 'Euros' – the football, not Brexit!"

She takes some chalk and then some red soil from the well of the car.

"I'm walking between where I grew up and where I live now. The one is chalky, the other red soil."

"You live round here?"

"Nearby. During the football there were all these red and white flags, I found them nationalistic and mean. Violent, actually. I didn't know what to do with them. Then I realised that my journey unpicks the flag, the red and the white..."

The image in the Valley of the Rocks, from 'Where the Rainbow Ends', of the green enclave in the Dragon's Wood protected by the flag, had been bothering me all day, but Helen B was taking it into her work and stretching it in a journey, undoing the flag cobbled from a red hair ribbon, a white shirt – she was unflagging the materials.

I turn down her offer of a lift, she slams the door and chugs off onto the busy road.

There is enough verge on the side of the main road here to get back to the turning and I take it. Long Lane. Once past a few farm buildings it runs off ahead of me, a long straight bumpy lane, almost a mile long. I really enjoy this now. Perhaps it was the meeting with Helen, it has shifted the walk away from being about me, and back to the materials. But I love the potholes now, and the rocks and the thick bracken and the empty fields and the excessive security signs – MOBILE PATROLS ALARM RESPONSE – and the sense that I am in the edgelands, here. The kind of lane someone would drive down to hand over stolen goods. Or discover a secret government installation. The late sun is making things golden. Where is the treasure?

Halfway down Long Lane, I see a group of the fringe walkers, organisers of the 'walk out', coming from a way off, carrying shoulderfuls of signs and fingerposts, dug up from around a nearby town.

"Can you do that?"

"Until we get caught."

We sit in the shade of a tree by the side of the lane. XXXX puts her flask in the middle, while the more impatient ones are already dragging the posts off, to gently hammer them deep into the field behind the hedge, with large stones.

"I can see you don't approve."

"No, I'm just documenting. I'm not judging."

"No names, you understand."

"Well, no...."

"So, why does it bother you? That we're damaging a little property?" It was not a question. "Is it public, is it private? Why is there so much effort to preserve all this uselessness? All this waste? All these ruins and hollow shells of private homes? All these fences round empty fields? Spaces for those who can pretty much guarantee that they won't have to meet anyone not like them? In a real city you only ever meet strangers! You know who will come to our signpost forest? Doggers, probably. At least they're not romantics."

She rolls a thin cigarette; her blue fingers peeping from clipped rainbow gloves.

"We've all been brainwashed, the most horrible, stupid things have been normalised; you see us steal a few signs and you're discomforted. Oi, XXXX, where's the black book?"

One of the hammerers breaks off and fetches from his rucksack a nicely bound book, something that probably once had a dust jacket. He brushes away some bread crumbs from its spine.

"Read it. You know. The bit."

"You like that."

The hammerer flicks through the pages. Stops where one is folded over.

"This was written in 1929..."

"49."

"OK. 49. But that's not recently." She blows a thin stream of cigarette smoke into a cigarette smoke sky.

"Whether I am a sensualist or a philosopher," he reads in a rumbling voice, like he is resonating with something in the ground under us, "in romantic terms an offshoot of Constable or Coleridge, I want to feel that the landscape exists, between me and the landscape; not between me and the landscape and a dead poet and the National Trust and a by-law and a new fence. I want to discover, not to be shown; to find my way by a map and my own nose, not by signposts; to be with myself, not with Gray, Wordsworth, Ruskin, Thomas Hardy, and all the pantheon of the dead, who are forced to make me see the landscape their way."

"Pretty amazing, huh?"

"That is remarkable. It's so acerbic. I don't think anyone would dare write that now. Who is it?"

"A poet. Geoffrey Grigson. Have you heard of him?"

I have to admit to this tall man that I have not. The woman with rainbow gloves extinguishes her cigarette between her fingertips and searches for a stone.

"Keep it." He passes me the book. "It's a first edition."

He turns on his heels and his large frame tips forwards and slinks off toward the hammering. There is already a thickening copse of car park directions, footpath signs, NO BALL GAMES, miles to so and so, even a 'Not A Play Area'. I follow him in among the signs.

"Excuse me."

He does not hear, or does not want to. I badger.

"What about the sentence that makes no sense? You could at least explain that to me?"

Bang went the stone on the pole.

"'I want to feel that the landscape exists, between me and the landscape'", I quote.

"Me", he says and takes another pole, standing it straight to the ground.

"Landscape," he says, and holds up the stone. Bang it goes on the pole.

Maybe Grigson had proposed smashing the very idea of landscape.

Bang goes the stone on the pole.

The forest of signs grows.

I lie down against the pile of 'liberated' signs and fall asleep.

I wake an hour or so later; the familiar faces have gone. Across the field, at the edge of woods, I can see something going on and go to take a look; I find a scene like a cross between cosplay for a not-yet-existing comic universe and the bit in *Fahrenheit 451* where people gather around memorisers reciting whole novels.

One of the storytellers takes hold of my arm and leads me to where they have some apples, tea, the remains of a risotto. I pass on the offer of a spliff and chew on an apple. The storyteller wants to hear about my journey; but I suddenly have the feeling that would be wrong and turn the question back on her.

"We'd just climbed out of the village of Coffinswell", she started.

"O, I've just come through there."

"Did you see the field of llamas?"

I had not.

"And then we came up a footpath overgrown with ferns up to your waist. We got to the middle of this field and a huge buzzard had flown over us. It seemed big enough to lift one of us up. I don't do much walking in the country, do you? It's weird. The bird made the air around us seem real; like the air was something you could hold in your hand. On the other side of the field was a track that ran out into a sunken path..."

"I was in one of those earlier."

"Not this one I hope. Chest high in nettles. There was a farmer there and he told us they used to keep the path clear but no one had been for a while. He said: 'it goes down to the bottom road. You can get through if you don't mind a few scratches. If I hear y'oller I'll know you's stuck!' Half an hour later we managed to get out of it – we had to crawl over a complete sheep skeleton, laid out like it was a display. We startled three foxes, five minutes later we were in a secret valley."

"A what?"

"Really quiet, like it holds the sunlight to itself. There's a big house and a kind of church there, a chapel for the house, I didn't hear what the others found out. Haccombe. A local told us that the champions of the local big families – the Champernownes and the Carews – use to race each other into the sea on horseback, see how far out they could get; then the winner would have his horse unshod and nail the horseshoes to the church door."

It sounds like the Parson and the Clerk story, guided by the Devil into the surf.

"...the maddening thirst for space..."

I say goodbye. The little copse of finger posts is casting long shadows.

At the end of Long Lane is a house with the sign:

The Round House
that was

It's a rectangular box, with a dog the size (and look) of a walrus sleeping on the porch.

A path through the trees brings me to a very tall wire fence. I follow it round to the gate of a large Centrax factory, makers of gas turbines. The shift has just turned out and there is a stream of cars out of the gate and backing up on the main road.

Centrax packages technology from different sources, including Rolls Royce, to sell as working turbines for projects like the production of floating power plants with the Bahrain-located Arab Shipbuilding company; these are barges fitted with power generation plants that are a popular means of supplying power to industrialising economies without permanent generating sites. This pattern of use may change though, as New York City is due shortly to get a massive power 'barge'. Power barges create the possibility of sailing a globalised industry from place to place in pursuit of the cheapest labour and last resources. Last year the German industrial giant Siemens AG – a company which ran its own factory, co-managed with the SS, at the Auschwitz death camp – extended its agreement with Centrax to co-supply packaged turbines to 31 European countries.

The Centrax firm, a business developed over 70 years by members of the Barr family, has just been gobbled up by the MB Aerospace company – MB's sign was already up alongside Centrax's at the gate – after MB Aerospace received a major investment from a private equity partner, Blackstone, a multinational based in New York.

Blackstone is one of the world' largest investors in leveraged buyouts. The company founders, Stephen A. Schwarzman and Peter G. Peterson, had previously worked together at Lehmann Brothers. The value of the company's total financial assets (AUM) is over $300 billion. The company name, Blackstone, is a cryptogram of the surnames of the two founders (Schwarz is German for "black" and Peter for "stone"); the result is oddly close to Black Peter (Zwarte Piet), who listens at the chimney of ordinary homes on behalf of Father Christmas, reporting on the good and bad behaviour of the residents. In response to the protests against the 'blackface' portrayal of this character in the Netherlands, the 'high-end' Bijenkorf chainstore has recently introduced its own gold-faced version.

I watch the workers stream home, and then overtake them on foot as the traffic jam backs up almost to the gate of the factory. I can see that most of the traffic is heading down towards the town and follow it. I am sure I can turn up a B&B. I look at all the faces above the steering wheels, framed in the windscreens, and hope things turn out OK for them. They are jellies in a vast ocean now. This little Devon town, run from an office in Park Avenue, Manhattan.

On my left, as I march down the hill on aching shins, there is another, smaller and more anonymous industrial building. Beside its solid steel fencing, almost hidden by a thick growth of shrubs and large trees, is an informal stone circle, hovering somewhere between ornament and (as I realise afterwards) ram-raid protection. I sit on the stones, thinking of them as some kind of kind of giant rockery, photograph them, and am quickly joined by security guards who want to know what I am doing. There is no signage, no KEEP OUT or PRIVATE PROPERTY, the whole space is low profile. Yet the feel around the stones is rather lovely, almost sacred, a haven of quiet next to a busy road. The guards are adamant that I am on private land, highly sensitive private land, though they refuse to say what is so sensitive about it. They accept my explanation that I am out walking and looking at things, and they are very keen to (as it happens) mis-direct me to a nearby hill fort that I have missed (in fact in the tree line at the back of the farm buildings on Long Lane). I am not turning back now, but thank them, savouring a last moment in the almost-fakery of the stone circle. I wonder if such confabulations might serve some better purpose; places for quiet contemplation. How brilliant it would be if neo-Druids would adopt the ram-raid protection of a cash-handling division of the Post Office as their new Avebury.

I complete the walk into town as the light fades and find a guest house on the Torquay Road, book in and fall asleep in my clothes on top of the bedcover.

Babbacome Downs Road, Beach Road, Babbacombe and Oddicombe beaches, Cliff Railway, Higher Downs Road, Hampton Avenue, Babbacombe Model Village, St Marychurch Road, Petitor Road, Coastal Path to the bottom of Watcombe Beach Road, with back to the sea take the right hand path after the toilet block, take the left hand path through the Valley of the Rocks to car park, Watcombe Hall, up Watcombe Beach Road, straight over Teignmouth Road into Moor Lane, turn right onto footpath parallel with Steps Lane, at the top turn left into Brunel Avenue, ignore the steps on the right and take the footpath on the right into Brunel Woods, sculptures on your left, to the fence of Brunel Manor, turn left and skirt Brunel Manor, until a back alley of wooden fences takes you onto Seymour Drive, turn left, bear right onto Padacre Road, right and then immediately left on Golden Park Avenue, right onto Brachington Avenue, right onto Barton Hill Road, bear right onto Great Hill Road, bear right where the road divides and take the small, quiet lane, at the junction with Claddon Hill turn left onto Honey Lane, where it comes out onto the busy road again, cross onto the verge on the opposite side and walk a few yards to the right, the hollow way Fluder Lane is on your left, take it and turn right at the end onto Footland Lane, take the right hand turn at Daccombe village, opposite New House Farm, and follow this unnamed lane until Coffinswell village, right up Conybeare Lane, just before it reaches the very busy St Marychurch Road take the gate into the field on the left and skirt the edge of the field on its permissive path, at the far gate turn right onto Blackenway Lane, and cross St Marychurch Road to the verge opposite, walking right and then take Long Lane immediately on the left, at The Round House take the path immediately ahead and turn right at the fence, skirt the fence and turn left onto Shaldon Road, Penn Inn Roundabout, Torquay Road.

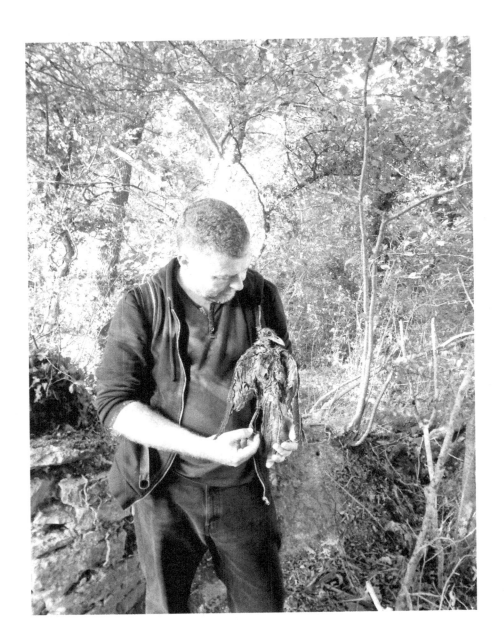

Chapter Eight: Newton Abbot to West Ogwell, Broadhempston, Torbryan, around Denbury Hill and back

Next morning, in a branch of W.H. Smith's, I sneak a look at an A-Z. All the way from Oldway Mansion I'd been tracking what looked like a very old route: Old Torquay Road, Preston Down, Cockington Lane, Old Paignton Road, Broadley Drive, Old Paignton Road (again, this time in hollow lane form), Cockington Lane (again!), Drake Avenue, Upper Cockington Lane, Dairy Hill, Collator Road, Kingskerswell Road, Great Hill Road (where I rejoined it briefly), Honey Lane, where I'd again joined it very briefly; all the time, without a map or any intention, I had been weaving in and around this ancient route. The more I look at the map, the closer I feel to losing any bearings.

I meet Tony the birdman, by arrangement, at Newton Abbot Railway Station and we set off down Queen Street together. We are going to head out for the church at West Ogwell. Although not a delegate to the conference, Tony has friends among the walkers and has made some performance walks himself; tipped off I was nearby, I think by one of the sign people I had met in Long Lane, he emailed and I picked it up at my B&B. For once, I am not winding my own way, but another's. We have a very specific destination, a route that Tony knows reasonably well, places to visit, and even a timetable of buses at our destination to bring us back to our starting point. Yet, nothing the birdman does is functional; and it is me who eventually forces the pace and suggests we escape from the loops we are making inside the town.

At the war memorial, sited at the end of what had perhaps been some main drag, now disrupted, I tell Tony (without crediting Salmon, sorry) that this whole place is described by W. G. Hoskins, the 20th-century landscape writer, as a "failed town": two 'manors' united administratively in the 17th century. Despite its industrialisation after the coming of the railways – Tony calls it "a Northern town in Devon" – the architects and planners never found a way to stitch the parts together. A place of bits, there are gaps to think in. Superficially, it's "Neutron Robot", homogeneity and alienation, with the anti-suicide grids armouring the multi-storey car park. But alienation leaves its own unspent excess of pleasure, and it lies about here in heaps.

The fishmonger's has little sharks on show, dogfish and Huss; they are not ready to sell the jellies yet. A bucolic 1995 mural in ceramics of 'Dartmoor Landscape' on the wall of the cattle market, generic and dis-placed, is ignored, its explanatory plaque obscured by a Parking Pay Station. We rise up the side of the car park, built over animal pens, in a glass-sided lift, afforded a view that just escapes bathetic. There is not much to be understood from up here.

The anti-suicide barriers would deter no determined climber, but they demonstrated concern and the suicides stopped. In the stairwell of the car park are huge cobwebs, and piles of dead flies, windows stuffed with breeze blocks and odd rectangles of painted surface. In the car park, once a week, a cattle market is held and beasts are brought for slaughter by the chequebook.

On our way into the Market Hall, The Walking Library is ensconced at one of the shaded outdoor tables. They travel with books in backpacks; selected and gifted by others, then share and shape their library again on the road. A visiting academic from Denmark is reading from Garnette Cadogan's article 'Black and Blue', about walking as a black male in Kingston, New Orleans and New York City: "some university staff members warned me to restrict my walking to the places recommended as safe to tourists... they trotted out statistics about New Orleans' crime rate. But Kingston's crime rate dwarfed those numbers... these American criminals are nothing on Kingston's, I thought. They're no real threat to me. What no one had told me was that I was the one who would be considered a threat".

I enjoy listening to the politics of walking in New Orleans, while sunning myself next to the burger stalls in a Devon town. But I had already noticed the cold, non-committal, 'temporary truce' stare of the man in the made-in-Malaysia England shirt, polyethylene terephalate stretched over his huge belly, as two young men coast by chirping loudly in Russian. The man is a walking (barely) stereotype: his weakness, nothing to do with his character but his social status, allows others to look on him as a sign not a signified, yet in the months after my walk people like him will repeatedly rock the establishments of the world with their direct democratic activity, from the US elections and the EU referendum to their abstention from Hungary's anti-immigrant poll.

I think of Helen B's attempts to get down to the materials of the red and white; that nothing progressive can come from these iconographies until their parts are unpicked.

The readings are completed by a local teenage boy who has chosen a Sonia Overall poem, 'inverted', about walking upside down:

> There are stars in the grass. You feel these with outstretched fingers. Your nails root in the soil, tickling the soft bodies of seeking worms. Your palms flatten. Your toes spring skywards. Your wrists beat with pressure, your knuckles rise and fall like viaducts.
>
> Your fused calves are an arching whip above your torso. Your pointed feet are a hovering scorpion sting.
>
> You look the laced boots of your companions humbly in the eye as you recede, a scraping suitor, from their presence.

You are a diver. The horizon swallows you."

It is as if the poem walked through me.

I have not physically felt a poem like this before, it has really caught me out. I would shiver at Mallarmé or Baudelaire sometimes, or at the turns in the stories of Villiers De L'Isle-Adam, but I had not been shaken. Now, changed by words, I will have to walk like Charles Kingsley's sea slug, a glove turned inside out, mouth, tentacles and all, falling inwards, and down into my stomach.

We move slowly out of the town. In the old market, its granite pillars and elegant roof host to intense displays of the ordinary abstruse, we visit eccentric stalls, on one of which Tony turns up a fine pair of faded Maoist pamphlets – "Against Liberalism" and "A Single Spark Can Start a Prairie Fire" – evidence of a Maoist cell in Newton Abbot in the 1970s. The conflagration was not ignited. During the 2011 riots there were arrests in Buckfastleigh as a result of attempts to organise looting online, and an 11-year-old received a "telling off" in Plymouth about a "Plymouth Riot Save Are England from the Government" Facebook page; among those confirming their attendance ("Going") were the Devon & Cornwall Police. They were the only ones to turn up. That thing I'd been told by the curator of a tiny Yorkshire village museum once: if you took things by percentages of population, the riots in villages and little towns, especially in rural areas, are always bigger and more radical than those in the great cities. But no one wrote about them, sheer weight of numbers counted, the historians were in the cities. Did that bathetic Facebook story express real levels of anger in these places? I doubted it; in the rhythms of my feelings of ease and agitations I felt occasional intensities of a deep bitterness and despair, underplayed by a stoic indifference and lack of confidence. When the Brexit result came, it was not a surprise to me; before I walked I had assumed that a 'natural conservatism' would make an automatic alliance between 'enlightened' pro-European people like me and those with less to lose, fearing they would lose even that. Before I walked, I had underestimated just how deep the despair had eaten, how little it was about rationality any more. I knew I was wrong before I was barely out of Paignton.

We pass an extraordinarily exotic building – the Passmore Edwards Public Library – the sort of place that tourists would visit if it stood anywhere else. Here, its Renaissance style looks oddly officious on a mini-plaza favouring the nearby Asda. It lacks all drama in the newly pedestrianised space, buffered by a bed of obstructive shrubs. The building's architect, the restorer of the Templars' (crusader knights, not local bigwig family) church at Temple (the one in Cornwall, not the Dan Brown one in the capital), had shot himself in the lavatory of a train as it entered Brownqueen Tunnel, a little before this library was built. How far are the psychological states of designers present in the realisation of their visions? How far intuited through the stone and brick and terracotta by passers-by?

After staring down at the maw where the Lemon goes under the houses, Tony speculates on a future walk wading beneath the town's foundations; we turn and follow the river, against the flow, along the side of Asda and under the A382. Cutting through workshop spaces we pass a wonderworld of discarded granite monuments and huge, thick marble baths piled one on top of another, great slabs of veined pink polished stone, fallen pillars and a smashed plinth with a few stone toes still intact. It is a world of material, a universe with its own laws and lawmakers. It is immediately ambient; it might be misrecognised as waste, but it is a forest of petrified symbols as full of stories as the cluster of signposts on the edge of town, and ruled, like it, by Absurdity, a mayor of misrule in office within the lulls in production.

We round 'Dip Demons' and turn left down a lane at the sign of a hollow man pushing a trolley: 5 M.P.H. LIMIT PEOPLE CROSSING. A door with a graffito: DALEK'S. Had the writer wanted to colour the building with the fiction of machine-monsters? Or, as the birdman suggests, is s/he asserting ownership? What would cause a person to be called, or call themselves, DALEK?

We pick up the route of the Lemon again. Tony finds a damp, folded sheet of white paper on the path and opens it up. It's the scenario for a horror film. Of course it is. The birdman's idea for this walk is for us to visit West Ogwell Church, a few miles beyond the town, the main location for a recently released low budget horror movie: 'The Borderlands'. So, of course, we would find the scenario for a horror movie.

If Froude can have his Law of Steamship Comparison, then I would like to have my Oak Law of Ambulatory Coincidence: whenever one or more people walk with a hyper-sensitised intention, each thing they find will connect startlingly to something else on their walk.

When the birdman got in touch, tipped off by his friends, he recommended that I watch 'The Borderlands' in preparation. I had found a reasonable wi-fi connection first thing and watched a bleary, pirated version on YouTube, with the sound on low. Horror films are not my thing, though this is a rather well-cast, 'found footage' movie (don't like those either). The movie follows the efforts of two paranormal investigators/debunkers from the Catholic Church and their agnostic techie, who "believes... stuff", and an entity reawakening under a recently re-consecrated church (enter the church at West Ogwell). Troubled by persistent bumps, groans and pixelations in the chancel, the investigators drive to a local airfield to collect an unorthodox exorcist, by the name of Father Calvino. In fact, I think they might have said "Italo Calvino" at one point, but the sound was too fuzzy to be sure; I wondered if this was a hint about 'hidden cities'. At the end of the movie the various investigators, for no very clear reason, though by then they have been driven to various degrees of irrationality, race around beneath the church, in spiralling tunnels, until they find themselves in a section that is softer, wetter and living. It closes up behind them. A sleeping, worm-shaped organism under the church – perhaps put to bed by Pope Gregory's instruction to preserve the sacred spaces of the pagans while replacing their symbols – has been wakened and swallows them.

For the birdman this resonates with the Cthulhu mythos – a giant dragon-like tendril-thing sleeping and dreaming in a hidden city, R'lyeh – the author of which is H.P. Lovecraft, all of whose identifiable pre-emigration ancestors lived in a small triangle of communities, at the centre of which is the West Ogwell church.

Tony does not come over as a fantasist. Most of our conversation is about bird calls, the loss of countryside skills such as making 'cut and lay' hedgerows and the malicious survival strategies of trees. I had no idea beech trees poison the forest floor around their roots. Horror or straight-up Gothic literature holds little interest for me. I thought it unlikely there really was some kind of Lovecraftian space just south of Newton Abbot, something that had oozed from his mythos into the landscape, but there might be something in the landscape – maybe a myth or an atmosphere or a monster – the representation of which the Lovecraft family had taken with them to New England and passed on to H.P.? Something still here.

We take turns to read aloud from the horror movie description on the piece of white paper; it's a school exercise. The final reel explains too much; Tony re-folds the scenario and puts it back by the hedgerow.

'Puritans' Pit', in the middle of Bradley Woods – remembered by the birdman as 'Devil's Pit', Devonians are obsessed with their Devils! – is a little way outside town. In the 17th century it was a refuge for dissenters who held their services here, posting lookouts to warn of the approach of the orthodox. Down in the pit, clambering over a NO ENTRY DANGER sign, it is hard to imagine anyone wanting to stay here for long enough to hold a service. Centuries of tree growth have put the pit in a dark, damp shade; it is like an ossuary full of giant green thighbones. At the bottom is a mouth to a tiny cave. The birdman climbs in. The whole pit had once been a limestone cavern, then the roof caved in. All day we talk of hollowness; chattering around the edges of an abyss.

Above us, we can hear people reading aloud from the same plaque we had found, almost buried in leaves: "A bible used for prayer in the Puritan's Pit survives to this day" (it doesn't say where) "and when held in the palm of the hand naturally falls open to Jeremiah 15: 'I will deliver thee out of the hand of the wicked, and I will redeem thee out of the hand of the terrible'". Naturally, just the right sentiment. But this is verse 21, and the Lord also says, in verses 7 and 8: "I will winnow them with a winnowing fork.... I will make their widows more numerous than the sands of the sea. At midday I will bring a destroyer against the mothers of their young men; suddenly I will bring down on them anguish and terror".

I suppose it's not surprising that the followers of a Maniac God are selective when they quote It.

Passing a giant limestone kiln operation, we emerge from the woods and into someone's garden. I love these public footpaths that take you through private rose beds and lead you up strangers' garden paths. On the gate is the sign: GATE.

The bridge has an enigmatic O NA on it and its own sonic ghost: the sound of a galloping horse returns without its rider, apparently. I am more unnerved by the prospect of meeting Lord Tebbit, an architect of Margaret Thatcher's miserable neo-liberalism, who lived somewhere here.

The birdman leads the way, we walk up quiet lanes with never a car passing, and up a footpath, the ground of which is secured with the broken parts of something carved and ornate and blue; something from a vandalised monastery perhaps, or a 1930s' petrol station?

At the bottom of a long falling lane – with tall, brutally sheered, once cut-and-laid hedges on each side – Tony bemoans how the loss of cut and lay skills has led to hedges so poor that many have been doubled up with wire fences – we cross a small stone bridge, beautifully constructed, very old, and then pause at a stile for the birdman to collect a desiccated crow, a fan of dark playing cards, the decay of which he has been monitoring for a few months. Dressed all in black the birdman is like the amplified shadow of the bird – "And what spoke that strange silence / After his clamour of caws faded?" (Ted Hughes) – then we bear right and up across the fields until we have a view, standing among sheep and red cows, of the surrounding landmarks. The birdman gives names to the shapes of yesterday; on one side, closer now, the round hill is Denbury Hill Fort, shrouded in large trees around its summit, and to the north-west, the two thick granite peaks are Haytor, its shaven surrounds clipped by ponies, cattle, sheep. Would this view have been a family memory the Lovecrafts exported, transposed by H.P. in his fictions of weird realism?

Denbury Hill looks to me like a belly.

We are connecting more and more deeply with the artificial dramaturgy of our walk as we more closely approach the main location of the movie. Movies, plays and novels can make 'worlds', not like 'real' worlds but with their own kinds of relations, their own kinds of ego, id and super-ego; usually cruder and, usefully, more symbolic than 'real' ones; I feel my familiarity with staged fiction is helping me here, but how much I am bringing and how much I am finding is too mixed up to judge.

We walk doubly now; partly in the terrain and partly in the imaginary vocabulary of 'The Borderlands'. As if our walk, rather than an original adventure, were a 'walk of interpretation', subjecting random things we find to the overbearing, but blurry omphalic 'green fuse' of the film: the marble treasure trove, the scrawled graffiti, the story of the sound of the galloping horse at Chercombe Bridge, a strange construction on the River Lemon near Bradley Manor, a kind of platform, possibly ornamental but with a smooth, cup-shaped stone set prominently in it. A pink pillow left in a vast stretch of playing-field grass.

The speculative realist philosopher Graham Harman has spoken of how enigmatic objects, unable to present what they really are, "can have gravitational effects on the internal content of knowledge, just as Lovecraft can allude to the physical form of Cthulhu even while cancelling the literal terms of his description". When I saw or heard the various things – pillows, stories, leaves, vistas – of our journey, I did not understand them and I could not translate them, but I did feel that they were all describable by the same gravity; there was nothing direct, but I felt an effect within the symbolic that was in some way common to these diverse things in this landscape.

When I later read Lovecraft writing in 'At the Mountains of Madness' about creatures as "truncated cones, sometimes terraced or fluted, surmounted by tall cylindrical shafts and here and there bulbously enlarged and often capped with tiers of thinnish scalloped discs" it was little different from "the mouth of the shell; a long grey worm protrudes, not the rightful inhabitant... finding the mouth of the Turritella too big for him, he has plastered it up with sand and mud... he turns mouth, tentacles and all, inwards, and so down into his stomach". Lovecraft like Kingsley, Kingsley like Lovecraft. Horror and zoology are challenged by the same things at the edge of description.

I'm not sure I'll be able to write directly about what it is that organises the pink pillow on the sports field with the spectral hoofbeats and the DALEK's green door; but a gravity has entered my feelings about the walk before we get to the church, and though I struggle to know why, I know my notes are different from here on.

The sky is a cap of blue. On the green hills, the animals are dots of red and white. In all the miles in view just two or three farms. There is isolation out here, long distances to ride or walk. Errands without motor vehicles would be measured in many hours. And all the time that hidden fort of graves is hunkering down under the high trees in the distance, and then further off the bleakness, model-like in the far, far distance, the double gateway to the vast expanse of moor with its bogs, its hairy hands, its black panthers, its artillery ranges and clapper bridges, its railway with rails of granite and its squealing winches still workable but chainless.

The birdman tells me how he made recordings of the silence in the church we are walking to. He sent them to the director of 'The Borderlands'. The director had not replied. The birdman is involved with a series of concerts of quiet music – I notice that Aeolian Hugh is among the composers performed – played in resonant spaces. Just as Bess Lovejoy, who now writes of the strange adventures of the cadavers of the famous, had once argued for darkness against the spectacle of oppressive brightness (a critique equally relevant to the exposures of a confession culture of 'tragic life stories'), so this quiet music movement has reacted to loudness, seeking out insulated spaces for interventions at very low volume. In the language of 'Spinal Tap', they turn the dial down to minus 1.

The birdman is steering us by various calls – chiffchaff, grey wagtail – interpreting the geography of a robin's defensive cries, different for threats from above than for threats from below. *Threats from below*. The robin – which navigates in relation to the earth's magnetic poles, by collapsing a quantum superposition in the materials of its eye which then react and turn its vision blue whenever it moves toward a pole – is a fierce prosecutor of boundaries. Not a bad companion for the borderlands.

In the movie, the techie character argues with one of the fathers that "pagans" have always been more grounded in their beliefs – they worship "what's there", the sun and the moon. And, presumably, the snake coiled under the hill. Hidden in the old BT logo, the Starbucks' Melusine, on tins of the Monster energy drink, the man-eating 'biscione' on the badge of Alfa-Romeo cars, commerce is seething with snakes. When I check out Blackstone... I nearly fall off the bed in my B&B: a snake beside a straight line!

The techie's improvised theology is an interesting play on a Hermetic idea: that what is spiralling above (priests out of control) is also spiralling the other way down below. Not because there necessarily is a monster at West Ogwell, but there is, 'down below', a space that is "what's there", that produces a resilient atmosphere, a something that has attracted first the pagan, then the Christian, then the filmmaker and now us. Not a physical snake so much as a coiling principle with some geological vessel that can hold together "various monstrous features", all the more powerful where the rocks are most exposed, or only thinly hidden. In its shapes a city or countryside forms its ambience – bellies, navels, throats.

All that is certainly true (or, at least, gravitational) here. Nestled among the Devon slate and limestone slabs around West Ogwell are spilitic lavas from subterranean seas, long ago subjected to metasomatic transformations, their original minerals dissolved and replaced by new formations. Among the slow cascades of small dead creatures, falling to the bottom of warm grey seas, was another metamorphosis: of hot rock changing in cooler water. The snake here is a traumatic geological memory curled up in pain like a serpent under the church, long ago oozing out of the ocean floor and transforming into a thing of clavicles and vesicles, a frozen and desiccated organ biding its time for waking and beating, an offstage member of the cast and crew of sweet Donna Haraway's Cthulhucene. Horror, acknowledging the power of 'dead' things, delivers a scenario for getting rid of the flagellatory Anthropo and putting ourselves fairly and squarely in the horror of the Capitalocene, guilty, on an industrial scale, of conniving with Cthulhu and conspiring with minerals in our own poisoning when we should be 'gathering up the trash' of the Anthropocene and what little the Capitalocene will leave behind with its wiped slates and scratch starts. In this 'horror', in which we play minor characters, we might finally begin to accept that there are no individuals, that oil is more in charge than oil executives, that we (and our fates) are inextricably bound up with other, more powerful organisms (jellies, the dictator-inheritors of our acid seas) and that our exterminism, in both its heartless and its kindly forms, obsesses on an elephant we can hunt or save, and ignores the fleets of grey seals and flotillas of jellies sailing to block up the inflow pipes of our nuclear power stations; they will only finish us if we do not include them in us.

I think that's what 'The Borderlands' is saying. To worship what is there. Not floaty ideas – fairy tales or surrealist writing – but the serpent actually in the stone. The atmosphere of a place is how we feel its organising principle; the point is not just to understand the serpent, but to arrange a date with it. Not cowering under a desk writing horror stories, eaten up with entitled disgruntlement and neo-fascist anxieties, but confident in the knowledge that we can handle this, that not only have we "always all been lichens", as Donna Haraway says, but that we are also made up of the rock the lichens live on.

The monolith monsters are us, and it is time to hybridise.

What a strange and quiet thrill it is to begin to recognise the landscape of the film in this gentle green space, fixed among the views of what an 'English landscape' is supposed to be. Rolling hills, a patchwork of fields, one or two farmhouses nestled under the protective windbreak of the combes, hedges, clumps of woodland, and the distant framing of the moor, the whole thing dancing 'ring a ring o' roses' around that pudding hill in its middle.

Although ahead is West Ogwell Church, there really is no West Ogwell; the church has been redundant for almost forty years and there is no dedication to any particular saint there. There is no recognisable village, just a few randomly scattered farms, and beside the church a large and old house that is as old and is not as old as it seems; a 16th-century manor house which passed to the Anglican church in the 20th century, became a retreat, then after the Second World War a Convent of the Companions of Jesus The Good Shepherd, an order of high church Anglicans, survivors of the bruising 'churchmanship' battles of the 19th century. In the 1960s the Sisters engaged in considerable construction work, expanding the convent, but moved out in the 1990s to consolidate their shrinking numbers elsewhere and the New Age moved in.

There is a Walking Room in the old house: now called 'Gaia House'. Back in the last field, we had passed a walker, presumably a guest of Gaia, who seemed loathe to make eye contact or speak. "Walking meditation", explains the birdman.

We make our way to the stile into the graveyard through a herd of red cattle.

At the bottom of the tower someone has painted out in white rectangles a five-letter word. SATAN or DEVIL, obviously. DAGON, possibly. DUMNA, doubtfully. Some animal has been digging at one of the graves. Inside, the chapel has a simple beauty. A very different, mediaeval elegance.

It looks smaller and more contained than in the film.

There is a heraldic plaque for a Mister Silly, Churchwarden.

And under the altar someone has placed a small 'fetish'; a forked twig and a piece of slate secured together with green twine.

The bible on the lectern is open at II Chronicles, chapter 4, a description of the creation of the Temple at Jerusalem, including the design of a massive ritual cleansing pool: "[T]hen he made the Sea of cast bronze, ten cubits from one brim to the other; it was completely round... and under it was the likeness of oxen encircling it all the way round, ten to a cubit, all the way around the Sea".

I thought of the red cows, South Devons, stood on a limestone sea bed, holding up an ocean of dreams.

In 'The Borderlands', the Fathers (including "Italo Calvino") and their techie access the mouth of the serpent through the door in the south side of the chancel, next to the 13th-century sedilia. I am ready to find that the door does not actually lead down to a serpentine tunnel; much more excitingly, though, is knowing how close the metasomatic stone is beneath my fungi-feet. In fact, the South Door leads directly outside the church again. Opening it and stepping through into the graveyard, as if perhaps into the spiral in non-visual form, I am especially pleased to find at my feet the curl of an empty snail shell, under the gaze of a sooty and melancholic face in the exterior wall.

In the graveyard someone has stuck twigs and feathers, in neat lines, into the earth of a grave; as if trying to grow trees and birds from the loam.

We walk down the drive past Gaia House. In the car park a sign designates parking spaces to GAIA AND STAFF CARS; I had not ever thought of her as a driver. A young and eager meditator has arrived on foot from Newton Abbot. We wish him well and follow the road to the left, past a wooden fence, each post of which is crowned with a disintegrating walking boot, an outdoor museum to thousands of miles of hiking. We cross a couple more fields, Haytor on the horizon to our right, and climb into a tiny lane opposite a five-bar gate with the legend – guaranteed to chill my blood with thoughts of bad monochrome sci-fi movies – GOVERNMENT PROPERTY. KEEP OUT.

In the middle of Denbury we turn left at the mediaeval Village Cistern, which has been topped with a strange table lamp operation to mark the millennium (any reference to "lava" is site-specific, but probably unintentional) and end up at the village green. I recognise a signpost that features in a scene from 'The Borderlands'. After a quick online search and some help from a guy running his dog on the village green, I ring ahead and book a room for the night at 'The Monk's Retreat' in Broadhempston.

Birdman and I (I have begun to think of myself as Robin) drink pints of Denbury Dreamer. We sit outside at the pub tables on the green as the sun goes down over the dominating mass of Denbury Hill. We talk of anomalous beasts, of a lynx loose in Newton Abbot in the 1920s, a tiger shot somewhere in Torbay in the 1930s, and the white vans that, in local foaftales and the pages of the Western Morning News, deposit sick city foxes in the countryside on a regular basis. The bald man, exercising his Staffie with a Frisbee, reprimands us for omitting the black panther on Dartmoor.

Birdman talks of how his watching sinister Morris dancers on a village green in an episode of 'Doctor Who' had deeply affected him as a child, and we speculate at length on just how far the sinister ambience of certain rural sites is a production of 1970s' children's television, rather than geology.

My taxi arrives and the birdman asks if we can continue the search a second day; he has another lens to see this landscape through. I agree. I feel secure with him. I would never have walked through that herd of cows on my own, I would never have made it to the Borderlands church without his confidence in the fields.

On the way to my digs at Broadhempston, the taxi driver, at my goading, produces a tale of ferrying two young women ("girls") from Totnes, armed only with a postcode which turned out to be a field; assuming that they were going to a party the taxi driver had apologised for his mistake, but, no, this *was* where the women wanted to be. They were "looking for fairies". Which surprised me; not that someone from Totnes (twinned with Narnia) would hunt for fairies, but that fairies were using the postcode system.

In the bar of 'The Monk's Retreat' I am delighted to find Angelique from the conference. Our meeting is unplanned; Angelique has decided to walk back to London alone. She is carrying a huge bronze-coloured flag which is now propped up in the corner of the pub.

"We'll fly it from the roof if you want," the manager says. "What does it mean?"

"It doesn't mean anything in itself, it's the least used colour on flags, some people think it means coming third, or something heavy, everyone has their own meaning for my flag, just as they all have different meanings for themselves. My quest is to discover both."

The manager pours our halves of 'Lady of the Lake' and 'Gold' respectively and disappears with the flag.

"It's not really about the flag", Angelique explains, "it's about what it does to the identity of my body; the flag is a kind of translator for the landscape I'm in and the landscape of my body changes depending on that landscape. I know I'm jumbling those two things, but my project is about jumbling those two things."

"Your project?"

"I don't mean project. I just do things. Sometimes I get paid for them, sometimes I write about them. My work is multi-disciplinary, I work across dance – I do body weather – and film, particularly. My mother is from Peru and I look absurdly like her and the flag is my way of being able to talk about place and identity without it always having to be through the medium of my skin. The first thing people ask is 'why is your flag bronze?' rather than why I am."

I ask her how her flag is being received in Devon, but she excuses herself from answering and wants to talk about what I am doing and about the fringe events I missed. I tell her about my theatre research and where I am seeing connections to walking artists and she tells me about the various fringe sessions she has been to.

"Did they discuss people who sabotage cars?"

Angelique laughed.

"No."

We are both tired. We finish our drinks and say goodnight.

Newton Abbot railway station, Station Road, Queen Street, Courtenay Street, Sherborne Road, Market Street, Market Hall, Back Road, footpath between Asda and River Lemon, workshops between river and Bradley Lane, Bradley Lane, footpath to left of Launa Windows warehouse, footpath following River Lemon, ignore the bridge up to Bradley Manor, footpath to Baker's Park, path through Bradley Woods, via Puritan's Pit and limekiln to Churcombe Bridge Road, Mill Leat, just before the junction with Littlejoy Road turn left down the

footpath, over the small bridge over the Lemon and turn right along the footpath through the fields to West Ogwell Church, past Gaia House, left at the road, pass roadside farm buildings and take the footpath on the right across a long field, through a hedge and across to the far corner of a second smaller field, out onto the small lane at the junction of Doughy Lane and East Street, follow East Street into Denbury, left into South Street, to the village green and Union Inn. (Taxi ride to Broadhempston.)

Maybe it is this sleeping in unfamiliar beds, but I am having very odd dreams. I am usually the director of some Symbolist masterpiece – either Ibsen's 'Brand' or Strindberg's 'Dream Play' (haha) – trying to realise their wonder-full dramaturgies with ridiculously thin resources: tins of talcum powder, hand torches, a few ice cubes and a three-bar radiator. But the theatres I am working in are extraordinary: a warehouse full of Spam, the headquarters of the Inland Revenue (how can I have imagined that?) and a flooded opera house. Professional humiliation is always followed by my retreating to some kind of grimy 'digs' or student accommodation, where I am sharing rooms with schoolgirl characters from the Ghibli cartoons and mini-skirted communards who complain about everything I do. In the dreams, I want desperately to see the theatre productions I have directed, even though I had forgotten to read the scripts or prepare for rehearsals, even though I know the productions have effectively collapsed and it is my fault. I somehow imagine that the plays will come alive on the stage. But I can never get to the performances; my clothes become incredibly tight and I fall into the road, or I turn up at the box office wrapped in a duvet and nothing else, imagining I can 'speak my ticket'.

Each night I go to sleep willing myself to dream the scene in Strindberg's 'The Great Highway' where the traveller meets two millers fighting over possession of the wind; just to see how a dream would stage that impossible contest, how it would cast the role of 'the wind'. I never do.

Next morning, I find that Angelique has already left, her flag is no longer flying over Broadhempston. Over coffee the birdman explains that 'The Monk's Retreat' had once been run by one of H.P. Lovecraft's relations, that another had been head of the church band here and that there were others nearby at Woodland. (A meteor had fallen there in the 1600s and Tony wonders if that event inspired Lovecraft's 'The Colour Out of Space'; I didn't know it). The last of the local Lovecrafts had died in the asylum just outside Newton Abbot, at Wolborough, where John Lethbridge, one of the first submariners, was buried in a wooden cask, surveying the wreckage of the dark deep, just as he did in life.

Slipping around the side of the inn – someone has left a pair of shoes on the roof of a car, it feels as if we are already picking up where we finished yesterday – through a short tunnel to the graveyard, we quickly identify, among many Palks, the tomb of William Lovecraft, second cousin to Joseph Lovecraft, H.P.'s great grandfather who took the family to the USA.

William's tomb is, pleasingly like nothing else in the graveyard. Indeed, like nothing else in most graveyards. It is made up of three large rectangles of stone, placed one on top of the other in descending size, the effect is of a pyramid without a peak, without a benben stone, a thing with no beginning, no birth, no creation. It is an end without a point. The bright white lichen is like guano.

Inside the church a box of Fuzzy Felt Monsters is stored in the children's toy cupboard. There are representations of various beasts on the hassocks – the snake in paradise, whale, swordfish, something like a cow crossed with a dog. On an old map of the parish, hung on the wall of the church, one of the fields up near Woodland is called Memory. That's what yesterday was about; looking for what in this landscape might have been carried to the US as a memory and then translated into gravitational prose. Today the birdman thinks we might burrow down under that.

We head for Torbryan.

Passing an abundance of Traveller's Joy in a hedgerow, Tony says its sap was used by beggars to raise blisters on their limbs; all the better to inspire pity.

As we pass down the footpath through the land of the Old Rectory, across to our right, on the other side of a pasture in the flat bottom of the valley, there are caves in the cliff face hidden by trees. Though we strain to make out the shapes in the green shadows we can see nothing. The birdman, however, has extracted some documents from the web. A report by a local man, James Lyon Widger, written in the 1870s, revealed his finds made over many years at Broken Cave. Part of what he found were Neolithic human burials; an old man, a young woman, one or two juvenile boys and two babies or foetuses. Another cave, that he called 'The Old Grotto', had accumulated to itself a "mediaeval" chapel, a reasonable-sized building with a ground plan of seven metres by three metres. That "mediaeval" was by no means certain: pottery found under the building had been dated back, if rather vaguely, to the Late Bronze Age.

One of the birdman's documents, a paper published in 1960 by F. E. Zeuner, Professor of Environmental Archaeology at the University of London, a colleague of the famous Gordon Childe, finds it unlikely that this 'Old Grotto' had been an official chapel. There was no mention of it in either diocesan or parish records; Zeuner suggests that more probably this was something 'informal', something comparable to a contemporaneous mediaeval chapel that existed in the north of the county where an altar was erected to "proud and disobedient Eve and unchaste Diana" (according to a diocesan edict) as part of an abounding worship of "heathen Latin and Germanic deities" that disturbed the church authorities, particularly as that site had been smiled upon by the local monastery. A description of its destruction in 1352 matches the state of affairs in 'The Old Grotto' at Torbryan: there was some looting of building materials, an engineered rock fall or talus now blocking the entrance. Perhaps at Torbryan there was, then, an image of a mediaeval descendent of Dumna, goddess of the Dumnonii people, here long before the Romans arrived, on a wooden altar?

There is no one in at Torcourt Farm, the owners of the land with the caves. In the orchard by the gate a huge apple tree, with fruit every bit as red and bright as those in the Garden of Eden on the Broadhempston kneeler, seems to be leaping, like a horse with a funerary plume, over the wall and off to Denbury. We call at the pub to ask how to contact the farmer. The birdman explains about the caves. One person has never heard of them; another, a trickster, assures us that the caves run all the way to Kent's Cavern, while an older puckish local makes obscure wisecracks. Discussing the bones of 800 hyenas found in a pit in one of the caves, the drinkers become very excited about dire wolves and I become confused as to whether we are discussing the Pleistocene or George R.R. Martin.

We follow the drinkers' directions up a lane to the farmer's barn. I shout his name repeatedly, but only his cows respond. "You were trying to conjure him up", says the birdman. I clearly have no magic in me.

Instead of the caves we check out the 15th-century Gothic Perpendicular church; its tower absurdly impressive and elegant. Its North Door, the door through which the Devil is supposedly ushered out during the baptism service, has been blocked up; maybe on the orders of Bishop Phillpotts, who disliked such baptismal magic. A copy of a 'Vinegar Bible' is on display: a 1717 edition in which "vineyard" has been wrongly rendered as "vinegar".

A crepe-paper dragon is slain by a two-dimensional St George with a red sword.

A sign that things, belief-wise, might have been slightly different here is the rood screen. Everywhere else I have been, the Anglican churches have been stripped of their decoration, even the decoration at the Catholic Church in Paignton was restricted to banners and statues; the swirling psychedelic wall patterns and instructional murals that would once have filled every inch of smooth space, coils of colour winding up every pillar, have all long been chipped back to bare stone or whitewashed over. Where symbols have returned they have done so nervously, conservatively. These are still chapels of the word, not Symbolist theatres. Yet at Torbryan, the rood screen is decorated with forty bright panels, depicting saints, long ago emerged from a whitewash disguise.

The one panel that strikes us both is St Apollonia's, a saint with a powerful presence in Devon. In a large pair of pliers she is holding a considerable human tooth. We recall the teeth of the cave bears and lions and the hundreds of hyena teeth that Widger found in the cliff behind the church. Apollonia, a deaconess in the Christian Church at Alexandria in 3rd-century Egypt, had suffered martyrdom during a hunting down of Christians provoked by a poet's (the Radovan Karadžić of his day) predictions of catastrophe. During her murder, Apollonia's teeth were systematically smashed; in the iconography of her martyrdom, the implication is that her teeth were pulled. Later I will stand at the West Door of the cathedral at Exeter and marvel at the carving of a saint, murdered by flaying, holding his entire skin; these reversals and messings with time suggest a metamorphosis of suffering into the symbolic means of self-transformation.

Is Apollonia signalling to us, through the whitewash of time, about the importance of cavities?

That night, part of one of my teeth broke off, next morning Tony emails to say his post included a reminder for a six-monthly dental check-up. Oak's Law of Ambulatory Coincidences.

As we walk along the lanes away from Torbryan, we discuss the recurring image of the hollow hill; the collapsed cavern that had become Puritan's Pit, the Old Grotto, Bulwer-Lytton's narrative of subterranean superhumans in *The Coming Race*. The birdman suggests that we walk to Denbury Hill, the omphalos in the valley, topped by ancient burial mounds; a hollow hill.

The Torbryan caves we had failed to access – later the birdman would speak by phone with the farmer's wife, but she refuses us; the caves are too dangerous, and, anyway, they are blocked with brambles now – were rediscovered in the middle of the 19th century by a local villager. James Lyon Widger had few resources, working as a draper's assistant in Teignmouth until his obsession with the caves became fulltime and he decided to live solely off his savings. He spent at least twenty years secretly exploring and excavating and collecting. Such was the volume of his finds – one cave alone yielding over a hundredweight of reindeer antlers – that the little cottage in which he lived alone itself became cave-like: "he had in his cottage six large drawers of trays, each about two foot long by a foot and a half wide filled with teeth of bear, rhinoceros, hyena, a few of the horse and of the wolf or dog. When asked about bones, Mr Widger replied that he had many *barrowfuls*" (John Edward Lee, no relation of the Babbacombe accused, surely not, no!)

Two contradictory drives (perhaps only contradictory to me, as an outsider here) seem to have motivated Widger. One was a desire to prove the literal truth of the bible's account of creation; a mission that would eventually deprive him of scientific funding and of the cooperation of William Pengelly, the key interpreter of the finds at Kent's Cavern, when Widger turned to him in the 1870s: "his intention is to explore it in such a way as to prove – Kent's Cavern notwithstanding – that the 'Antiquity of Man' is not greater than our fathers supposed". By then Widger had been excavating across five decades, making his first cave find at just twelve years of age, in 1835. The Windmill Hill Cave at Brixham, the find that would turn the evolutionary debate, was not opened up until over twenty years later.

The second drive, seemingly incompatible with the first, was the place of the underground in the local folklore of Widger's own village. In his memoir, Widger describes his listening to "old men who had scarcely ever been outside the Parish boundaries... well stored with legendary lore of hobgoblins that had from time to time been seen in the immediate neighbourhood". He was particularly impressed by the account of one of these men who, returning from playing fiddle at a "country hop... saw a Fairy Queen and her attendants dancing within one of their circles, so he scrambled over the hedge (or I rather expect he fell over) and advanced to where the little ladies were whirling around (probably thistles swayed by the wind), he was then requested to play his violin to them ... He also said that they resided in the rocks close by".

Widger was persuaded by his father that this was an over-imaginative, alcoholic folk memory of a "former time" when "people lived in such places [the rocks] and their only weapons, such as arrow and spear heads, were made of flints".

Impressed by both folk lore and lay palaeontology, Widger made his first venture into Dyer's Wood in search of his first cave, where "after all my father had said to the contrary I could not entirely divest myself of some misgivings, for I had heard from different sources that such little ladies were really in existence". Why such an accurate guess for a place to start? Were the cliffs inside the wood, the "rocks close by"? Was the fairies' ballroom that long flat pasture between us and the caves?

Walking out from Torbryan we follow the lanes, vividly aware that the first late afternoon dullness is just beginning to creep across the sunlight and that these are the lanes that had become, for Widger, narrated into the cluttered dens of fiends, hobgoblins, mischievous beings, Puck-ish things. Beings that maybe cannot daunt the walker who "labours night and day" to produce themselves as pilgrim and for who "then fancies fly away, he'll not fear what men say". Yet something in Widger continued to "fear what men say" of another world. Once in his first cave he "halted with throbbing heart", stopping in "fear and trembling and to listen for any sound that might be inside". The devout Widger was also the superstitious Devonian, drawn not to the open road, but to the hollow hills. Such was the impact of the old men's stories that he soon "found that every lane had its nocturnal visitor so that no thoroughfare was left free by which I could return home after dark without encountering something supernatural at a particular spot. So when benighted outside those limits there was no alternative but to take a steeple-chase course over hedge and ditch until I reached the homestead".

Could you find a better example of the production of space than Widger's fields?

The lanes are generators, at times they are like tall green screens, at others they dissolve in a fluttering of wings or a shake of the wind. In Strindberg's 'To Damascus' trilogy, the LADY says: "don't speak of the elves; it makes me sad" and the STRANGER replies "Frankly, I don't believe in them; yet they're always making themselves felt". It's not about arguing with people's belief systems, but staying sensitive to how what is believed makes itself felt.

As we climb and the height of the hedges diminishes, we can see again the pattern of pastures, hedgerows and copses that Thomas Sharp, the planner responsible for the post-war reconstruction (destruction) of Exeter, identified as a constructed "'natural' beauty... of the highly idealised landscape of painters like Claude, Salvator Rosa, Poussin and others... an imitation of Nature... modelled for pictorial rather than dragooned for monumental effect".

Yet for Widger these fields had become a labyrinth across which he would find transgressive routes, seeking solace for his troubled orthodoxy in the darkness underneath the fields and hills, by which to read the scriptures in the ivory letters of teeth and bones. His loneliness makes some sense of the Newton Abbot Puritans climbing into their damp Pit. But we keep to the lanes, where the only mischief is of the motor vehicle kind: two cars pass us in quick succession, both driven by the same person. Twins? Doppelgängers? A moment from a Tracy Fahey story.

I like the idea that we might be walking through a Poussin realised by Devon farmers and monitored by clones.

We come close to fields near Ippelpen where the parish magazine I find in Denbury church reports on the latest finds from an extensive dig that has been going on there for years. Close to a length of Roman road, the archaeologists have uncovered a community of the Dumnonii who had set themselves up to service the road users "rather like a 'Granada service station'". The site was first discovered by detectorists who recovered a hoard of Roman coins. Despite this initial find, and the assumption that this signalled an adaptation of the Dumnonii to Roman culture, the consequent failure to find anything comparable to similar but culturally compromised sites in other counties means that now: "we are wondering whether the Dumnonii... still retained their traditional identity, rather than becoming entirely Romanised". So, what made the difference? Dumna?

The birdman takes a call from the BBC; a falcon has been shot.

The belly of Denbury Hill is soon in view, but to get to it we have to walk the lanes in a circle, almost circumambulating the base of the rise "widdershins" before we can approach it. Entering the hill via Denbury itself, a village of furiously high walls, and passing the Union Inn once more, we then cut up a dark and green-smelling path, almost overgrown above our heads, climbing high out of the village. Halfway up the birdman picks a wasp sting out of his arm. We have a brief view to the Haldon Hills, the Lawrence Belvedere glaring like the Eye of Sauron in the evening sun, until the path turns us out onto the wooded hill fort itself, then snakes clockwise outside the ramparts and, finally, with one last shake of its trail, deposits us into the inner space and up the twin burial mounds within the fortifications.

The fort was built by the Dumnonii, shortly before the invasion of the area by the Romans, who largely seem to have left them alone. The tribes gathered under this name took their name from Domnu or Dumna – called by Henri Hubert, the French sociologist and close friend of Marcel Mauss, "a very important and vague goddess", Queen of a Deep which never feels very far away here, even in the woods – so it is no surprise that they had appropriated into their fortifications the twin stone and earthen breasts left by their ancestors on the hill top a thousand years before.

On one of the breasts is a nipple rock, made of granite. By the drilling mark this was a possibly hippyish addition made in the 1960s or 1970s. On the second mound, there is an ashen aureole, remnants of a camp fire, in which we make a sigil-face then scrub it out for fear, my fear, that someone might take it seriously. As well as the unpleasant aspect of making a fool of others – and though I do appreciate the arguments of Rod Dickinson and Rob Irving that hoaxes are a kind of art – I just feel that the world is too full of the unintended consequences of hoaxes not to ever undertake them lightly; up on this hill I cannot help but think of 'The Report from Iron Mountain'. Purporting to come from a US government think-tank, this 'report' concluded that a long-lasting world peace would not be in the economic and political interests of a stable US society. Intended as a satire on the US's permanent arms economy, today it circulates mostly among right-wing groups and militias as evidence of government conspiracy and the necessity for violent resistance to democracy. I would not want to be responsible for accidentally triggering a reprehensible cult in the 'Lovecraft Triangle'.

On our walk yesterday, in Bradley Woods, the birdman had raised the question of conspiracy theory and its place, if any, in radical walking. I wondered if conspiracy was not a kind of space rather than narrative, a space of sur-reality or parallel reality; not something neutral or flimsy, but more like a physical empire with its own troops and ambitions and violence. Like dreaming, conspiracy theory is futile where logic, interpretation or empiricism is concerned, indeed it is dangerous to try to explain it or co-operate with it. To subject it to scientific analysis or expect it to render up anything meaningful about the real world is a fool's game; a game that will *make* you a fool. It is a space where the subjective and the objective are separated and yet look as if they are the same; a room of dreams in a house with too many rooms.

Inside that nonsense, the anxious can find every fear they secretly desire, safely shorn from actual events, intuiting by the general shape of things the gravitational pull of shapeless things; apparently entangled with aliens and monsters, when, instead, they are looking at themselves in the mirror of their fears. Conspiracy is fantasy's false flag operation; and now it is taking over the real world.

That's why I kicked the ashes away.

For those overwhelmed by information, conspiracy seems to organise and explain things without need of recourse to verifiable facts or reliable sources; showering the world indiscriminately with drivel and peer-reviewed science, until no one has the energy to explain the difference. While its believers rarely bother to explain themselves, and are always wrong in detail when they try, they are right to have intuited that for a good while now there have been no reliable sources; when a former Education Minister can 'ad lib' that people are tired of experts, then the days of respected expertise are over. Even the mainstream media only check a small proportion of their sources.

The 'experts' characters in the geo-opera in Torquay were exemplarily embedded among the great unwashed; what they said was consistent with science's best understandings. But such expertise no longer applies, because everyone is waiting for the limestone bones to speak directly to them, without mediation, and the 'great washed' will not put up any more with the exclusion of their superstitions from mainstream discourse on the grounds that they are "an intelligent draper with little geology". Many supposedly left-wing liberal critiques of these tendencies – commentaries on Sarah Palin's speech patterns, for example – strike me as nothing more than snobbery about drapers.

Conspiracy theory does not help us with actual conspiracies, of course. But what it helps with is the non-rational understanding of what the absenting of the rational looks like. It is a map of what terror aspires to in the absence of rationality. It is the horror movie of "wipe the slate clean", "that makes me smart", "howzabout that then, guys and gals?" and "I just want you to know that when we talk about war we're really talking about peace".

In conspiracy theory, every citizen, no matter how stupid or poor, is redeemed by their victimhood; not because they are victims (some are, some aren't, conspiracy theory doesn't care), but because when they become conspiracy theory's victims they will do so without any way to object or even to know that they could object. Conspiracy seems to be our new empress.

Conspiracy, with all its myths of the theft of agency – alien abduction, the conspiracy of experts, the ubiquity of surveillance – correctly identifies the people in their weakness, pins them, paranoid, angrily entitled to their dissatisfaction; a mirror of those with real power who believe that for them, by entitlement, all things are permitted. The powerful – the new geo-political business class of Putin and Trump – think they can 'climb every mountain' no matter what the mountain wishes.

We have to recruit the mountain. The hill. The rock and dirt belly and breast.

In the face of the Gogmagog of conspiracy, it's no good to keep resorting to logical, materialist, empirical criticism. It doesn't work any more. Instead, we need to trust in what Ralph Waldo Emerson called "the recoil": that sensitivity to the dull intelligence of ordinary things and the maintenance of a fierce individualism which will help us find a good way through. Neither bowing down to the entitled without objection nor riding riptides of information brought in plastic bags, but jealously protecting the irrational creativity of our subjective lives – and I'm including redneck Trump voters just as much as Lucy Irigaray in this – while allowing *things*, dumb stupid and solid things, to work on each of our behalfs.

A new kind of ecological movement; not one about preserving aesthetically pleasing wilderness, but about getting the wild to invade us.

There was, of course, no 'Lovecraft Triangle', nor is there any real evidence of a landscape here that reappears in the prose of *At the Mountains of Madness*; what was powerful, though, was how everything was leveraged by *pretending* that there was. Not so much the fuzzy felt monsters in the church at Broadhempston, but rather the fallen cross on the small wooden stage beyond the graveyard wall, beside which lay a huge pile of excrement. Not so much our failed attempt to reach The Old Grotto (even if it had succeeded and we had subsequently revealed new evidence of a revenant of the 'Old Religion'), but rather the non-marking of the gate to the way through the grounds of the Old Rectory to get to Torbryan at all (like kids on tough estates taking down road signs so that only locals can find their way). Not so much that old story of tunnels linking one place to another, but the locating by the barmaid of our probing after local legends within the mythos of 'Game of Thrones'.

If we take the leap of her association and deploy it knowingly, then, by *knowingly pretending*, we can beat conspiracy theory. By sceptically, honestly and openly *pretending* we can inoculate ourselves against conspiracy theory and immerse ourselves in how things and people, in the particular, right up close, tell their own stories. Not how they fit in with spectral or paranoid narratives. By *pretending and immersing*, we provoked the recoil of real, solid things. That is the way to the radical walkable ground that giddy theory has compromised and poisoned.

Widger, persecuted by the old men's hobgoblinisation of the lanes of thought, had taken to the fields. His response was exemplary. Not to follow the Old Ones' lanes of haunted thought, but by a creative steeplechase to leap from field to field, sustained by the multiplicity of things built layer by layer, held up by the "recoil" of the much older things both within and without us and beneath us.

We need a new kind of ancientness: not about myths and legends and romantic and ethnically divisive 'forefathers', but about taking certain social forms and anti-magical worship in solid things, and placing them as torques and tyre levers in the wheels of today's slippery and Spectacular narratives.

Our searching for serpents in old churches, the felt monsters, the redness and extent of the apples in Torcourt Farm's orchards matching the apples on the tree of knowledge on the hassocks, the tale of tunnels snaking their way to Torquay, all this "*pretending* that there was" has put the fields in place for our climb up Denbury Hill, the snaking path up the tail and then around in the spiral to the two tomb-breasts and to slide our own vulnerable layers within the fragmentary layers of 3,000-year-old burials, 2,000-year-old ramparts, 20th-century stone additions and 21st-century campfires (with what tales?) We make shapes in the ashes, combined in a sigil-pattern: a jellyfish spider with a beak and a single eye, like the single 'eye' of John Lethbridge's oak diving suit, laying down splayed sticks for its oiled leather cuffs.

Even up here, its top shaded by huge 200- or 300-year-old trees, Dumna's deep was never far away. The limestone bones speak clearly, not of Shaver people or Vril, but of the bottom of a real old sea.

Later in my B&B, searching online for hints to the meanings or effects of this deep oceanic soaking of the land, I discover a mythos of the Devon coast that neither Salmon, birdman nor anyone else apparently acknowledges, hiding in plain sight, written by one of the most famous of all mythos-makers: H.G. Wells.

In his *The Sea-Raiders*, on a beach just north of the Exe, a human corpse, one of those four suicides perhaps, is found in the process of being devoured by 'indescribable' animals, of a kind with those sea beasts that "must to a large extent remain unknown to us", octopus-cum-jellyfish, their body like a face, ready at any moment to break up into a riot of clustering tentacles. The hybrids of *The Sea Raiders*, like Lovecraftian speculative realities, resist description; single organisms woven together in an assemblage, like slime mould or lichens, moving as one to turn a seafloor into a forest of arms, animating the metal spinney of signs, transforming a victim into a cluster of faces.

Wells's story speculates that the arrival of these unknown animals may be due to a starvation migration. And there it is again: the unholy and enormous appetite of the migrant, its blazing joy in surrogate cannibalism, triggered by its 'stumbling' on a fresh shipwreck.

The racism at the heart of what H.P. feared.

The horror within the hollow mountains of madness is the shadow of Dumna, in turn the shadow of the shadow of Starbucks' Melusine.

Coming down the hill I jump when I see a black shape move suddenly, and even more at a green ivy creature which the birdman sees too.

We share additional pints of Denbury Dreamer and contemplate the nature of the Dumnonii and what or who it is they might have worshipped. Salmon has written a whole section of the guidebook about them, furious at the local heritage industry for beginning Devon's history with the Roman Invasion; but what he has turned up is dismissive. They were described as "a loosely organised tribal confederacy... lacking political cohesion... economically backward and culturally isolated". Why 'backward'? Because they issued no coins? Because their response to the Romans was "peaceful submission"? Because they made an alliance with the Romans and fought with them at Hadrian's Wall? Because they did not use storage pit agriculture and Belgian cremation burials; because they weren't someone else? Because a pre-invasion Roman visitor had described them as being naively welcoming towards strangers?

As a result of their policy, if that's what it was, the Dumnonii were mostly left alone by the Romans – "the Roman military largely withdrew from the South West to fight in Wales" – and they, in turn, left the Romans alone, ignoring the abandoned city at Exeter when the occupiers withdrew to Rome around 410 CE. Rather than centralised units – the hill fort at Denbury is an exception to the rule – the Dumnonii mostly lived in scattered settlements, more like the layout and social structure of West Ogwell today than clustered Saxon villages like Cockington, let alone towns or cities, with "firm evidence for industrial or commercial production... very limited indeed. Although South Devon possesses a number of potentially valuable industrial commodities... there is little evidence that any of it was exploited much beyond that needed to meet local requirements"; in other words, they did not conform to the expansionist, scalar, commodity-based, growth economy of present-day post-colonial capitalism – "surplus production does not seem to be part of the Dumnonian way of life" (Branigan).

The Dumnonii do not fit within the parameters of either feudalist or imperial, colonial or capitalist normative history.

If they did indeed worship a Thalassocenic goddess, celebrating the pressure her inhuman oceanic magic exerted on their histories and welcoming a power inimical to their own interests, it might explain their dispersive and ecologically sustainable social relations, their enthusiasm for gaps and a discreet welcome to the strange. Now that would be a Lovecraftian speculative reality with its tentacles rooted in hard rock and violent sea.

That night – having booked a room in a converted barn just outside the village – I dream I am to change my life, wholly. Not in a comforting or continuing way, necessarily. I walk with a new friend and then say goodbye to her forever, hugging her tightly, a soft whale fat on the hard display stand of her ribs. I pass through a series of rooms where charity workers and then arms dealers are meeting, as if I am throwing off both good and evil. I wake under the barn's heavy beams not knowing what it is I am supposed to be becoming.

The Monk's Retreat, Broadhempston churchyard, turn right out of the churchyard and then left on the road signed for Denbury and Woodland (not the Torbryan direction), ignore the turn left to Woodland and Ashburton, at the Waterford crossroads carry straight on, after about a kilometre the road dips down and then climbs steeply and flattens out after a sharp right and then a sharp turn to the left and along the bottom of the flat valley, on the other side of the valley bottom the road takes a sharp turn to the right and then to the left, then go through the gates on your right, and along a narrow metalled drive, this become a grassed footpath, (the hill with the Torbryan caves will become visible on your right), follow until you get to another gate at the village of Torbryan, through the gate and turn right onto Torbryan Hill and immediately right to the Church and The Old Church House Inn, then retrace your steps and turn left up Torbryan Hill, at the angled T-junction turn right and immediately take the footpath on the left across the fields, through the farm, turning right when you get to the road, at the next junction bear left, enter the village of Denbury, when you see the Union Inn on your right, bear left on the narrow road which then bends to the left, this is Shute Lane, at the staggered crossroads take the left turn down Woodland Road, ignore the turn right down Denbury Down Lane and take the footpath immediately on your left up to Denbury Hill. Return by the same footpath, right along Woodland Road, right down Shute Lane, right at village green to Union Inn.

I walk back into Denbury and meet up with the birdman again. Since he lured me out of Newton Abbot it is only right that he completes the loop with me.

We begin with the enigma of a huge wall, in length and height, which has been bugging both of us. The wall, in parts at least, seems to have been made in two segments, a new layer added to an already high barrier. The birdman has a tale about a resident unhappy to have their tennis games overlooked; but it might be about somewhere else. We trespass inside the large arch with PRIVATE on the door, him more confidently than me, and find a second wall within. The birdman explores one arch while I find another to a garden off to the left. In the garden, now packed with huge trees, nothing much grows at ground level, a neatly paved path winds to a blue door in a far wall. There are a great number of walls in this complex; as if its ground plan might have been laid out during times of armed conflict or fears of invasion and secured again, more ornamentally as these divisions were internalised.

Feeling cowardly, I join the birdman's trespass; he has found a manor house, a converted barn and between them a sound-looking ice house, with a modern door which stands open. There are two large cars parked. I expect an anxious or angry owner to emerge at any moment, but no one comes.

Later, adding to the repeated instances of the incursion of the sea, no matter how far inland we go, I equally nervously follow the birdman up a vertiginous drive, rising from the side of a country lane. This time someone does come; a woman emerging from her garden. We have climbed onto her property to admire a sailing boat stranded at the top of the drive; as if poised for a launch down the tarmac slipway. "We're waiting for the Flood", she jokes. I am surprised she is so relaxed with our invasive inquisitiveness and explains that the BOWLING on the stern is a place, near Glasgow, from where the boat was fetched. WID-YIN, the name, is Scots for WOODEN. She says the boat is her husband's, but immediately on purchasing it he had started up a new business and this has eaten away all his time. Coming on it along a country lane, sat high above the road and the drive like its slipway, there is something apocalyptically surreal about it; the people in the hills waiting for the coming waters. Later, arriving into Abbotskerswell, the birthplace of John 'Babbacombe' Lee, one of the cottages has a large wooden koi carp pool, decorated with dolphins, a sea horse and a Cthulhu. In the reeds around the pool, a plastic elephant hides his face, a premonition of slaughter in Exeter's museum.

Backing out of the manor, back through the arch, we wander up the street to see where the blue door might lead. There is a narrow entrance to the churchyard and we take that. Inside, a yellowish-stone boy scout salutes us; he is drowning not waving, a memorial to an Assistant Scout Master from the village who died swimming in the waters of Torbay aged 24. We follow a set of tiny footpath signs, below knee height, zigzagging through the gravestones, to a dead end (sorry) in a reserve area with only a few burials. Over the fence, an angry goose is flapping its wings and a huge shaggy goat with a single curled horn lies malignantly. The birdman wonders if the signs are for the tiny fairy folk and we chat, idly, about survival peoples, branches of evolution that once developed, isolated but in parallel with early humans. I am surprised he has not heard about *Homo floresiensis*, the tiny hominin whose remains have been found on an island in Indonesia. He refers to Richard Freeman, the Exeter cryptozoologist, zoological director of the Devon-based Centre for Fortean Zoology, who goes seeking relic hominids like the Almasty. He has a story from the late 1940s, via a friend, via Jon Downes, the CFZ's founder, via a doctor at a psychiatric establishment close to Dawlish of just such a relic turning up, taken from nearby Dartmoor, and brought to the hospital one night, naked and angry, only to be removed, following telephone calls from "Devonshire Police Force, the Lord Lieutenant of the County, and one from an individual associated with the then earl of Devon... and the Home Office", taken by van to a secure part of the London Underground system. All are sworn to silence.

Are such tales, with their echoes of movies and conspiracy theories, like Widger's fairies and hobgoblins, a clumsy attempt to acknowledge what weird plant-animal-mineral-alien-hybrid monsters we all are, in our ordinariness. I am so suspicious at how the discoveries about Neanderthal culture, their music, their ornamentation, and their flower burials suggestive of abstract thought, have come so quickly after the discovery that two-thirds of the world's humans are the descendants of Neanderthal/human inter-breeding. Is the characterisation of the Dumnonii as essentially primitive and of no real contemporary interest the product of a similar fear and ignorance and transference of contemporary values? The assumption that a different culture must be primitive, brutal and ignorant? The Dumnonii minted no money, they seem to have borrowed some coinage from others, but mostly they had a non-money economy. They built no temples but, from what few accounts we have, worshipped at small unexceptional sites like small groves of trees, or streams or springs. The assumption by archaeologists and historians is that that puts them, on the unspoken sliding scale of civilisation, way below the temple-builders and money-changers of the Roman invader.

But what if their culture was somewhat different from this transference of our lack of imagination – perhaps it is significant that what often stands for imagination (fantasy, horror, gothic) is actually expressive of a lack, of a fundamental failure to empathically imagine a real 'other' – and that they, in contrast, had developed a rich culture of things without requiring their visual representation or their textual authentication? What if – given our own shift from a text-based and empirical culture to a digitalised one in which logic and verification have begun to vaporise from the sheer friction of the movement of visual spectacle – they provide us with a non-money-based, non-image-based, but conceptualising and ecologically immersed and dispersed living? So, just as the literature and arts of the Greek and Roman elites (and even, in its more pagan and esoteric expressions, of the Egyptian elite) are ideal models for a text-based Renaissance and Enlightenment (and their final-thrash conspiracy decline into decadence), perhaps the Dumnonii are the ideal model for a post-text, post-Internet, post-Anthropocene world? An end to the progressives' worship of cities as the motors of the best change, and an end to 'green' fantasises of communes and post-industrial communities (as highly vulnerable to exploitation and hierarchy)? Neo-Dumnonian meshworks might enact a dispersal that was not *away* from the cities or *alternative* to them, but was within and across their borders, a systematic 'loneliness' of social visiting and medium-term journeys, of limited and localised digital communication and deep corporeal motion, of nomadic identities under the artistic control of the nomads themselves rather than of algorithms, travelling in companionship with their many selves rather than defined in their bodies or borders by any single meaning.

Among the graves in Denbury churchyard is that of Lieutenant-Colonel Charles Hudson, who – as well as commanding troops during the Archangel Campaign (the British intervention in Russia against the Bolshevik Revolution), leading the Iraq Levies (a British colonial force comprised of Iraqi minorities), serving as *aide-de-camp* to George V, and wining a Victoria Cross in 1918 when leading a rag tag detail of headquarters staff to recapture a position lost on the front line to the Austro-Hungarian army, demanding (and getting) the surrender of a vastly superior force and carrying on his attack despite a bomb exploding on his foot – was held at least partly responsible by the author Vera Brittain for the death of her brother, Edward. Hudson had been ordered to keep from Edward Brittain the fact that a letter of his had been intercepted, revealing that he had been having sex with men in his Company and he faced a court martial; Hudson disobeyed, told Brittain, and some believe (including Hudson and Vera Brittain) that Edward Brittain's subsequent death in action was a result of his purposely putting himself in harm's way in order to avoid a disgrace to his family.

Inside the simple tubular building of the early mediaeval church, pinned on the West Gallery, is an extensive needlework in seven panels; the middle one a generalised introductory image, but the other six, moving from left to right accounting for the history of the parish from its prehistoric past to Domesday, and then accelerating as it reaches the recent millennium. The contrasts and leaps are revealing; though their authenticity is based on no more direct a set of connections than the birdman-Freeman-Downes-doctor's extended foaftale of a Dartmoor relic-human.

The earliest panel shows the Dumnonian hill fort, with its twin burial mounds still prominent but already surrounded by Saxon farmsteads, with the Saxon centralisation of the village well under way. Torbryan caves are represented by a hyena and a fabric elephant; there is some kind of spring with a building around it and then in the darkness of the caves a naked figure holding up a long black stick seems to be conjuring a star from a bowl; the upper half of the person has brown skin; the lower half of the person is greenish and trails to the side like a tail. There are scenes of pastoral idyll.

In the next panel, dated 1285, the manor in which we trespassed has appeared, along with its fortified arch, with a side door (still there) for when the main gates were shut. The church is equally dominant. There are small strips of farmed land, and almost everyone pictured is working on some small distinguishable plot. In the distance lies Haytor. In the next panel, undated, a transformation has taken place: the Enclosures. No longer are the people associated with particular patches of ground, but they are isolated and specialised. The land itself has disappeared from the village and is divided into two large areas for grazing and for arable; the manor house is overgrown and empty, the church has receded, the burial mounds have been obscured by trees, and in the next panel the shape of the twin mounds is lost.

Bunyan Calling, written by Mary P. Willcocks, a Devon intellectual who was born on a farm just north of Modbury but lived most of her adult life in Exeter, suggests that driving *Pilgrim's Progress* is an anger against these Enclosures and a sense that a 'birthright' had been lost. That the ecclesiastical authorities connived at the sale of that 'birthright' in exchange for a "mess of pottage" (the establishment liturgy of the Book of Common Prayer), allowing Eden to be turned into a City of Destruction. The journey of Christian is a flight from this dispossession towards a new kind of anti-property: of liberation, abstraction and light.

Willcocks sees that when a piece of work strikes widely it does so because of the relationship it makes with particular circumstances, not by vapid mystical well-meaning; for Bunyan knew that devils have direct access to the world. He had seen them in scenes involving himself and others "tossed up in globes of fire"; so vivid that he wondered if he should become a devil and, so, avoid victimisation.

Like Bunyan, Willcocks understands that "most men have felt at some point in their lives, 'o, that a man would arise in me, that the man I am may cease to be!' ... to feel this is to realise what Bunyan meant when he talked of the City of Destruction, and the need to leave it". To transform oneself by a journey. Is that what I was lured into? Some kind of Symbolist trap? I can feel the layers of association piling up so thickly now that I am suffocating.

Like Bunyan I am becoming "instinctively haunted by the urge to escape into freer air... his dreams and visions show the claustrophobia which comes from a hidden memory of the birth struggle from the womb into the light. Only a man with such a memory could have seen that mountain with the wall and the narrow gap of light in it through which he has to creep from darkness into light". Maybe the small door in the manor arch could play the same symbolic role; that after all the great ways are blocked there is still a last chance to sneak in or sneak out.

In the final panels, physical work seems to fade away; spectacle and leisure dominate, which is not how it looks to me peering over the hedges, with farmers chasing sheep into pens, loading bullocks, rolling with their tractors and roaring down the lanes on the giant wheels that threaten to crush the walker without the driver even noticing. These later panels show the hunt, maypole dancing, carol singing; the Second World War airfield becomes a prison between one panel and the next, the twin peaks of the hill appear and disappear once more, ramblers replace the collective harvest.

I feel as if all the figures in these panels are running in my brain. Oh, I am very familiar with the pandemonium of research. Not just from my doctoral studies, but from the years of preparing programmes and press releases on artists and performers of whose complex work I often had little direct knowledge. I am skilled in grasping a crucial detail from a seething mass of ephemera clamouring for attention. I am cautious against those tendril leads that can splay the subject across multiple disciplines and genres until everything means nothing and time runs out and into its own buffers. This is different; the chaos lies not outside me, but inside *and* outside.

There is something very different about researching from a library, or a screen, to researching on the road; everything is so intense and when those huge tractors with wheels twice my height, as thick as oak trees, are lunging at me from around the corners of lanes, the levels of sensitivity and awareness from which I never seem to switch off are so intense that the only reason I sleep so well is that the walking drains me so completely to the bottom of my soles. All affective moisture is siphoned out of me and everything that I hold solid is vaporising to lubricate a next step.

In the church porch is a notice:

If you are here in a working capacity:
1. Do you need to be here alone?
2. Should you have help?
3. Have you told someone – where you are? What you are doing? How long you are likely to be?

We cannot get into the glass-walled vestry in the South Transept; but we can see a huge obelisk-shaped memorial to someone connected with the sea; there are stone maps, a stone sextant, a stone anchor and winged stone skulls. The woman arranging new flowers around the altar cannot tell us whose memorial this is; in fact, although a regular here she has not noticed it before.

The bible is open on the lectern: "The floods have lifted up, O Lord, the floods have lifted up their voice".

She asks if we are walking through and recommends that we visit the church at West Ogwell, which she believes to be a beautiful but troubled place. It upsets her dog if she takes him in there.

High inside the vestry, over a mounted sword, is an ornamental helmet with its visor down and on its top a metal leopard. Or possibly a hyena.

Outside we head off beside the high wall, passing a poster for 'Inventing Utopia', a play about the cultural and agricultural experiment on the Dartington Estate; written by the Devon theatre writer and director Nick Stimson. The birdman expresses his ambiguous feelings about Dartington; a place of artistic and architectural experiment and the development of intensive agriculture.

Beyond the road to the prison is a massive flat field – presumably the old airfield. I imagine Father Italo Calvino landing there. It is so green; the birdman says such colours are a result of fertilisers; Nitrate Green. I feel stupid and naive to be so fooled. I am not comfortable, walking in ignorance. The birdman finds a narrow corridor of hope between the long planes of solar panels and the flailed hedges; scrub is returning through the grass with the prospect of an emerging diversity of wildlife along such channels. "Diversity emerging at the margins", he says, "as ever".

We pass an Equestrian Centre decorated with almost-Ferrari silhouette horses.

PLEASE <u>SLOW DOWN</u>! FREE RANGE CHILDREN AND ANIMALS. (Obscured by ivy.)

We follow a briar-filled 'green lane', fenced on one side by a tall wall of corrugated iron, to a dead end in a kind of cattle pen; with a view to two tumuli. Back at its start, a Red Admiral is sitting on the gate post. I realise that, in all this green, there have been very few insects.

We eat very good pies at Two Mile Oak. At the garage opposite, beside a giant gold Pontiac, an MG is for sale, a telephone number scratched into its red bonnet.

Just outside Abbotskerswell, we spot a Nothing. A view across a field to a gap in the trees. Or what appears to be a gap in the trees. There is something like a wall, but not a wall. Then above that is something like, but not, a dome-shaped spill, perhaps a vertiginous slag heap, or maybe a leafless tree that only appears to be solid and silvery, but with a giant shadowy hole halfway up its side that must be the size of the MG and the Pontiac together. It looks approximately like things, but exactly like nothing. It is the Abbotskerswell Nothing, like the one – a patch of emptiness – that appeared in the 1800s in nearby Trusham.

> *Would you let the ghosts in? Dare an instant memory to take charge?*
> *Would two recollections explore each other equally honestly?*
> *Make fighting look like loving and the thump of sweet nothings on wood?*
> *And then there's still the moment to come just before a world begins,*
> *An orchestra of conductors waiting for musicians to arrive, or magicians*
> *Rearranging clouds; at the gate of the park a woman sits,*
> *Carefully watching her lives, like chameleons escaping from their cage.*

I leave the birdman at the café, finishing his latte and treacle tart, and head off alone again. The café is an anomaly; very few of the villages I am passing through have anything similar; but its friendliness and connection gives a hint of what Lutyens's modern village might have looked and felt like.

I am sad that the upper story of Church House, filled with model railways, is locked. We could have tested some of our theories there.

There is a simple two-road route back to Newton Abbot where the B&B still has a room for me tonight. I do not mean to be delayed. But at the top of the hill is (another!) long wall; at first I am irritated and turn away, considering a footpath across the fields that must connect to Newton Abbot. No, I will play safe. I carry on along the road beside the wall and it opens up to an arch, its ironwork gate padlocked.

REQUIESCANT IN PACE

Beyond are strange shaped crosses. I have the feeling that I have been here before.

I find the entrance to the complex, a 19th-century monastic building with a large church; all around it are modern residential wings that were probably added fairly recently, but preserve a 'cloistered' feel. I march in, hoping that if I look as if I know where I am going, I am less likely to be challenged. I stride around the edge of a croquet lawn and into the trees; in the general direction of the graveyard. It feels a little odd, as if I am acting in a play. Or taking part in a historical re-enactment. It is dark in the trees and I can see a powder blue cardiganed figure walking on a parallel path. I pause a moment and listen to the crunch of her slow tread fade away. I carry on down the path, close to the wall, when the woman in powder blue suddenly cuts across the path in front of me and disappears again into the trees by the wall.

I unfreeze. Close to where the woman disappeared a small building is emerging from the woody gloom. It is a kind of green, like a formica surface under fluorescent lights, very artificial, like an unearthly glow, a strange mixture of fabrication, banality and magic. It shines in the last of the day's light, in the smallest of clearings.

I go to try the door, just in case.

Wow. A single chair faces an elevated statue of the Virgin Mary. It's a chapel and its inner walls are like a veined organism, a mesh of serpentine root-like lines made of cork bark. I sit on the tiny chair and enough light bleeds in to illuminate the startling brightness of the statue. I am overwhelmed by blue and white.

Above the statue is a stained-glass window with nine points of light. The same number in a cloverleaf window behind and above me; three circles, a triangle with its corners at the centre of each of the three, the centre of the whole thing repeating the configuration in a triple-petalled flower that completes each of the three circles.

It is a while before I notice her foot, stood upon the thorned stem of a rose bush, three pink roses around the hem of her robe, a fourth on the hem, and between her feet a spring, a gushing flow of foaming water from the mouth of the chocolate brown rock on which she stands.

The gloom of the trees, the glowing institutional and unreal green, the rich darkness inside the chapel and the brightness of the surface of the statue; a hypnotic rhythm of light and darkness.

Worried about being caught and embarrassed, I exit. This is as far as the birdman's example can push me. Closing the chapel door, I head for the cemetery, where the iron crosses with their forked-tongue ends are arranged in exact rows. Dead nuns and priests: the last marks of a monasticism that has almost disappeared now, leaving a legacy of timetables and terms and summer holidays and TV schedules and disciplines. Caroline Levine uses the word "portability" to describe how "techniques of organizing bodies or objects spread quickly because they are simple, iterable, efficient ways of imposing order on heterogeneous materials". Was this not the experiment being conducted on me?

A woman is coming, in a red coat, shining in the evening light. An elderly lurcher slopes by her side, then runs up and nibbles my fingers with the last of its teeth. I explain my project. She is friendly and helpful, like the woman with the ark and the one in the church; I had expected suspicion and exclusion. These women are more guides than guards. Though their interest is also a means to gather information; friendliness an efficient means to security. One of those portable techniques.

She explains that the Augustinian order, here until the 1960s, were a teaching order that then elected to become a closed one. The priests lived in a separate part of the priory, while the nuns had their own eight-sided chapel (now a snooker room) for when they did not have the exclusive use of the church, which is now the communal space for the residents of what is a 'retirement village'. When male maintenance workers visited the Priory, the nuns would turn their faces to the wall to allow them to pass by. When I ask if the nuns were ever seen by the locals, the woman says "O *yes!*" as if she is about to impart some scandal: "they went to the village... to buy chocolate!" When I mention the chapel and how well looked after it is, she says she re-painted the statue herself, yet I omit to ask her what she makes of those roses and that gushing spring. As I walk back to the Priory buildings, I spend another moment at her 'Chapel in The Woods' marvelling at its brightness.

Back on the lane I am shocked by the darkness. I have no torch and none of my clothes are bright enough for a motorist to see easily. I had not intended to stay so late, but the woman's conversation had been so polite and engaging. A car passes a little too close for my comfort and I decide that the footpath across the fields may be the lesser of two evils. I backtrack swiftly along the lane and take it. Away from the nunnery wall and the hedge, there is more light in the field and a dull huge moon skulks in thin clouds. I make my way down the red scar of path, diagonally across the first field to a stile.

I can almost see the light going, it's that fast. The fields are slipping away from me. I feel real life slurring. I hurry across the second field, slipping on the bottom step of the stile. I throw my arms out wide as if to fly, but stay upright. Earlier in the day I had spoken with the birdman of the disgrace of falling; now I can barely stand. I want the day to be over; I am willing to trade dullness for safety. The third field is full of bullocks and I make my way through their stuttering shapes as they jitter across the gloom. One strikes another with its head; they are powerful if, individually, timid things. I hope they are not the aggressive strain of Nazi auroch cattle that a Devon farmer has just thrown off his land: "they would try to kill anyone" – these have the same looking horns. Nazi cattle!

What is going on?

The last pair of bullocks shamble off, after a brief panic, and I clamber over the stile and into deep darkness. The footpath is now set through woodland and I am grateful for the reasonably sure surface, cushioned by a fall of leaves. I try to distract myself by wondering what a Dumnonian woman would make of that statue of the Virgin Mary in the chapel; would there be some recognition of its spiritual or magical nature, or would it appear to her as a representation of an ordinary woman cutting her foot on rose thorns on the way to the spring, raising her eyes in exasperation? I wonder what she – Dumnonian or Virgin, either – would make of me? What would they see? An ardent researcher and heroine of her profession, an idiot, a bad mother? I refuse to look at my phone, I refuse to turn it on. I plunge deeper into my aloneness in the trees.

If you are here in a working capacity:

1. Do you need to be here alone?
2. Should you have help?
3. Have you told someone – where you are? What you are doing? How long you are likely to be?

The Dumnonian woman might recognise a cross as having some significance; those parallel lines on the incised stone in one of their huts might have conceptualised a path, so they would have understood a crossroads. Like the eight-sided chapel bringing together infinite circles and the earthly square, so the cross might be seen as a meeting of differences. We had been at many crossroads today, birdman and I, and every time we took the route of least resistance, of greatest utility, of least enquiry. I felt ashamed and that my fear, which is all I had now, had repeatedly held us back from the wonders that lay in the caves and grotto and ice house and dig and prison we never trespassed into. I am dull; that is what this route is telling me, dim, without a bright shining light, without a critical torch to hold up to what I see, stumbling through dark trees and fearing to follow treasures through the tall walls and flailed hedges of my nervousness.

I bottle again when I see a playing field through the branches and climb out to that; relieved and infuriated by its dull rectangles and staple-shaped goals. On a rough drive behind some houses, the ghost of James Lyon Widger looms out of the darkness at me, as if from the mouth of his cave. He should be carrying armfuls of my bones, but I have left nothing behind, nothing has survived into legacy. Flailing to live in the moment, I have disappeared from the future, a thin sheet of darkness sliding un-witnessed down the puddled and potholed drive.

No crossroads, but a roundabout. I run over to the central 'reservation' and let the occasional cars make their own decisions.

On the *dérive* the walker allows the ambience and atmospheres of the different possible routes to guide them one way or another, but I feel nothing. I am the O at the centre of the roundabout and the roads are indifferent to me. I take Decoy Road, just for the sake of the name. The very slightest glimmer.

Then I see myself. I confront myself.

In 2006, ten years ago, a series of 'Atmospheric Walks' were made around the line of Brunel's Atmospheric Railway; the routes were made up by the walkers as they went in search of 'atmospheres'. I have the map of these walks, printed and distributed for free to local libraries and schools and clubs and pubs to encourage others to make their own atmospheric explorations. The text of the map reads:

> *"each walk turned up its discoveries – an eel making its way upstream at the bottom of a Newton Abbot garden and nearby a Cecile Oak in the bowl of what had once been a 'Decoy Pond' for luring ducks, a quiet and timeless lane above Starcross, a cut-out Basil Fawlty in a Dawlish hotel window."*

There is no such thing as a Cecile Oak. There is a sessile oak (its acorns do not grow on stalks, but directly on the twig) and that is what I am looking at right now on the side of Keyberry Park (which is not a park, but a street). A little bowl of green that was once where ducks were lured for strangulation. On the lip of the former pond is the oak tree, slightly but pleasingly lop-sided.

I am a spelling mistake. I am destroyed in the moment of finding the Decoy. But I carry on; the travesty far better than the feeling felt earnestly before.

When the walkers arrived here, sketching and photographing, an irate resident rushed up to them. When he found they were not developers come to "take our last bit of green" he invited them all into his garden for tea and cakes.

I am an event on a walk.

In the lamplight I can see a strange thing. A low, planked fence surrounds the former pond. From the pavement, a set of concrete steps descends into the bottom of the pond. However, there is no gate in the fence to allow the pedestrian from the pavement into the basin.

Walls, hedges, fences, corrugated iron sheets, padlocks and 'CLOSED'. Yet people encountered are more often guides than guards. We have allowed ourselves to be architecture and planned and built into a prison of ourselves; when really we have nothing inside but darkness to protect.

I cut down a narrow and shadowy alley. I have nothing to lose now. I believe in others, though. Perhaps I can adopt 'Celia Fremin' as my real identity.

When I get to the B&B I speak to my daughter for a very long time, feeling my map of the cosmos wobbling around, lining up in relation to our special love. I am not going to keep on about it.

South Street, East Street, left down South Street and along the wall into Denbury Road, ignore the left turn to HMP Channings Wood and turn right at the staggered crossroads for Dornafield and Ipplepen. (Many of these roads have no pavement and though only a few are narrow, the walker should beware of traffic, particularly large farm vehicles and be ready to attract the driver's attention.) The road turns at a right angle, to the right, at Rydon Farm, and then to the left, at the next T-junction turn left, at Two Mile Oak pub cross over the main road onto Widdon Road, beside the garage, then at Gulland Cross take the left fork signed for Abbotskerswell, at the next T-junction turn left, this becomes Slade Lane, Laburnum Close, bear right at Orchard Café up Priory Road, The Priory Retirement Village, take footpath near to, and on the opposite side of the road from, the gate to the nuns' and priests' graveyard. Past the red cob barn, around the edge of the next two fields, into Decoy Brake woodland taking the path straight on, off to the left across the football pitch to the drive behind Kingskerswell Road, take drive to the right onto roundabout and turn left up Decoy Road, right into Keyberry Park, take narrow alley on the right and bear left onto Keyberry Road and under railway bridge, left up Torquay Road.

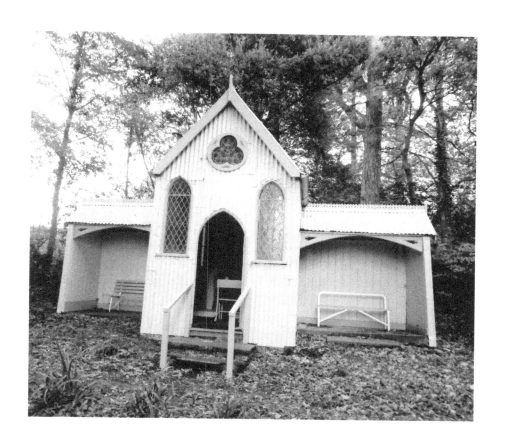

Chapter Nine: Newton Abbot to Teignmouth

In the morning, at breakfast, I discover that just beyond my B&B on the Torquay Road, counter-terrorism police have sealed off the road – a man, described by passers-by as a white male with long hair and a long beard, has been detained after a 'suspect device' was found on a crowded London Underground train. The suspect, tasered and arrested in Holloway (it's all connected!) Street in London has been traced to the address nearby and the area is secured, folk evacuated, and a house is being searched; a "non-viable" device has been recovered. The teenager's defence counsel says it was all a prank on the part of a young man who has a form of autism.

Getting out of bed, I look at my feet; they are shaped similarly to the Virgin Mary's, the second toe longer than the big toe, a syndrome called Morton's Toe. I do not know myself. The stress-bearing work of walking is usually taken through the big toe, but the Virgin Mary and I spread this work to the ball of the foot. I am surprised I have no serious blisters. I have bought some blister plasters at Boots, just in case.

I arrange to meet Jane at the Dream Church.

On the way, I retrace a little of my route last night, stopping to read a plaque I had no space in my head to take in.

> OPPOSITE THIS SPOT WAS
> PENN INN PARK
> 1935-1985
> CREATED BY PUBLIC GENEROSITY
> DESTROYED BY CORPORATE INTRIGUE

Protected by a Perspex panel, the sign has been professionally engraved in what looks like slate. Across the road, in what I assume to have been the park, is a Sainsbury's and a McDonald's.

I use my phone for once and find a photo and a postcard with multiple images of the park and its swimming pool from the 1950s. I walk through the supermarket car park as if through the rockery, past McDonald's as if it were one of the park's cottages and then down an underpass beneath the giant flyover and through the swimming pool, now ringed by a jammed-up traffic roundabout.

Before the roundabout, I find a magic space; left over by the destruction of the pool and park. It has morphed into irony and is trapped behind low brick walls, and accessed by bending under the boughs of coniferous trees. Inside this funny space are the frames, but not the seats, of two benches. The frames are made of pebble-dashed concrete; the benches are oriented to a view of the busy A381, but even that has gone, hidden by the trees. It feels like no one ever comes here. I love it.

Last night I felt it was as if I was disappearing; I am perversely comforted to find that, this morning, the world – at least this world – is no less contingent than I am.

It seems that word of my quest is getting around a few of the local networks. Jane is a dancer who has worked with the Crab Man.

It's a Dreary Dream Church, really. I am shocked at the contrast between its presence and the story of its making, which I tell Jane.

"...that no man may buy or sell, save he that hath the mark".

The dreamer, the Reverend W. Keble Martin was from a line of bankers, priests and officers (at least the men were); his mother was a member of the Champernowne family who owned the then decaying Dartington Hall. Keble Martin had been the vicar at Coffinswell, appointed so by Miss Carew of Haccombe, a shady residual power in the area, guarded in a secretive valley. He becomes famous at the very end of his life when, in 1965, after a lifetime of painting wild flowers in watercolours, he publishes the best-selling *Concise British Flora* at the age of 88, with a foreword by a wildlife conservator infamous for killing crocodiles, wild boar, stags, a tiger. Keble Martin writes in his autobiography that "Nature is good, beautiful and happy", though it was clearly lacking in something, despite its contentment, because "only personality can make or appreciate beauty". Nature without us is lessened and depleted, slack and inanimate, colourless without Keble Martin's paintings. I had got some grasp on his formulation of "personality" from his characterisation of the Boer War as "an unfortunate business... two white races fighting in the presence of the black".

Which brings me to his dream in 1931. At the time, Keble Martin was part of an Anglican pastoral-evangelical mission to the working-class residents of a suburb of Newton Abbot called Milber, which is where we are now. It was built on early neo-liberal lines, without any of the usual disciplinary public spaces – chapels, charities, communal halls – that might soothe upper-class worries about working-class folks' inchoate gatherings.

Later on in the day, Jane and I will call in at the Coombe Cellars, an inn balanced on the edge of the River Teign and famed for smuggling, like every other building along this coast, as if that solves the problem of history. Around a table a group of middle-aged men are gathered: freemasons or undertakers. In its isolation there is a sense of the place as a venue for 'informal' economy. Against one of the tables a signpost has been rested:

PLEASE BEWARE OF UNEVEN GROUND

On the TV I can see from the subtitles that commentators are discussing the possibility of a new civil war on American soil.

What's going on?

The conservative press here, just a few months after the murder of an anti-Brexit Labour MP, have labelled a group of judges "enemies of the people". Nationalist Brexit politicians give dog-whistle 'warnings' of "political anger" (meaning street disturbances) because "if people feel voting doesn't change anything, violence is the next step". I think I'm talking about 'derivative fascisms' here; all-out free markets hitched to misogynist white nationalism. And while all this is falling out, the best that the liberal 'chattering classes' can do is to openly discuss ways to ignore the choices of the 'great unwashed'.

What's going on?

The immediate cause is relatively simple to deduce: the central poisonous problem is the systemic disenfranchisement and disengagement of those stinky ordinary people. That's not new. I don't think my Dad ever thought anyone took any notice of him, nor of his Dad; that's without starting on the Ma's. But the immediate motor provoking reaction and threat is not, sweetly, sited in either the US or the UK. It's the defeat of the Arab Spring and the integration of that democratic movement into the dominant militarisation of the Middle East. When that happened, any hope for a radical leadership (in the sense not of individual Bernie Sanders-type leaders, but the leadership of the people) fell out of the world and left a massive hole in global hope, and in came anger and resentment to fill and sculpt the void.

In the past, there existed in the US and, to a greater extent perhaps, in the UK (I don't really know, I'm guessing, I am no expert on America) some big collective structures that restrained reactionary violence in oblique ways. During the industrial era both societies developed huge institutional and even democratic entities – many of them hard fought for – which large aggregates of individuals (and, yes, this is alongside segregation and 'colour bars' and many other more subtle exclusivities) immersed themselves in.

Since I have been walking I have seen *nothing* of this in the towns. In the villages the notice boards are full, even when they are appealing for more participation, but in the towns if there are community notice boards they are empty or thinly blotted with pronouncements from authorities. I see a few of the old halls of historic collectivism, but not a single new building that celebrates the principle of solidarity. There is some evidence that charities are still fairly lively – but this is mostly their commercial arm, their shops, stitched into a shadowy, low-paid, retail world – and there is the odd plaque about the Rotary Club and so on, but the ideology-producing structures like freemasons' lodges and mass conservative parties are gone or withering; the few mass, middle-class, membership organisations (the National Trust – plenty of evidence of them) are consumer-based more than participatory (with some problematical volunteering). The massive vacuum of meaning and mattering left by the divorce of work from things (alienation is one of the few things now distributed on a more egalitarian basis than before) is complemented by the winding down of the churches. Where there is evident growth in church activity, it seems more likely to fuel violence – the Halloween-baiters and clown-fearers of Torquay – than sublimate it. The vibrancy of minority faiths seems to fuel the disgruntled idea of 'lack'; the majority's fear that the lesser 'other' is having more fun than they are.

Resentful lower middle class folk (painfully aware that their kids have now missed out on the easy money of post-Big Bang deregulation) rattle around with no organisations to be disciplined by and to discipline by, dependent on leisure and commodity-satisfaction to frame their mattering and meaning. At the same time, with the hammering of the collective working class, the once big unions that once gave opportunities to be involved, disciplined and even democratic and powerful are almost invisible. I see no marks of radicalism or collectivisation and little of mutual support in the working-class areas of Paignton, Newton Abbot or Torquay.

Broadhempston Community Shop, yes. But in the towns? I see some despair and I see skilled workers suddenly finding themselves managed from Park Avenue, New York. I see individualised fragments running after zero-hours jobs in a race to the bottom. And I don't even feel that I am different from them any more. And I'm much better off. Before my partner and I split up, and my decision to follow my love of 19th- century dramatic literature, I had a properly remunerated post as a bureaucrat in the creative industries. I behaved myself, I promoted radical work, but that was in my job description. I gave structure to radicals and in return the structures I worked for gave structure to me. Now, I'm looking at the academic institutions I want to work in; they treat teachers and researchers as entrepreneurs and students as customers; matter and meaning seem mostly irrelevant, when matter and meaning is all that they should be.

Any real power to create significance is dissipating in the hands of technologically savvy man-childs and shock jock commentators; distributed on the servers and across the platforms of companies whose priorities are warily exploited and sustained by a thin and non-authoritative layer of politicians and managers who struggle to explain their legitimacy. The 'reality-media rich' can only give very partial cover for the disappearance of the old regional patriarchal-philanthropic rich whose names I see everywhere engraved into dressed stone plaques on almshouses, memorials, hospitals, road signs, church heraldries, schools and parks; where some of these institutions are still going, they are mostly privatised.

Against all this vaporisation a tremendous appetite for direct democracy is discovering itself. Isn't that a good thing? Yes, it may be a kind of 'X Factor' or 'Strictly Come Dancing' democracy, of quick votes, and a refusal to be talked down to, talked down from the ledge or silenced by betters and experts, whether they be High Court judges or Craig Revel Horwood, a refusal to be calmed by the machinery of representative democracy, a refusal to be dissuaded even by the facts. And whirling it all around are the strange conduits of a globalised social media, so that ideas gather and disperse, surge and swell in ways that do not conform to the former strictures of educational, political or even broadcasting 'decency'.

This is all a volatile force; which means we do not know where we are going. On the one hand, we are walking into the conditions for a new generation of rough democracy and self-determination; on the other hand, this is (and we are) going to be exploited ruthlessly by demagogues and authoritarians armed with armies of algorithms. If all else were equal, this would be a precarious time; but nothing is equal and these volatilities arise primarily in two societies that have never confronted their histories of slavery and empire. If there is a way through to something that is at least safe rather than savage, then it will involve a wholesale transformation and democratisation and disciplining and de-neoliberalising of institutions and the unrigging of democracy. And it will begin with confronting its own racism in each of these respects.

But, mostly, I feel like I am walking through the last days before the latest of the many tiny apocalypses that stretch back a long, long way. And though my Ma and Dad thought that they were leaving behind everyday catastrophes and humiliations, I loved the funny resentments and sharply ground axes of aunts and uncles who were still going to Skeggy and eating steak and ale pie in Torremolinos. I never thought they were bad or lesser people because they didn't know a Muscadet from a muskrat. I could always get angry on their behalf, and now I am getting angry on my own. Out here on the river beds and hollow lanes. They intensify things.

PLEASE BE AWARE OF UNEVEN GROUND

...Keble Martin describes how "the Padre tried to check the bad behaviour of some young people from the town and there arose an element of personal opposition in some quarters". Keble Martin maybe gives away the source of the tensions when, first complaining about his unjust beating as a child he opines how "in these times when boys really do sin with their bodies, they should surely suffer in their bodies. A good caning every morning would do good." Out of this mix of discord, sinning bodies, a fantasy of colonial brutality inflicted on the local inferior class, a troubled Keble Martin dreams of how he is "preaching in a new church building from the chancel step. The church was filled with people, and was of a curious pattern... there were three diverging naves in front of me, one unfinished. A man came up the centre aisle to assault me. The warden and sidesmen came promptly and apprehended him, they conducted him down the North nave which was full of people, and cast him into outer darkness. When the congregation had left I walked out by the central nave, and could see through the arches into the lateral nave."

Keble Martin's dream was drawn up as an architectural plan by his brother, Arthur, and a church with three naves was eventually completed and consecrated in 1963. The font is positioned in the North nave, presumably so the door can be opened and the original sin of a young oik's nature cast out into the darkness of the Milber estate. Fixed in architecture: a nature in need of caning.

Today Keble Martin's dreamed church is part of the See of Ebbsfleet, an enclave within the Church of England that refuses to recognise the sacramental ministry of bishops who have ordained women; in their Christmas Message for 2015, after citing the Paris terror attacks and the drownings of refugees, they present, as the most distressing prospect for grief in the coming year "the disfiguring of God's image in the world". Despite their anachronistic theology, they are bang on message with the Spectacular economy.

The Dream Church is not the only architectural venture of Arthur and William Keble Martin; in 1909, with other pals, they built a small informal and roofless chapel from the stones to hand on Dartmoor. Some of the walls remain, plus a rock with a cross engraved in it. When the Ordnance Survey introduced a grid system for its 1-inch maps in 1931 the grid reference for the chapel turned out to be 666 666.

We walk round the exterior of the dowdy Dream Church and I help Jane to look through the windows. It is a hiccup in the dozy complacency there is around churches; the stumpy Norman fortified towers, mediaeval simplicities, 18th-century elegances, sleepy melodramas of the neo-Gothic; the Dream Church exposes what horrors of twisted thought and the subjection of distant bodies to suffering they abstractedly incarnate.

What is a river?

What is a bed?

Where is the bed in the body? Where is the river there?

As a dancer, Jane brings an attention to bodies I have not felt before. Perhaps ever. In our feeling for our bones, in the moment, when, walking away from the Mare and Foal Rehabilitation Centre we talk about the insecurity of the head on the neck, where our flexibility, our bending to the strain but also our reaching out from the strength across the chest, comes from and exits out of us.

Jane talks of the chest of the horse, not its most beautiful part, but the strength of it, the nexus, the junction of its motion and the power of its front legs. I mention to Jane that thing about how, until photography, there was a cultural mistake about the order in which a horse's legs move when at a gallop, how all the 18th-century paintings are wrong – both front legs thrown forward, both back legs thrown back – but Jane wonders whether when at full speed that could ever be true, for a moment. She 'flies in the face' of science...

At each moment we are more than we are. There is always a little of 'Sir Constant' in our walk.

I think this comes from walking with a river, too. The river takes on a personality that you hardly notice, although you fear its rising. Like you fear the rising temper of a lover. There is always a third person on the walk. At the end of the day Jane talks of being on Budleigh Salterton beach the day before, and I remember reading how Princess Diana had taken to walking there with one of her *beaus*, discreet security service agents blending into the pebbles.

We are on the edge of the Teign River for much of our time together. She is the third person. The to-the-side. Ablative river. Sometimes we get a little too close and go in up to our boot tops.

After leaving the Dream Church we are trapped for a while in the maze of Milber, following alleys that bend us back to starting points or end in garages. There are few landmarks. Sedate, even quaint, it is hard to think of this as the space of 1950s' juvenile delinquency.

How much do these houses cost now as a percentage of life income compared to when they were built? Where will the next generations live?

Eventually, we escape along a footpath into a long wedge of giant trees that divides one piece of suburbia from another. Jane stands in the split trunk of a tree, the green mouldy and symmetrical roots become the twin tails of her mermaid. A wooden seat is greasy, scored with swirls, loops, sharp gouges and parallel tracks, like Dumnonian scrapings on a stone from one of their hut sites, doodling across time. Is this what Helen B is doing; drawing lines that join up eras?

The trees push us out by the defensive stone circle protecting the Post Office's cash monies – I don't tell Jane in case we stop and attract the attention of the security guards, not sure how I explain a second visit – and into another wodge of suburbia. Across from a house with twin golden lion gateposts a parodic neighbour has erected a pair of plaster terriers. On the edge of this half of the sprawling dormitory is a new build of Barratt Homes, discrepant half walls of limestone too orderly to soften anything, and beside all that, an enticing maw of hedges and that rural otherness that is always a quick remedy around these little towns. We dive directly in.

Why do people find the suburbs boring? I have read a few warnings against walking in them. They might have sprawled first by the sheer impetus of urban growth, but after a while that sprawl was planned. Strategists looked at the space of death in Hiroshima, Nagasaki and in the Japanese and European city centres ruined by massive conventional bombing, and they saw that bombs dropped on the middle of a contained and crowded city killed everyone. In suburbia, even after nuclear war, a few people at the edges might just manage to bring up soldiers to strike back a generation later. So the rings of suburbia are formed by the waves of atomic blast and the organisation of the next war after that; just as the orientation of mediaeval villages were shaped by the Devil in the North and the crucifixion and resurrection at the crossroads. The homes we pass are armies waiting in dust form; particles at rest now, individual souls never quite sure why they feel existentially uneasy, faithless and incomplete, yet ready to receive their post-apocalyptic reason-to-be.

At the bottom of the hill there is a private road and Jane insists that we take it, because that's what "you would do". I am a little nervous; it is all very fenced and orderly and signed. I prefer the anonymity of the lanes. It is a service road to some kind of business or charity, I cannot even tell from all the signage whether visitors are encouraged or deterred. There are CCTV cameras, for sure, but nobody around.

We wander by the car park, plenty of cars, examine a huge stone milling base that is broken in three pieces and has been left as a sculptural trace, but no one comes to ask us what we are doing. Jane wants to feed the horses with grass. I am nervous that we might upset the unseen power. Or the ponies' stomachs. We pass an "Equine Admissions" entrance, and hang about outside "Reception", but still no one comes to invite us in or tell us off.

Behind the reception building a view extends to a long, curvy valley of mares and foals. The shaping of the ground here is so voluptuous, unfolding in grand bends of green. The equine tenants shift gently in the late morning sun. The day shines, the valley just settles back. I feel my rib cage unclip itself from anxieties and all my flesh is held together by hedges and tape. This space of wonder is all just three minutes' walk from the last Barratt Home, but space is not equal. It is only at Jane's insistence that we have mildly 'trespassed' without a good excuse – she invokes the fiction of all this – and there is a kind of art walking here: making your decisions on the basis of an imagined walker, or a walker who is not there. What would the Peace Pilgrim do? What would Garnette Cadogan do? What would Heidi – in her *Lehr- und Wanderjahre* – do? The valley is privileged by its re-purposing as a place of rehabilitation, as disciplined but de-militarised as a hospital, a place to be avoided by those 'without business' here, but not to be feared. The officious detail of signage and corporate landscaping keep away those without a fictional provocateur, cupping the near silence of the valley in its thick green being. To have climbed a gate and entered this space would have been to destroy it; for once it feels enough just to look.

We get to the river and start down its exposed and uneven bed. Jane wants to light a fire.

The river bed is part of the 'Templer Way', after the super-rich Templer family whose business exported granite from a quarry on Haytor to London out through the estuary and along the Channel. Their original fortune, however, came from India; James Templer made millions constructing docks at Madras and other government buildings. He returned to England in 1745, a 23-year-old magnate. It was the same siphoning that floated Robert Palk, who became Governor of Madras a generation later, returning to erect his white triangular folly to imperial surplus on the Haldon Hills within the 60,000 acres he had purchased with his spoils. The tower was later occupied by two brothers, suspected of Nazi-sympathies as they persisted in keeping lights burning during the blackout, a beacon to Exeter for the Luftwaffe.

A yellow metal sign lies in the marsh grass.

Jane and I talk about flight. About when people did that thing of standing round a table, pushing down on someone and releasing them; did they really rise up into the air? Jane thinks they might have. Can you defy physics if only a little bit? I like the craftiness of that negotiation, but, really, if you are going to levitate you should be able to soar like Peter Pan, Silver Surfer or the Human Torch.

We stand on a wooden landing stage with a few of its planks missing. I am scared to death. Actually shaking, but I don't want Jane to notice. She runs to the end of the structure and balances. This is something 'Sir Constant' is luring us into. The landing stage stretches maybe twenty metres across the mud and over what remains of the river left by the retreating tide. The planks are slippery and inconsistent. The structure is narrow.

"Look at this", Jane says, bracing herself on the final plank. "It's sloped, so if I step on it, it changes the whole feeling in my body". She steps back. "On here I'm solid and fixed, but", and she steps again onto the sloping plank over the drop to the deep mud, "this sends a feeling right through me. You try it."

I wonder if she is one of those fairies, one of those Torbryan hobgoblins. Jane is lovely, but there is an impish mischief to her. As I inch towards the edge I can hear myself saying the words in my head "and then, against my better judgement..."

Under the stage the mud is liquid soft; signs on the bank warn of its deadliness. If I fall off now, it will close over me, there will be no thesis-based publication about the Symbolist Quest, no school nativity plays, no signpost that I was ever here. I read girls' adventure novels when I was young, boarding school trash, I remember the fear of the swamp. I feel the quicksand, the irresistible suction, force without muscles or tentacles, soft things drinking me alive, and brown slime pouring into my mouth, into my ears, into every opening. Ugh.

The upside is the dreams.

I put one foot on the final, slippery, angled plank. I keep the other on the last of the flat ones. I feel the fear pushing blood to places that only usually tingle this intensely in infatuation and at the imminent prospect of its reciprocation. I am amazed at how this old and rusty, rotting iron and wood structure, in this place of cold sunshine and dampness, is taking my body, is playing with its feelings. This is just the place doing this; an unreliable erotic partner subject to tides. The moon has something to do with it too; its orbit comes closer to the earth today. We can see her big in the blue sky.

I tread warily but quickly back to the bank. Jane is still on there, hovering on the gap-toothed jetty above the enigma of the mud. I long for her to come down.

We walk in pyjamas, telling each other our dreams. Jane has this repeated and amazing one where she bounces off surfaces, and I have one where I levitate like I'm rising into heaven. Jane uses the springiness of surfaces to propel her body through space between planes, while I float gently upwards with my arms raised very slightly by my sides. I have to control my focus so that my feelings keep me floating; just as when I ride in boats I allow some part of my concentration to keep the boat afloat.

Half a mile after Coombe Cellars, at the Arch brook, a sign declares our route "out of bounds" for the National Flounder Championships. Although at times walking the loose stones of the riverbed is like competing in the National Stagger and Stumble Championships, we decide that this sign does not apply to us and flounder on. The river bed, sandy and uncertain, has become more like a thin pile of small boulders, capped now and then by big gloomy Pontiac-sized sandstone chunks, turning into silhouettes in the dampening afternoon shadows. There are houses above us on the small cliff, evident by their ruined staircases; one of iron, torn in half by rust, under the sightless gaze of an empty CCTV casing; a wooden one choked by ivy and its own rot.

We climb up a set of narrow grey steps and pass between holiday camps. Swathes of empty mobile homes are full of stripped mattresses; boiler-suited maintenance staff are working their way through stuff. On those mattresses, bodies have lain and dreamed and taken flight with all the intensity of my excited fear on that gap-toothed landing stage, slippery with a layer of green living stuff.

Coming down the lane I talk with Jane of my growing suspicion about the exotic gardens I keep passing by.

In a field, I see what looks like a giant firework rocket, five metres tall.

We arrive among signs of what might have been a religious community. House names – THE HERMITAGE, THE PRIORY – abut what seems at first to be an old, perhaps mediaeval church. Yet something does not feel quite right. Other than the names there is nothing obviously religious about the houses. The simple red sandstone box church building is too precisely shaped to be mediaeval, none of the sympathetic working to the eccentricities of the materials characteristic of old buildings. Inside, the font is very old, maybe Norman, but ruggedly out of place. Jane and I take turns to read a poem-prayer in Wiltshire dialect, from a book balanced on a dado rail by the lectern, about a god who "left no footmark on the floor". The author, unable to afford a cross for her garden, uses an apple tree with "stoopin' limb, all spread wi' moss" as her mnemonic.

The graveyard, much older than the church, is like a drunken crowd reeling out of an early morning night club. Jane picks her way among the stones as if dancing with partners.

On one of the crosses, straighter than the rest, is a wonky logo:

ARTURFUQIL

LIQUFRUTRA backwards. Of course it is.

On the death of the occupant, William Newcombe Homeyard, the Vicar of St Nicholas refused his widow's request to put LIQUFRUTRA – the brand name of the cough 'remedy' from which Homeyard had made his fortune – on his stone. I imagine the reversal was a compromise; hard to believe the clergyman wouldn't spot such a simple ruse. I am rather admiring of the vicar's anti-commercialism; but Salmon has a quite different interpretation. He says that Homeyard's LIQUFRUTRA started off under a different name: 'Mother Job's Liquid Fruit Cough Cure', advertised as the herbal recipe of "an old crone of the 17th century, burned as a witch". The change to LIQUFRUTRA came after a coroner's indictment of the liquid as fraudulent, and its claim to cure tuberculosis ("consumption") a dangerous and premeditated deception of a vulnerable public on Homeyard's part.

When 'Mother Job's'/LIQUFRUTRA was lab tested, it proved to be water, sugar, mint, garlic and something never satisfactorily identified but most likely the greasy part of an onion! Apparently, you can still buy the stuff, but now they've added guaifenesin. It is made on an industrial estate south of the Exeter to Plymouth railway line, not far from the farm where Mary P. Willcocks was born.

Against the back wall of the church are stacked three varnished crosses (four metres high) and three wooden stakes (a metre and a half each); discarded props from a passion or procession.

Leaving the churchyard, just by its lych gate, the car parking space I had thought irritatingly ornamental, made with broken ceramics and pebbles, is something more complex and interesting. Jane and I walk around the space, trying to give a name to the different symbols. On the wall is what turns out to be a 'master's square', a square within a square within a square within a square; each square arranged diagonally within each other, producing sixteen triangles; not unlike The Chalkers' description of the Plymstock 'Da Pinchi Code'. (I only got most of this after trawling the web.) Within the innermost four triangles are symbols I recognise as those for the gospel writers: ox, lion, eagle and angel. In the other twelve are bloom-like lead frames each holding something; perhaps twelve minerals with symbolic meanings? I don't know. In the centre of the centre square, on a ceramic tile, is an eight-pronged wheel, with another eight prongs in pairs around the four corners of the square, while wending across it are four kinked symmetrical forms each defined by two parallel lines.

On the bricked floor of the parking space are symbols set around a Kabbalah 'tree of life' (recognise that immediately): these seem to be mostly astrological (Aries, Taurus, a highly abstracted Sagittarius bow and arrow that flummoxes me at the time, and so on) but others include yin/yang, an ankh symbol of life, a six-spoked wheel of fire, and a pentagram which puts me in mind of Bunyan and Sir Constant and the symbol on the shield of Sir Gawain with his five perfect senses and fingers, the five wounds and Mary's five joys; here, however, the single point of the pentagram faces the master's square which suggests the primacy of spirituality, whereas, if the two points are upwards, they represent the horns of the lusty material goat thrusting aggressively at heaven and the dominance of the earthly.

This all put the mad goose and the dirty one-horned goat in the Denbury churchyard in a new light; the goose abruptly raising the points of its wings against heaven, while the goat gently turned its head, eyeing us up, while screwing itself to the spiritual. There is a mediaeval Marian M, the "M" made of two "V"'s, Virgin of Virgins, and an image for Virgo with a head and tail suggestive of a serpent... I feel tempted by the kind of sloppy conflation of symbols – Melusine equals Dumna equals Mary – I really hate. But I can't pretend I'm not tempted.

When I put the images up on Facebook later, a 'friend' comments that the combination of symbols is characteristic of the Hermetic Order of the Golden Dawn. Hmm... Someone else posts that these are symbols of a spirituality of light generated from an "eccentric pivotal point", not the sun, not the centre. Could we be talking about diffraction here? My correspondent guides me to a Plymouth University astronomer called Percy Seymour. When I look him up he seems to have been a fairly conventional academic, studying magnetic fields around planetary objects, until he suddenly "flipped" and began to interpret *everything*, including human personality, as subject to the magnetic and gravitational fields of the sun and the planets. This is great fun, but I am sceptical about Seymour's arbitrary scaling; how could he be so sure that we're not miserable gits because of the electrical charge of our washing machines? Or the gravitational field of our condiment set? Why Saturn particularly?

In Shaldon, Jane and I pass a house with a black ball hanging above an archway haloed by twenty-two black beams of light. We knock at the door, but the friendly young woman there has no idea what it signifies, and though she tries to think of someone who can help us she cannot. Later I ask the local museum and they reckon it was recycled from a demolished Christian Bible Chapel that stood nearby; a miniscule Devonian offshoot from Methodism which early on recognised the ministry of women – who they called Female Special Agents! – before the sect disappeared altogether in 1907.

The walk across the bridge over the Teign, almost half a mile long, opens up the vistas to the river valley and hills. Behind us, above Shaldon, a bunker is found under the grass between Long Lane and Sharper Lane: a cannabis factory growing weed on an industrial scale, a stairwell hidden in a stable block. Hollow hills!

To the left is the path we just trod.

In front of us is the figure of Teignmouth and on its back, like a fin or a tick, is a tower; looking like the stereotypical Scottish castle by the loch.

To our right are the docks, where coals from 'Communist' Poland were brought in to break the 1984/5 miners' strike. 'Communism', a conspiracy of various nationalisms, a vodkacola requiring no meetings or committees, a conniving of enemies to fool their armies about the nature of their enmity. George Orwell was right about both sides of the wall.

Just beyond the docks is where an inadequately prepared 'Teignmouth Electron' launched in 1968 on its way to becoming wreckage on a beach on Cayman Brac; a fanciful entry into the 'Golden Globe around-the-world race' by its impecunious pilot Donald Crowhurst.

Crowhurst was almost brilliant, but acted like the real thing; like Joanna Southcott, or James Bathurst. When he stood for the Liberals as a local council candidate in the early 1960s his manifesto was designed like a computer printout; he briefly dabbled in the paranormal. His plan for winning the 'Golden Globe' race involved the building of a cybernetic boat but, although he installed some gadgets, he ran out of time before he could install the computer that was necessary to run them.

Crowhurst must have known, as he launched, that he would either give up or die. Instead he discovered he could mislead. While making his own journey around Einstein's 'Relativity: The Special and the General Theory' – intuiting relativity in his body – he radioed an account of a third journey in which he was ahead in the race, though the 'Electron' was actually going round in circles in the Atlantic Ocean. When accidents to other competitors scuppered his plans to drop back slowly to an honourable third place, he found himself facing the prospect of sailing into Teignmouth victorious and subjecting his log books to the kind of scrutiny that would quickly expose him as a cheat and a liar; and this just as he was corporeally experiencing the Great Truths of the physical cosmos. Either the shame or the tragedy of his position overcame him, or perhaps the option of realising a fourth journey; he seems to have picked up his boat's chronometer and stepped off the boat and into the sea.

Like him, we do all feel gravity; not as a force pulling us towards a greater mass but rather we feel the idea of it, the geometry, the curvature of time-shapes in the universe. When we make ourselves free, we are in free fall.

The Crowhurst-overleaping of a self has happened a few times along this coast: Pete Goss's 'Team Philips' catamaran built at Totnes broke up in mid-Atlantic in a freak storm in 2000, Simon Chalk tried again in Teignmouth, building the 'Spirit of Teignmouth' in a workshop on The Den, just behind the promenade. Chalk never got to launch his boat: "political infighting, negative press and small-mindedness" did for him; there were people trying to "stick a knife in his back". The project, reportedly, left him a million pounds in debt, his 'Route 66' night club closed and he went bankrupt. His trimaran left Teignmouth on the back of a lorry. The global, blue marble 'planetarity' drinks these folk alive.

SUPAWASH
WE DO DO DUVETS

You would have thought that having gorged ourselves on symbolism in Ringmore we might have kept to a straight and narrow path, but somehow Jane and I get trapped on a few centimetres of cobbled kerb on the main route through the town, hanging on to offputtingly aggressive railings until we can race across to a traffic island with its own complex cobbled patterns of circle, stars and triangles; rarely visited, it is succumbing to colonising moss.

I say goodbye to Jane who heads for the station with promises to contact the Crab Man for me, while I long to see the sea again. I head towards the beach.

No one knows if Donald Crowhurst stepped off the boat because by personifying relativity he had reached a point of sensual inadequacy, slithering like a slug down the blade of a curved universe no longer able to detect the wrinkles in matter, to get a hold on things; he did not love the darkness he found inside himself, but recognised it as a useless god rather than a resource from which to make himself anew.

The bad faith in Teignmouth, the suspicion and exploitation around Crowhurst's quest had already poisoned his joy; and this canker grew not just around the local investment in Crowhurst's doom. There would be a succession of ill-advised relaunches of the town: a topless restaurant, an attempt to host Nude Miss World, the expulsion of people with learning difficulties from a specialist hotel, the deal with the Polish dictatorship to unload 'scab' coal. The town bowed to the thin myth of individualism, with its strictly reactionary rules about what rebellion is.

Since his drowning, as it will be with the middle-aged men washing up on its beaches now, the county attempted to forget Donald Crowhurst. As far as I know there is no memorial to him here. Chalk or his organisers omitted him from their exhibition of local seafaring, mounted on The Den during their ill-fated construction of 'Spirit'.

But this place is changing.

In some of the other towns, change feels like decay, or the drying out of former things, but there is something in Teignmouth that is seizing on its decline and turning it on its head. I find a trail of sculptures made of driftwood and other trash washed up on the beach, there is a new theatre built on the ground plan of an old one and the silent Riviera Cinema, cold and dead in the heart of its large building behind a restaurant and under a penthouse flat, has been briefly opened for the shooting of a film about Crowhurst with Rachel Weisz and Colin Firth.

A huge rusted anchor covered in poppies has become an accidental ankh. A blue door eyes it: AUDI VIDE TACE, a shortened version of the Latin motto "see, hear, and be silent if you know what's good for you". A large burst of Traveller's Joy by the main through road. The winged roundel in the stained glass of the Biggles Bar is like a flying eye. The omens are good.

COUCH
DRAPER

The branch of W.H. Smith's is still open, I buy a new notebook. In its doorstep are pin marks for missing metal signs:

BOOKSELLERS
LIBRARIANS

There's an independent bookshop, a book about Donald Crowhurst in the window, but I've missed its opening hours.

I cannot resist turning down THE STREET WITH NO NAME. It comes out on a triangle of raised grass on which sit three stone shapes. Despite its evident use as a dogs' playground, with a drinking bowl and a plastic racket strewn in pieces, the grass worn by paws, there is a certain power to this place. The *cylinder* is what remains of the market cross (marking a right granted by charter in 1002), and the *sphere* of *granit rose,* sat on an octagonal base divided into eight triangles which are in turn divided in two, is a gift from the twin town of Perros-Guirec. The *wedge* is a plaque describing the other two shapes in the charged space of French Street (destroyed by a French invasion force in 1690, rebuilt by public subscription); the three shapes shimmer. Even the positioning of the scraps of torn red racket seem to signify something.

In Dawlish Street I find a shop that is no longer trading, but not yet tidied up. Through cobwebbed windows, a semblance of order, stacked shelves and files, overflowing boxes and spaghetti confusions of tumbling wires. It is hard to tell if the clutter is what tripped up the business, or if this was its modus and something else ended its operandi. Even among piles of alarms, wires and paperwork, there is the sea. Or something like something like something like the sea; a print of a scene from an aquarium. The ocean is repeatedly internalised and symbolised; not simply as a history of people's work or their physical relationships with it, but that they are drunk alive by it; it is inside them as they are inside it. And that is monstrous in its way.

I find the doorway of the church where Crowhurst was asked, and refused, to pray for the cameras. Inside, the building is cavernous, designed by the same architect as the Riviera Cinema and St James the Less where an eight-sided 'lantern' (like a crown of light on the top of the roof) is mounted on eight thin, cast-iron pillars over an octagonal nave. In both buildings emptiness prevails. Though both are heavily ornamented, there is a sense that things can float.

A tablet for two sailors who drowned:

WITHIN SIGHT OF THIS CHURCH.
READERS, BE AT ALL TIMES READY, FOR YOU KNOW NOT
WHAT A DAY MAY BRING FORTH.

Whitney Houston's 'I Will Always Love You' booms around the church; a sound test for a funeral:

If I should stay
I would only be in your way
So I'll go but I know
I'll think of you every step of the way.

The Bible is open at the Book of Brexit, the chapter concerning the false freedoms of sovereignty: "foreigners shall no longer use them as they please; they shall serve the LORD their God and David their king". Put even more eloquently in the Marriott Edgar monologue that would once have been heard in revue on the end of the pier:

And it's through that there Magna Charter,
As were signed by the Barons of old,
That in England we can do what we like,
So long as we do what we're told.

A '2' has fallen from the frontage of the pier, it is now dated "1865 – 016"; which is what happens when you let nostalgia go too far. On the pier I find an ancient machine for telling fortunes and a primitive bagatelle thing that dispenses love hearts from a representation of the Palace of Westminster. Outside there are games, like Paignton's, wrapped up like artillery. I look at the murky grey sea and wonder if it is as dead as it seems.

My indulgent reverie is disturbed to a reality that is more fantastic. Far up the beach, a dancing line of Charlie Chaplins is weaving through the last remaining 'sunbathers' braving an early evening wind that blows a hymn in Gujurati. These are the processing Chaplins from Adipur! I thought they were in the spoof programme, but they are obviously real! Prodding the sand with bamboo canes, lifting black bowler hats, led stiffly by Ashok S. Aswami – I presume it is he, laughing louder than the rest, a survivor of threats from nationalists and fundamentalists 'offended' by his worship of a clown; too close, perhaps, to representing their own problems. I run down to the promenade, but the procession of funny walkers has gone. I run up and down the sands, my trainers filling up with grit and shells. I follow the prod marks of their canes, running in circles, like a credulous Dawlish hunter out to corner the Devil. The 'sunbathers' are too busy rolling up their towels and packing away their folding chairs to bother with something so haunting.

I take solace in the town. In the fabulous juxtapositions of ceramic tiles that some of the B&Bs have glued up around their entrances: Loch Ness monsters (a whole school) and Urquhart Castle (looking just like the tick part embedded in the silhouette of Teignmouth) beside Ermita Virgen de la Peña, kangaroos with the *Tour Eiffel*, elephants and sheep dogs, Las Vegas and a writhing ectoplasm of fixative, a suckled devil, where a tile has fallen off. But much, much more in the depredations of weather and creative vandalism that have reworked the paintings hung on hoardings around a derelict space on Brunswick Street: a moody silhouette that scratched eyes and tusks are turning unearthly, colours escaping frames on the backs of raindrops, wood grain re-emerging through a painted wave, a psychopathic camel striking down a slippery rhino on the pier, something lizard-headed made of bleached paint and chipboard, a variety of floating geometrical solids, a torn minimalism in a breeze-block niche, and a sharp-faced martinet head on a slug's body with "HAZARDOUS AREA DO NOT ENTER" across its maw. It does not surprise me, but it does delight me, when I look through a gap in the chained wooden gates to see that behind all these rampant images, and powering them up, are two discarded, life-sized white plaster horses. One still rears, while the other is fallen on its side and draws its legs up to its body defensively. They wriggle and jerk among a pile of ladders, chairs, plastic sheeting and pallets; as if two stallions in the painting and decorating business have been attacked by creditors and left for dead. I am beginning to love this town!

I check into a B&B in the street where Keats contracted tuberculosis from his younger brother Tom: "I would have taken a walk the first day, but the rain would not let me, and the second, but the rain would not let me; and the third, but the rain forbade it. Ditto fourth, ditto fifth, ditto – so I made up my mind to stop indoors, and catch a sight flying between the showers: and behold I saw a pretty valley, pretty cliffs, pretty brooks, pretty meadows, pretty trees, both standing as they were created, and blown down as they were uncreated."

Lying on the bedspread, following the cracks in the ceiling, I get to thinking about "uncreated" and what that might look like in general...

In her book *The Secret Life of God: A Journey Through Britain*, Alex Klaushofer describes how, for some Christian mystics, "God – the divine, groundless ground, Source, whatever you want to call it – is not an object among other objects... but an aspect of experience that defies human powers of comprehension". I think that what Klaushofer is failing to describe in theological terms is a 'chora', a space of potential for some kind of becoming. In the mystical tradition, this is a space you don't get into by simple faith – this is the great mistake of those 'born again' lightweights – but only by a prolonged *negativa*, "a loss of faith or meaningless misery as an intrinsic part of the spiritual journey... Despair is a... necessity". We are at present going through such a dark night of the soul, collectively as a divided society, globally as a divided world, both paradoxically.

Under the integrated Spectacle (in which slippery images work across both public politics and private markets) it is necessary to assume despair and overleap Romanticism's optimistic "abyss of fusion" with nature (Frédéric Gros) in favour of the kind of desolate "abyss of faith" that St John of the Cross identifies as evidence that a connection to something unrepresentable is 'taking place'.

If Mary P. Willcocks is right about Bunyan being right, then the despair we are experiencing is just the latest Enclosure of our mattering and meaning. Despite the massive surpluses of the Empire, these were never shared, I've seen the evidence of that; the hatred and fear was redistributed democratically, but not the wealth, a 'colony-at-home' was established in people's hearts. So we must leave that 'colony-at-home', skip work, skirt mass entertainments and make our own ways, whenever we can, pilgrims on any and every road. We should ask for legislation in favour of self-discovery and write it into law that private property is its binary opposite. Pass laws to allow any pilgrim wearing the pecten or winged eye or sun-and-rose to enter any space without penalty. That would make politics interesting and repopulate the paths. The villages would respond, in tune with Lutyens's vision, with new inns and cafés.

How come the walking artists haven't written a serious manifesto, a proper strategy for millions to walk? To make a change?

Walking with Jane today, that "everything else but" of Mallarmé's "that defines the thing itself", was our bodies. Until Jane joined me today, apart from in the cold seawater with the psychoswimographers, I had been keeping my body safe, not really walking with it. But she put my body in with the horses, shaking our necks, fronting up the strong chest, making me shake involuntarily on a gappy landing stage. So no surprise then that what all this bodiness threw up was a firework display of "everything else but" symbols in a parking space, symbols I am now hunting down...

Such whirling displays of symbols, freed from the burden of working for metaphors, will generate a revelatory dynamic, I know it, a whirling planetarium of invisible movements riding on faint motions of meaning, like shady meetings on wasteland viewed through dirty windows, they will reveal a human machine detached from any single subject or sense but thrilling to everything. Our attractive enemy.

The objects are in charge, linen referees,
Mirrors teach and concretes police, saws cut
Streams of words from mental trees,
Branches fuse and blow, and lips mime to
The rumble of the body's deep cave system. But things
Are more powerful than that. They transform and imitate,
The blade becomes a looking glass, a stone a child,
Soft muslin a winding sheet, while a hammer conducts gangs of nails

And a television becomes a smoothing iron. Then it all changes again:
Chalk into a token of some ancient currency, the camera
A way of stitching up friends, and all this time the things have been caught
conspiring
To put legs in relation to legs, and arms to arms, and trunks to fraught
ground.

There is a limit to how much you can learn by talking to yourself, I say to myself, perched on the edge of the bed in my rented room.

I fall asleep and dream I am dragging a ruined white horse over the missing planks of the landing stage.

Torquay Road, Keyberry Road, cross to supermarket and turn left through McDonald's car park, to Torquay Road and turn right to underpass (Penn Inn Roundabout), take exit to 'Milber', Addison Road, Laburnum Road, Silverwood Avenue, alley to Beechwod Avenue, Rowantree Road, back to Silverwood Avenue, right at Pinewood Road, take signed public footpath on the right into Penninn Plantation, path to crossing Marychurch Road at junction with Aller Brake Road, path into car parking space, down to and right along Belgrave Road, which becomes Swanborough Road, alley on right to Twickenham Road, left to Shaldon Road, right along Shaldon Road and cross over Shaldon Road at the 'stone circle' outside the Post Office money collection depot, Riverview, Moorlands Close, Tor View Avenue, right along Oakland Road, right onto Windsor Avenue, which becomes Buckland Road, turn right down lane at Mare and Foal Sanctuary, left at T-junction down Hackney Lane to river, right along Templer Way (on river bed – only walkable a couple of hours either side of low tide), right up steep stone steps at Devon Valley Holiday Village, left along Coombe Road, Ringmore Road, Torquay Road, Bridge Road (over Shaldon Bridge across Teign), right along Bishopsteignton Road, Bitton Park Road, Higher Brook Road, Lower Brook Road, Hollands Road, Regent Street, Esplanade, The Street With No Name, Dawlish Street, St Michael the Archangel Church, Promenade, The Den, Den Crescent, Carlton Place, Bath Terrace, Brunswick Street, South View, Northumberland Place.

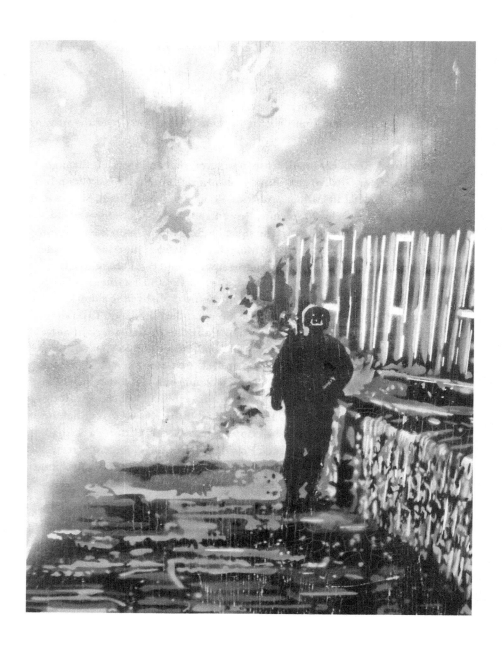

Chapter Ten: Teignmouth to the Lower Haldon Hills and on to Dawlish Warren

In the morning I head towards the river again, thinking of walking the river bed on this side. There are solid workshops here made of corrugated iron, sitting on a concrete promontory 'reclaimed' from the river; as if it had ever been anyone else's *but* the river's! On the outside wall of one of the workshops is a display of maybe fifty boots and of a similar number of potted plants, the boots rotting and the plants sinking their roots into them, flowers of bright red and purple growing from their ankles.

A large freighter is docking, navigating the running tide. It strikes me for the first time that these are really serious docklands; in a few moments I run up against a sign to tell me that I am in the River, Beach & Arts Quarter and that it requires something as solidly anachronistic as dock work, torqued by objects when so much else in global circulation is soft or digital, to prop up the fantasies that are sustaining whole shops here. In one of the gothic art shops a salvaged dalek top has been reconfigured for a more basic weapon, with stabilisers and caterpillar tracks, rusted to chocolate: AND MECHANICAL BEASTS ROAMED THE BATTLEFIELD.

In the back of a Land Rover filled with rope and compound pigfeed sits a tiny, smartly-suited and bow-tied mannequin, with one eye red and the other green.

DANGER
AT CERTAIN STATES OF THE TIDE
WARNING   WARNING
DEEP WATER   SHALLOW WATER

They are determined to scare you.

In the underpass a plaque describes the study of the arts, crafts and cultures of many regions of the world conducted by local children before creating a mosaic of numerous tiles celebrating the multicultural society in which they live. Unvandalised, without graffiti, it is a murky fragmentation of symbols, in the dim light of the subway; perhaps too unreadable to have provoked a response of any strength of any kind. Yet, studied for a moment, it is as potent, here in the passage under the main through road, as the car parking space in Ringmore. I am beginning to learn, that in these Devon towns and villages, the magic is shared between the ritual spaces and the most abject of the everyday; they each push out into excess, with the 'historic' becoming almost entirely fanciful and the ordinary triangulated somewhere between humiliation and invisibility. I love these towns! The big northern cities are so explicit, but Devon towns are so subtle and bittersweet.

The symbolic roundabout looks incoherent from behind the pavement railings. The eight-sided church is locked. I imagine the massive void beneath its 'lantern', which has the look of a Tardis shuffled through a double-exposure. I keep going up.

I think I may have mentioned that Devon is not flat, it's a weave. The undulating hills, the threading together of villages and towns, the line of the coast are all held up by a scaffolding of travelling stories. Not stories about travel, but stories that travel, that tendril out, that creep under the ground they prop up. The whole county is a hollow hill held up by the pillars of its fiction and the props of its anecdotes. At times, I feel as if I am walking without my feet touching the ground, because there is so much between me and the earth. What I have not always been able to find in dreams – a realisation of the Symbolist mysterium – I am swimming in, being walked in, climbing in, falling in, all in this anywhere.

The sign for 'The Traditional Building and Conservation Company' has been screwed across and obscures a ghost sign palimpsest; "traditional", then, in the sense of ignoring the heritage of what is conserved.

A bricked and plastered-up former doorway. In Abbotskerswell, I noticed that a terrace of houses had once all had gateways and steps up from the road and that these had been blocked up in favour of a single entrance, and I had wondered whether this reflected a very, very long process. Because I thought of that dispersed community around the West Ogwell church and that it could only be sustained by the regular visiting of one by another (which perhaps explains the heightened mythic status of the loner in those times, unlike today when they are Kafka-boring-normal), hence the excuses like plough plays and mummers and carol singing and All Hallows' Eve and the stranger knocking at the door on New Year's Eve with a piece of coal and the back door opened to let the old year out; and that that was still reflected in the details of later Saxon villages, but was finally brought to a withering shrinkage by the advent of common television. Individualism no longer based on a meshwork of routes of common visiting, but a solitary or familial relation to the machine.

I pass the entrance to a school, with a memorial stone to a VC-winning baronet, whose final decision as an acting major-general of an Indian infantry division was to blow up the means of retreat for two-thirds of his division, placing them in the tender race-supremacist mercies of the Japanese army. He was made a privy counsellor in 1962. Behind the stones an extraordinary cob structure rises and threatens, octopoid, a dolphin-like predator, a back to front neck, like the violent camel of death inflicting suffering on the fallen rhino in the simulacrum on the hoardings of the Brunswick Street waste ground. Troubled and troubling shapes.

When I look back, a huge WELCOME TO TEIGNMOUTH pedestrian bridge frames the Ness on the other side of the estuary: a headland pierced by a tunnel that appears in Siobhán Mckeown's 'The Devil's Footprints' movie about the odd legacy of techno-militarist innovators on this piece of coast. I am not sure where it is, but I cannot be far from Babbage's house. Just before the grim gateway to The Yannons, the grey tick tower where Vivien Leigh and Laurence Olivier romanced, I turn right onto the service road for the Live Fitness Centre, surprised to find that I am passing the Police HQ for the region. The road swings around the gym into a car park with a disastrously neglected mediaeval ruin in one corner, the sad remnants of its heraldic badge above broken windows (a square tipped on one end with rods piercing the centre of each of its four sides). The building is sealed with alloy doors. Beside it is a long and tall wall, yet another! There is a door set into the angle of what seems like some enclosed space, but there is no sign. I am lying on my face trying to get a look under the warped door when a voice asks whether I would like to look inside. It is not, surprisingly, a sarcastic one. Once again, the welcome. The alloy doors have opened and a middle-aged guy and his younger assistant are following me up the footpath.

"What is it? I can't see anything really."

"Come and see."

He fumbles with a key and eventually the large door wedged into the corner of the two walls swings inward and a slightly puzzling, but large space opens up. It looks like a badly attended giant allotment.

"A kitchen garden for the big house that stood where the gym is now, our store is its barn, you must have passed us!"

The man shows me around and explains his plans for the walled space; to regenerate it as a garden for children to come and learn horticultural skills. He describes the massive bulk of brambles and buddleia that they have carried through the corner door. But there is something odd about this garden. Something that should not be here, that does not quite fit in. For though there is a pattern to the space, partly spectral and partly the work of new planting, there is an anomaly at the centre of it; a nitrate-green panelled construct wrapped in a turquoise plastic sheeting roof.

"Ah, yes, ah. Well.... do you want to see?"

Of course I want to see. What could spoil a garden?

The man retreats to a kind of greenhouse affair where he has an office, while his younger assistant shifts uneasily. The man returns and the padlock is released and clumsy panels pulled back. Inside the dome is a heavy, brassy telescope. The structure is just big enough for all three of us to squeeze in. The man explains that the lenses have been removed until the structure can be properly secured against theft. There is a CCTV camera but it pretty clearly is a shell. Like the telescope.

"It was opened by Patrick Moore, Sir Patrick Moore, the..."

Sir Patrick Moore the xylophone-player, founder of a hopelessly unsuccessful anti-European and anti-immigration party, and ufo-hoaxer, covert co-author of *Flying Saucer from Mars*, pseudonym: Cedric Allingham, vouched for by Lord Dowding (then former Air Chief Marshall of the RAF), the whole thing looking like an official disinformation exercise. Moore, a good operative, died denying that any of this was the case. He was surfing the Adamski wave of contactees, on behalf of his handlers.

Flying Saucer from Mars is subtle and sinister. Rather than setting out to wreck or even parody the ufo-obsession – which is what I'd expected from the arch-sceptic Moore – the book simultaneously promotes and guts it; in other words, it demonically possesses it, takes charge of it. It even copies and parodies the rhetorical dishonesties of pseudo-science books: "though the theory of the lost continent of Atlantis is largely discounted, there is no reason to doubt the reality of Saucers seen in ancient times", "are there still people who remain unconvinced? No doubt there are. But there are still those who believe in a flat Earth."

Were Moore and his book part of a 'mirage' project for turning the minds of sceptics and believers alike to mush? A para-political strategy that goes way beyond saucer mania and is now what we call 'post-truth' – the cultivation of the inability to have a sensible public discourse about anything? While dullards in power grind on.

Deep breath. I turn and exhale along the top of the kitchen garden wall. The idea that there is a lensless telescope at the centre of this huge skewed trapezoid is strangely gratifying; particularly as its absurdity now floats on some social funding for ecological education. I presume that bureaucracy will quickly kill such excess dead. But I hope not and thank my guides and hosts sincerely.

I accidentally trespass through some kind of facility, climbing over a low breeze-block wall into someone's drive and head back to the main road. I am trying to avoid churches and graveyards now, but I get sucked into the cemetery by an angel with missing hands. Tussocks bulge from graves. In the heart of this older part of the cemetery is the busted symmetry of a funerary complex, a central building with two chapels: one relatively sound but with boarded windows, the other wholly ruined, roofless and full of nettles and brambles. I manage to find a way through, a remnant of some animal track, crouch down and have a pee.

In the modern part of the cemetery is a stone that stands out from all the others, dedicated to:

A Man of Two Worlds
Who Offered So Much
From Science to Art
You had the Midas Touch

Then the chemical structure of an amino acid, Serine, two fists between which there is a cord, and an eight-pointed star, a regular octagram, the line of which completes no other symmetrical figures until it returns to its starting point. The line is not quite continuous, but at two corners does not meet; the artist's modest refusal to even suggest perfection. Salmon says there is a memoir dedicated to this Egyptian-born sculptor and businessman, or rather to his relationship with the author, his lover, the abrupt ending of which precipitates her into a fugue, which reads like a more intense and less dispersed version of my own: "I don't recall travelling... Sounds were out of place: a child was laughing, but I heard crying; a woman was talking to me but I heard a man's voice saying the words. Sights changed colour and definition constantly in front of my eyes... someone inside was screaming to get out, but I had to keep her locked away... I could almost see the shape of feet and hands under my skin".

I slog up the aptly named Breakneck Hill and its tunnel of bracken, then turn sharp left. I have been walking uphill all morning, from a couple of metres above sea level. Although the tops are heavily wooded there are momentary views back to the far side of the Teign and, further off, to the cliffs that sustain the Bishop's Walk. That seems a very long way back.

There is a laminated sign, a WARNING that the police are monitoring the area and CONDUCTING REGULAR VISITS TO DETER ANTISOCIAL BEHAVIOUR. Dogging, presumably. The sign looks far from official, of a kind with the REVOLTING! one I find a little further on that threatens imprisonment for fly-tippers. I wonder why there is such excitement about gatherings of consenting and anonymous adults having sex in remote spots like this; is it the collective nature of these events? Is there some sense in which they transform and taint the spaces in which they meet? Or transgress the appropriate and conventional individualism? I have certainly heard people speak of it 'spoiling' a place even if there is no material residue. I can't say that the idea of dogging either excites or disgusts me; I feel the same indifference as I do to, say, pigeon racing, yet there is something extraordinary to the moment in one of the Wrights & Sites' '4 x 4' videos when the camera very briefly, surprised, settles on a tree in Haldon Forest draped in a thousand used condoms. I realise I have turned inland towards those woods...

I take a left turn onto a hollow way; it is shaped beautifully to the ground, but leads me quickly down to a very busy road without verges, so I backtrack to the upper lane. Above the hollow way two strong ropes, one blue and one white, bear a black tyre and an orange ball, the ball sits within the tyre, gently spinning as if it is a planet trapped in its orbit, or an uneasy sun within its black halo.

Then it gets nasty. Passing a whole shower room, smashed and then dumped in the road, and a broken wing mirror, into which I peer and separate, I turn right onto the busy road I have been avoiding. There are tiny slivers of verge into which I can press myself, but then even they run out and for a while there is simply a solid earth wall and trusting to the last moment reactions of the car drivers. I wave to the oncoming drivers and trust them to move out a little. When an ambulance, all lights and sirens, comes racing towards me I dare not signal, but press myself hard into the earth and hope. Halfway into this peril I pass a well or spring housed in a small red sandstone structure; like the tiny truncated footpath, this suggests that the sheer volume of traffic, with nothing to accommodate it, has attenuated things up here, a place to race through not ever reside or be attentive in.

Finally, after a couple of close shaves, I see a turning up ahead on the left, the stream of cars from behind me has dried up for a moment and I sprint the last hundred metres to safety, follow a quiet lane uphill and then take the public footpath across the golf course.

It is rather as though I am some disgraced and obscure relative, for whom the family have constructed a private path hidden from all; I walk in a corridor of bushes most of the way across the course, until it opens up and I can relax into the view to the horizon of Dartmoor tors over the valley dip. Once on a road again, I jump a narrow trench and take a well-trodden track from a gravelled area, meeting a young woman walking her dogs who tells me that if I keep going I will see the airfield.

"There are four old blokes up there at the moment, flying their planes."

I expect to see Cessnas or something, but these are model planes with huge wings, circling high above the unrelenting gorse, riding the thermals. And instead of the runways, control tower, arrival and departures, radar, wind sock and so on, there are four men in folding chairs sat in the middle of a levelled area within the mass of tearing gorse. I find a narrow path through the spikes and cross their mown strip.

I come to them and stand watching one launch his plane and steer it upwards. Two of the others are deep in conversation about the extra lift from air passing over a hill; I think they are talking about the Bernoulli Effect, but I resist the temptation to femsplain. The men ignore me; they know I am there. Finally, the youngest of the four, the man who has just released his plane, acknowledges the awkwardness and comes over to chat. Then they all join in. They explain that this had been a military base during the Second World War.

"HMS Heron 2, but there's nothing left, there are a few bits of concrete from the old control tower in the corner but kids ruined that."

"Weren't no good as a base, they had trouble with mixie."

"What's that?"

"Mists, rain."

Same as Keats.

Between complaints about dog walkers, for doing quite what I am not sure, I learn that this was once "Devon's airport, before Exeter", that "the king" had landed here – the all-purpose king, I suppose – and that Frank Muir, a figure in light entertainment, had been commanding officer ("His brother lived near here.") What I find out later is that long before the war and the king (two of those markers that define and police what *is* the historical homogeneity), the airfield was famous for its women pilots, ladies of the local gentry who seemed to regard planes as a mechanical development of the horse. The air shows they participated in as stunt fliers and parachutists attracted crowds of up to 10,000 onto this windy moor.

Not four old chauvinists.

Standing on the top I can see the huge valley that I came through with the birdman and then the tors up on the moor and then further round, the Forest where the Lawrence Tower is and I'm not sure I want to go there, all fairly remote, will there be B&B's? Will there be any walkers from the conference, are most of them not urban-based and heading for a city?

I break off the malfunctioning conversation with the armchair pilots and head back the way I came, treading over myself. Tracking down a mown path I can see that some way off to the right, in the gorse is some remnant of the old airfield, dark orange rusty, a square metal stump. At the trodden junction back to the road there is a fainter track and I take that. Like the walk of disgrace across the golf course, I am surrounded by gorse, bramble and thorns; it is a while since anyone walked this and I have to repeatedly tread down the sharp stems of brambles and wild, maybe blue, roses, near impossible to get through. Gorse prickles work their way through my jeans and a thorn tears the fabric. The gorse is not cutting me, but pricking just deep enough to touch the nerves; the feeling is almost *jouissant*. I am losing control. I have come too far to want to turn around and do this all again, but there is no prospect of escape from the striking, tearing tunnel. I press on. At times the thorns hold me for a moment, until I am able to shake them off; I am scared of losing my balance, too far from the pilots for them to hear a cry for help. An arm of bramble drops across my shoulders and I stoop to avoid its uninvited intimacy. It starts to rain, a thin rain, and I realise how unreal the weather has been up until now as if my liberation from routine had brought out and raised up the light, and now as I pay for that with a crumbling centre and a flapping purpose, the moistness descends to mulch things even further. I stumble and scratch my fingers reaching out for support; underfoot it is no longer trampled grass, but low gorse that hides the humps and dips beneath. I wobble. Where the walls of thorns close in I hold my hands behind my back, poke my head through to the light and let the spines scrape across my anorak, like fingernails down a human blackboard, until surrendering myself to the darkest, thickest wall of bramble and the thinnest birth canal – "that mountain with the wall and the narrow gap of light in it through which he has to creep from darkness into light" – I stumble out into an expanse of knee-high gorse with the rusty metal structure poking a metre above its spines. I am no nearer. I have circled it. Now it stands on the edge of what is visible; the thin rain becomes a descended mist, the ancient airfield is lost to view. A 'mixie'.

There are no short cuts. And no path. I can turn back through the thorn tunnel, something I refused to do some time ago. Or I can take my chance on the gorse, guessing at what might be underneath. It begins to strike me – or puncture me – that reality up here (up where?) is a pretty thin curtain. I can poke my hand right through it and feel beyond, and yet I cannot get anywhere. Nothing tears; as if I am reaching around the side of a stage curtain to feel for an audience or a way out. But what I touch is scary; another curtain. Curtains all the way down.

I imagine a tiny dog pulling at the 'mixie', and the haze bulging violently as if someone were struggling to stay hidden. If the curtain fell back I would expect to find a pathetic old man, sat in a folding chair, twiddling a joystick on the control box balanced on his crotch, socially-inept and passive-aggressive. Instead it reveals a terrible curtain-god, a mist-evil, full of fear, worry and hatred, nitrate-emerald translucence and glowing, radium-bright, roaring tongues of Pentecostal flame;

burning off the mists so I can see direct into the rawness. A thousand faces flicker across the same white skull of low cloud and I recognise every effing one of them; and as the curtains close again, I catch a glimpse of his uniform, embroidered in blood with a million symbols and 'no entry' signs one over another.

I panic, reaching urgently into wet blankets of vagueness. I am losing touch with my body; who is the operator and what is the operation? I can hear my bones creaking in my boots as I stumble down the hidden holes; perhaps I am a surgeon, or an editor or a piece of earthmoving machinery the size of a baseball pitch, come unintendedly to self-consciousness and now rearranging the terrain.

I get a sudden rush of power and exhilarating joy.

I feel myself floating off with the symbols. Coming apart like the three men in their geological costumes; disappearing into the murk like the four men in their folding chairs. It is hard to concentrate on levers and shovels when your brain is dancing with a 'mixie'.

It is incredibly banal. An H-shaped stump. The peeling black paint and rusted bolts fail to coalesce. I am shocked by its refusal to speak its precise purpose.

Who mined the materials in the land of Oz to build the Emerald City? I'd read that question in Darran Anderson's *Imaginary Cities*; part of a more important one about how the significance of work is made to disappear in art. Art's proposal, that everything that is, is based on something else made up, is its lie. The more I move my fingertips around in the 'mixie', the more unsure I am that I have a hold of ambience, a hand on the scenery... I am scared of pulling the whole thing over. If I am sensible I can change things backstage. When the 'mixie' clears and the curtain lifts, things will be OK.

A couple chatter on the mown path. They are a few metres away, but they cannot see me, even now the mist is lifting and the sun burning through. But I can see them, hear them. Know their business. There is no wild to be lost in. As early as 1949 Geoffrey Grigson wrote that there was "hardly a wild, lonely place from the Pennines to Land's End where one might not find a wooden leg".

I expect every black rubbish bag to contain body parts.

I kneel down beside the orange stump, at a loss to make any sense of it.

Between the two uprights of the rusty H, in the far valley, I can see Denbury Hill. The stump is a frame.

> *The sterile sea lapped to the door of an empty fish shop.*
> *Moss stood a foot deep in a library.*
> *Victims clustered at the windows of perpetrators.*
> *The graveyards were full of penny falls.*

I spread the poem of the woman from Cockington's Front Lawn over the rusty H, but its letters move around like smoke particles in a beaker.

I am sub-atomic on the hill top. A tiny thing of tiny things that have all lost their thingness together; there is no separation, only flow. This is what everyone says is good; but this is evil too – eood, eiod – or maybe mostly gvil, gool. I feel no choice; only swimming and spitting and crawling up through a grey wetness, and being smacked backwards and forwards between the arms of the carousels, a single lightbulb in a sterile room turned on and off repeatedly, spearheads smeared with antiseptic. I give up making sense and feel my way back to the path, calves prickling.

No words describe. (I hate that. Usually.)

I don't know what any of it means. Mostly I see crowds of pineal glands swimming like seahorses in a cage, like the waggle dance of honey bees. All swaying to the illusion that when we close our eyes we are unique inside.

I can see clearly that the glands are doing business. Trading on the serotonin market. I get it! The filthy swill that the pineal glands are trading in, awash with tiny endocrine demiurges, is a soft fertilising system, all the time inventing more and more filth to be cleared away. We should be proud of our waste. Not the corporate shoals of pink Vanish (haha) that wash up on the beaches, but the excess of us, our pearls, that's what the mist is. The overcast skies. The dullness of the dead screen. Our genius put in its place. The grit, small coin, marble chip that catches in the gears of the big earthmoving machine and changes its direction, bit by bit.

By almost giving up and fearing to turn back, I have discovered, in the most unpromising of places, the missing control room, apparently smashed up by kids, the bathyscaphe in the basement of ideology, and I have been allowed to touch its switches and joysticks.

Like a woman I heard about earlier from a taxi driver, looking for fairies by un-focusing her eyes, I can still see the swill all around me, its prejudices and identities, but also a darkness, a filth that is pure shadow, splashing everywhere and everything and I easily find my way back to the road.

I walk out of the last of the mist.

"I thought I came here once, on a quest. My name is Alice."

She looks about me, then through me, and disappears into the miasma.

I want to get off the tops and off the roads, but have no sense of direction so head back along the road that was so dangerous before; this keeps happening. Quiet lanes and cross-country scrambles that loop you back to dangerous roads. Waiting for a break in the traffic, to cross from one verge to the other, it strikes me that somewhere on this journey I must cross routes with the journey in *The Unlikely Pilgrimage of Harold Fry*, Rachel Joyce's novel about a late middle-aged man who spontaneously sets off to visit a lost love on her death bed up North. Starting from his home in Kingsbridge in South Devon, he passes through Exeter, so I must be near his path. I had not liked the book, it's a sentimental *Of Walking in Ice*, yes the narrative is wonderful, but the further north its pilgrim gets the less the author seems to know or care about the places, the less she has bothered to find out about them; someone at the conference mentioned re-walking its route. How could you do that? How could you plan a fugue?

Making the same mistake, I try to find another 'Sir Constant' later, in charity shops, as if you could repeat an accidental find. The only interesting thing I come across is a fundraising publication, I forget the charity, called 'Secret Invasion': a collection of stories based on the Cthulhu mythos and other eldritch literature and set in Devon. One story is drawn in comic form, penned by Steven Trickey it says; in one of the panels of the strip there is a road sign:

EXETER 12
DAWLISH 5

I looked it up on Google Maps. Twelve miles from Exeter, five from Dawlish. It's exactly where I am now. Where, here, a jellyfish-crustacean-venus-flytrap-all-in-one ambushes a delivery driver and takes him hostage, feeds off him, turns him into "a vessel": "DON'T DELUDE YOURSELF WITH RIGHTS YOU HAVE CONSTRUCTED YOURSELF ON THIS BALL OF MUD YOU SO ARROGANTLY COVET AND CLAIM AS YOURS... WE... I... WAS HERE FIRST". The monster is a fish-vegetable version of the throwback on the moor. It empties the driver's head of foolish ideas and carries it into the sea at what could be Saltern Cove.

I come to a public footpath and can at last get away from racing traffic; deeply relieved.

I should not be. It feels wrong almost from the start, and yet it *looks* right. Once through a generous tube of bushes, things open up and I can see down the long green valley to the sea far off. I can see buildings nestling in the bottom of the valley and the hint of a more substantial community beyond that. My cutting inland has been fruitless as far as finding more walkers, I am beginning to struggle with the meaning of my research; when that happens, I know what happens, I start to become its subject. So I am pulling back, I am heading back towards the sea and the towns. That is where I have felt best. I loved Teignmouth, everything I knew about it from Salmon was bad, and everything I saw and felt was its dealing with all the stuff he obsessed on. It felt like redemption.

The wide, twin-furrowed track cuts downhill through bronze bracken and blackened stalks, ruinously beautiful. Then a small wooden post points me off this wide track and to the right and the path seems swallowed up between ferns and long brown grass. But it's not as bad as it looks and I easily pick out the track as it descends through small, isolated, silvery-bare trees, then through ferns up to my shoulders. Underfoot becomes less sure, large flint nodules roll about under each step and twist at my heels. Then I climb down through what might have been an orchard; there are tiny apples on the path, but mostly the trees are young oaks. The canopy keeps out much of the returning sun and I feel chilly for the first time, a chilliness that comes both from inside and from outside and meets just under my skin. Goose pimples arise.

There is a very, very deep, fenced, chasm to my left. I can hear water running at the bottom.

The fallen leaves give the extended grove a hazy glow and I should be enjoying its unexpected beauty, but I fear what lies beneath and to the side. The land falls steeply away again and I climb a stile, beside a trunk of tree that has grown over and around a line of barbed wire. Another hybrid monster.

The wide, green dome of the field means that I have no idea if there are other animals in here with me. Nazi cattle, for example, any of them. So, I keep close to the left-hand edge of the field, parallel with the chasm, ready to climb over the barbed-wire fence, mindful that there is a void there, not far into the cover. My knees hurt, the repeated thumping of the descent onto unsteady flint bits; the field is no easier, steep and ridged. I can see a farmhouse at the bottom and beyond that a bright pink cottage trailing white smoke. The land falls away even more steeply, to reveal a small sign in the grass:

> No public
> right of way
> beyond
> this point

Perhaps it is my exhaustion, perhaps it is the way that the word "beyond" is separated from the rest, but I feel alphabetically sick. I sway at the thought of re-reading the hill and its steepness. I feel very tired. As if I might just roll into the abyss. I cannot stay here, the field is sick too and being here is reinforcing the cycle. Backing away, there is a little gate in the fence. There *is* another way!

Maybe there's a bridge over the chasm? Maybe the stream disappears underground and the void closes up?

I open the nondescript wooden gate and pass through; boggy underfoot, a little overgrown, but I do not expect the black railings. Or the sign, ripped in waves of warped wood:

Lidwell Chapel

There clearly had been some explanation underneath the title, but it has gone to the dampness. The railings form a rectangle around a single stone wall, with an arch at the far end; presumably the west end of the chapel. So I am standing almost on the altar. Although I can see where people have entered, and there is a metal gate, it must have been some time since its last visitor: the grass and shrubs have almost completely retaken the floor of the chapel. I really do not want to trip and fall here. Few come here. I am too scared to even turn on my phone to see if there is a signal. I look but I do not go in. I feel drawn, but I resist. I try to leave and work my way around the railings, but there is no path beyond the chapel. If I try to make my way through the trees, I will head blindly for the chasm on a carpet of leaves.

I trip on something in the leaves, but somehow stay upright. It's a metal box and I wonder if this is the treasure that has been drawing me, testing me with anxiety and strange feelings of dread. I pick it up by its handle and unclip the lid which falls open to reveal a closed aperture. A trap for rats. I drop it into the leaves and back off wiping

179

my hands on the branches. I force myself to go through the metal gate into the chapel; to avoid the abyss. There is nothing else to do but to arrive and to leave as quickly as possible.

There is a carved wooden floral cross on the West wall, but the tip of its shaft is a simulacrum of a morose and weeping owl-god. I try to find the source of all the water, but fail. "Lidwell", so presumably there is a spring here, the well of the Lady. Have I got too close to the subtext of this journey?

On the way out I notice that someone or something has scored through the cross on the white noticeboard.

Calves burning, I climb back up the path. Very relieved to find that there's another footpath running parallel to the busy road, I take it. When it ends, after more beguiling vistas down the valley to the possibility of pub lunches or flat whites in beachside cafés, it is at a quiet road and I gratefully accept its invitation.

A few minutes later, aware of a vague shaping in the trees I follow a faint trail around a gate and enter a clearing. All the weirdness of the day disappears as I enter what is, unmistakably, my place, the inner circle of an old hill fort; this is the same feeling as on Denbury Hill, but now I recognise it, I come home to it. I am as fake and sentimental as Harold Fry; but it's a sentimentality that I have been able to fake only here, a unique, site-specific self-deception. I want to stay but leave immediately. I am researching; there is no point hanging about learning what I already know. I am manic with tiredness from climbing hills. I ought to take the road signed down to Dawlish, where cafés will be open, where there will be chips and sauce. But I cannot resist the fingerpost that points to ASHCOMBE TOWERS. Will they be good or evil?

They are probably evil, I decide.

Ashcombe Tower (not sure why the signpost pluralises it) houses Adolf Hitler's personal telephone.

Later on, when I get some reception, I find that the Lidwell Chapel has accumulated all sorts of grim fairy tales; murderous hermits living off (and on) lonely travellers; archaeological records of numerous bones found in the well at the east end where the altar would have been. The same as at the pub in Torbryan, there is a story of a mysterious speleological link, of the silver treasures of Teignmouth carried up here during the raids of the French, thrown down the well, only to re-emerge at the Ness. Or sometimes they emerge at Kent's Cavern, which would connect the Lidwell Chapel to the The Old Grotto at Torbryan caves; a web of hollow tales.

There is a drive in people to connect everything up; and I think it is a very healthy one. Given the qualitative shift in the occupation of the whole of life by relativism, by the post-truth of popular politics, by global mediatisation, "totality" is a virtue again. It doesn't matter whether it's Arthur Kubin's 'The Other Side', Grant Morrison's 'The Invisibles', Hope Mirrlees's 'Lud-In-The-Mist' or the Duchess of Newcastle's 'Blazing Worlds', it *outflanks* the Spectacle. It sits over the ever-present Spectacle and leaves a little space of excess, of difference, by which it threatens to impregnate the whole. It's what Bruno Latour calls "plasma", where "the big could at any moment drown again in the small from which it emerged... as if at some point you had to leave the solid land and go to the sea".

The wrist is the brow of the arm,
And two triangles are wild in the room.

The trees flanking the road lean in and stretch their ultra-long branches.

Ashcombe Tower is flying a flag of St George. I imagine Helen B painting around it in chalk and breccias, until the flag disappears.

A woman overtakes me, dressed in a heavy tweed jacket, apparently not noticing that I am sneaking looks over a disused gate across the lawn to Ashcombe Tower. She is striding down the road, but I interrupt to ask about a possible footpath.

"O", she says, "I have absolutely no idea about a footpath" in the tone of "I have absolutely no idea why someone like you exists."

Later I make way for her cream Land Rover and she smiles, friendlily. We are more made by our circumstances that we like to pretend.

Without a footpath by which to cut back to the Dawlish road, this is now a long walk; a new valley opens up far, far ahead, with a wide estuary, a whole new territory; this is a rhythm of walking terrain that I have never felt before, the unfolding of huge valleys over long hours. The road begins to head downwards and I lose the vista.

I wonder if the extraordinarily green moss in the middle of the road is due to a fertiliser spill.

The road drops down and down and for a while I am walking along the very bottom of the valley, drinking in its green flatness, with staring horses. I cross Dawlish Water (this is where the devil hunters are reputed to have come). Turning sharp right, I climb up the other side of the valley; I am walking reflected. I pass a corrugated iron garage overwhelmed by a huge yellow-leafed plant. Then, a field of greenhouses. The boggy bottom of the valley. A piece of RSJ, painted like an Everton Mint, protects the corner of a cottage. A large complex that makes me think of the treasures I did not find in the rat trap.

I pass a pair of young middle-aged country women in smart specialist-shop clothes. I say "good afternoon" and one says "hellurrgh" and I wonder if that is the correct address for strangers on a lane. I think it must be dreaming of the chips in Dawlish, but I can feel the one on my shoulder growing.

A massive uninhabited house. A couple of lights left on for security.

A branch twists back on itself, and then twists again. The tree of Z.

As I come into Dawlish, a wall on my right has ASHCOMBE in huge letters and a broken sign points to THE R. Behind the wall, in an enclosed terrace, after hearing a "suspected yoga noise" two days previously, two neighbours called on a retired shop worker to invite him for a cup of tea, but found him lifeless and "swaddled" in bed linen and home-made dresses, his face covered in a number of stockings with eyeholes, cotton wool in his mouth and ears, mouth taped over and head wrapped in polythene. The former shop worker was turning himself into wrapped goods.

The road ahead is crossed by a bridge built to provide a way into town for the Hoares, the banking family, original and present owners of Luscombe Castle, above the heads of ordinary citizens. The Hoares who own the land across which there is:

No public
right of way
beyond
this point

I avoid walking under their snooty bridge. I am not sure why I find the name Ebenezer Pardon so funny.

The pillars of the Hoares' mausoleum are being turned by the wind into candy spirals. A pile of untouched pillars is stored in a corner; an oblique comment on the depredation of lines.

The gravestone of Major-General William Sage of H.M. Bengal Army bears crossed sabres and the places and dates of the Battle of Nepaul (1815) between the Nepalese and the British East India Company after which a third of the territory of Nepal was lost to the British; the taking of Ghuznee (1839) as part of the invasion of Afghanistan to prevent the Russians securing an advantage in that country (that campaigns continues); and the relief of Saugor (1858) where 'the doctrine of lapse' by which the British East India Company annexed any princely state whose ruler died without a male heir was opposed by the army of the great warrior princess Lakshmibai, the Rani of Jhansi.

In a memorial garden the branches of a monstrous and magnificent tree, wider than it is tall, protrude thickly parallel to the ground.

There is a fabulous parliament of dogs in the park; the pets serve as delegates and go-betweens for their owners who are engaged in loud and friendly debate. I squeeze through six people and their four dogs on the narrow bridge. "Not the best place to stop and chat," one of the owners apologises. But of course, it is the very best place in the world; our proximate intimacy is a marker of a default trust in the equanimity of people and animals.

Bingo in the pavilion; at the bottom of one of its pillars a Banksy mouse with walking stick looks on as a monster raves behind the bars of its cell.

At the Shaftsbury Theatre, the Dawlish Repertory Players are performing 'Waiting for Gateau'. "A group of weight watchers are stranded overnight in their gym by a blizzard..." I have an irrational wish to see this.

A mosaic on the Tourism Information Centre includes an accidental Dumna; fishes for eyes.

Dawlish Water collects in pools before running into the sea, where a sign warns against bathing too close to its discharge. A black swan with a red beak is sat upon the water. Not unlike mythogeography's advocacy for a Fortean science based on anomaly rather than consistency, black swan theory promotes the significance of 'impossible' events that 'come out of nowhere', arguing that unpredictability is a given due to the nature of small probabilities, and challenges the general assumption that hides the prevalence of uncertainty and the significance of rare events from the majority. I pass under the railway track and turn left down the prom, past two old guys with cider cans; I am tracing the 1855 Devil's Hoofmarks backwards.

This is where in 2014 the water ripped out the sea defences so that the railway track was left in mid-air, hanging by its rails; with an estimated cost to the local economy of £1.2 billion. Now, there is a call to rebuild the line on a causeway thirty metres out to sea at a cost of another half billion. What could possibly go wrong?

...not to protect it from the sea, but from the collapse of the cliffs. Some of these orange-red cliffs are whole sand dunes from the deserts of 300 million years ago. Later in the RAMM I get to see the fossilised burrow of one of the tiny crocodile-like creatures that careened under these dunes. I love that it is the hole that is fossilised and not the sand.

The 'ghost house', the ruined state of which Salmon shows in photos from a trespass, has been refurbished; in the failing light the empty white villa, between rentals, seems even more ghostly than in dereliction. The sea is flat and grey. What if we have so colonised it, so exploited it, that, in despair, the life has emigrated?

Just as he imagined Devon's sea water counter-colonised by giant jellies, so H.G. Wells feared an invasion of the skies. *The Horror of the Heights* has an ace pilot who always flies with a shotgun in his cockpit, after the suspicious crash of a fellow flier – "And where, pray, is Myrtle's head?". Climbing, one day, to over 40,000 feet into an "air-jungle, as he calls it, exist[ing] only above the south-west of England" the pilot encounters "long, ragged wisps of something". Looking upwards, he struggles, like a speculative realist, to describe what he sees: "conceive a jelly-fish such as sails in our summer seas, bell-shaped and of enormous size – far larger, I should judge, than the dome of St Paul's". As below, so above. This is the horror of the coming monolith, what Steve Mentz calls the Homogenocene. Or maybe not coming, but come; perhaps there are already jelly-giants in the shadow biosphere; we just don't see them because we only look for kinds of life we already know.

Passing Langstone Rock, I see the chunks of granite sea defence supplemented by clinker from a blast furnace; from one dark orange piece a head forces itself out. Up on the cliffs there are lights. I follow the road under the railway and up the hill to a hotel where 1960s' chalet-style rooms have encased an American-Colonial style villa. I book in and sip a Muscadet in the bar, savouring the iron pillars on the veranda.

You became monumental, mostly planned,
A garden architecture resolved around
A good strong column, your crime in a hedge only mentioned
When the models were developed a little later
In a dark room. Then rowing out was not so easy
In the flood, and miracles happened smoothly,
Releasing the moment of beauty, only briefly, and then misunderstood.

Northumberland Place, Queen Street, Teign View Place, down small street beside New Quay Inn, Northumberland Place, Somerset Place, Fore Street, subway under Higher Brook Street, Exeter Street, Exeter Road, turn right into service road for Live Fitness Centre, past the gym and into car park space, turn left along wall by mediaeval barn, turn right along wall, then (trespass, possibly) right across grass below a mostly wooden building, and over low breeze-block wall into Yannon Terrace, right into Exeter Road, right into cemetery, crossing Higher Buckeridge Road into modern part of cemetery, exit cemetery at north corner onto Exeter Road, Breakneck Hill, left along Holcombe Down Road, right onto Higher Exeter Road/B3192 (extremely dangerous, with little verge; there is a fair amount of traffic on Holcombe Down Road, so you should be able to hitch a lift to the next turning), left at the sign for Teignmouth Golf Club, almost immediately take the right fork, at the golf club take the footpath on the right across the course, at Little Haldon crossroads take the road ahead signed to Exeter, cross onto the former airfield (now overgrown) by jumping over the narrow trench to the left opposite an informal lay-by, follow the winding track and bend around to the left and out into the open space where a 'landing strip' has been levelled in the gorse, retrace your steps to the road and carry on left along the road, at the junction turn right along the Higher Exeter Road/B1392 (this time there is a verge most of the way), then left at footpath sign, at the gate take the footpath straight ahead, at the wooden marker with yellow arrow take the path to the right, down through a grove of trees, over gate and around left-hand edge of the field, at sign "No public right of way beyond this point" turn left through gate into Lidwell Chapel. Retrace your steps up to the gate with three footpaths signed and, through the gate, take the right hand path, at the road turn right, then left and almost immediately right onto Luscombe Hill, there is an (unofficial) entrance to the hill fort on your left, by a gate, at the hill fort turn right and use the 'permissive footpath' to the junction of Luscombe Hill and the Port Way (take the Port Way/Greenway Lane, signed ASHCOMBE TOWERS, ASHCOMBE), follow this for about two and a half miles, after the row of small cream stones and having crossed the river, turn right signed for STARCROSS, KENTON and then shortly after, at the Dawlish Water junction take the right-hand turn onto the Ashcombe Road for about two miles into Dawlish, bear right at the entrance to Empsons Hill along Aller Hill, after re-crossing Dawlish Water turn left along The Newhay footpath, right through the churchyard, left along Oak Hill and Church Road, right into Barton Crescent and immediately bear left into Overbrook, into the park and turn left and cross bridge over Dawlish Water, follow the path downstream into Brook Street, Alexandra Road, Brunswick Place, cross bridge over Dawlish Water, across The Lawn, cross Brookdale Terrace and Station Road and take underpass and turn left along promenade to Dawlish Warren, Beach Road, Mount Pleasant Road.

Chapter Eleven: Dawlish Warren to Exeter

In the morning I wander down the hill towards the beach. Just before the Creep, up a driveway to my right I can see now, in the light, the railway carriages that cause Salmon to wax lyrical: converted rolling stock on amputated tracks arranged in a holiday park, each with beds and living rooms and showers, by the side of the working railway. The place is run by the Great Western Staff Association, but something has happened since Salmon wrote his guide as there is a large AUCTION sign tagged to the entrance gate. I ask at the coffee kiosk and the woman tells me that the carriages need extensive repair work the owners cannot afford. 'Camp coaches' were introduced in the 1930s and run by the big railway companies, but when British Rail ceased running them in the 1970s the Staff Association took them over at Dawlish Warren. Love the idea of living in a train that never moves! Maybe I should go to the auction? The roofs look rather liverish. Has anyone recorded the dreams from those bunks?

Under the Creep and the whole place becomes bizarre; I had missed this in the failing light last night. This is a holiday resort, where thousands and thousands come every year; yet the place is more like an industrial estate. There is a series of steel units in which are retail outlets and a slot machine place. And there's a pub. Salmon says that not that long ago there had been rickety sheds, including a 'Psychic Hut' where you could get readings.

> There is a kind of mild pageantry here,
> A rumour of killers in their spare time,
> Of kazoo bands and trying too hard too soon,
> The twirl in the playground, the charge of bayonets in the park,
> The first time you see that there's an "infant" in "infantry".

On the front is a line of brightly coloured beach huts and while most are inhabited by picnicking and sunbathing families, the first three have been commandeered by artists for a project called 'Buffer Zone', named for the area just behind the beach huts which lies between the industrialised 'fun zone' and a serious ecological nature reserve. I pop into the huts. I am struck by some fragments that I assume to be parts of a large crab's shell, but turn out to be plaster casts of the holes the artist has found in the sand, dug by birds and worms. The series of short video pieces is wonderful;

my favourite is 'Bush Dance': a fixed shot on a large windblown bush, it looks 'wrong' somehow, then two of the artists emerge from within the bush, wearing seaweeds and leaves, they sway. End of segment.

In the far distance is a town with a beach. I ask one of the holidaymakers and they tell me it is Exmouth. I decide that's where I'll go. I set off down the concrete promenade, and when that runs out I take to the dune paths. The sand is soft and hard going at times. Eventually, there is a way down to the beach and I take that just to walk on firmer ground.

The tide is on the way out and it is already leaving behind it seaweed and shells on the strandline. Once I have spotted one piece of plastic I am surprised by just how many of the seaweed clusters include a length of fishing line or the remnants of an item of clothing or a fragment of plastic bottle. I find a long thin translucent strip of something; possibly artificial, but I am not sure, it is encrusted with the work of tubeworms and when I peel it open there is some kind of sea slug sheltering inside.

I come to a groyne with a sign requesting walkers to keep off the beaches for three hours either side of high tide to protect the birds gathering on the shore, so I am back on the soft sand paths. They take me a little higher than before and I can see across the water to villages on my left beyond the links with its players marching from green to green. A World War Two pill box is tucked into one of the fairways.

A train darts along in the distance like an unnatural W.O.R.M.

Something howls like a giant owl and I expect to see a mountain-sized bird perched on the far hills.

Such is the intensity of the reserving on this nature reserve, there is very little room for nature. So it feels. The paths are fenced, there are signs of wrapping and propping up of the dunes everywhere.

Then the dunes thin and there is water quite close on both sides; the whole thing seems to relax, the dune expands and the management recedes. I find, amongst the marram grass, tiny oases of unexpected small trees and plants that are more like a back garden than a remote and bleak duneland.

Up ahead two rangers are policing the path, they ask me to stick within the red posts. That's fine with me. I ask them about the Warren and they explain that these days it is a very different shape to what it once was, even in the recent past. It is always changing. At one time there were around sixty houses built on the sand. Obviously had no foundations, but what about the sanitary arrangements? There would have been no plumbing, surely? This, apparently, was a weekend community rather than a shanty town; built on an extended beach for which no MP had constituency and on which no authority levied taxes. When I point ahead to where I imagine the houses to have been, one of the rangers explains that much of the land of this libertarian paradise has gone completely, swept away by the same storms as took the houses. I look out to where he gestures and it is an odd sensation, imagining the unfounded houses hovering just above the deep blue water.

I press on until it dawns on me that I have been completely stupid. The dunes are not taking me to the next town. On my right is the sea, on my left is another stretch of water that is growing ever huger. I am on some kind of narrow arm of land which is going to come to an end and the two bodies of water merge. But I am so far along now that I decide to carry on to the end and then turn back. The wardens' red posts are leading me into a part of the Warren which is its quietest and bleakest, first through something like moorland with meagre mossy growth and then almost a desert.

I see only one other person, a way off. He is not on the path, he is returning from the very end of the spit, the place the rangers have asked us not to go. I wonder about his motives. Why would he choose to put his priorities above the survival of the birds? Maybe his survival is connected with this place, wrapped up in the sands just the same as the gabions, fragments of Royalist fort and bones of Dutch sailors' bodies? One of the men I had passed, seated on a bench on the prom... I'm not sure of course, but I worried for him; his eyes looked inward to something bigger and more troubled than the sea.

Is this the 'wild'? There are no houses here any longer, no mark of human presence except the red posts; it is more complex than the more managed parts. There is more detail here, more texture; an austere and windswept world. A large flat channel, dry now, where the waters must sometimes cut the Warren in two.

I check my watch. A way off on the far point of a prong of sand there are hundreds of grey plover, oystercatcher and curlew. The three hour 'buffer zone' for the beaches is just about to pass. I sit down and let ten minutes tick by.

I walk down to the end of the spit. Everything has been bleached in salt and sun. Driftwood is silver. A fish is dried like an old slipper. Bleached wrapper on an empty food tin, faint Cyrillic alphabet. No bridge, no ferry. Just the boiling waters where the river catches up with the outgoing tide and pulls it down.

I read Salmon. Should have checked before. There is a story about a figure in a machine, a generation before the Wright Brothers, before Bleriot, seen climbing into the sky on the Exmouth side and fluttering down on the dunes.

On the water are boats with bright red, blue and yellow liveries; a dredger, a ferry boat and something else. And over a short stretch of water, what is presumably an estuary, Exmouth begins with its long terrace of large white houses. I can see people moving along the front. And a huge snail-like thing, glowing slightly, blurry and remorseless, seemingly pursuing them; moving first one way then another. I think I know what it is. One of the walkers from the fringe conference had left to recreate Monique Besten's walk where she collected every piece of plastic she found and tied it into a huge bundle around her. From what I can make out, the bundle is already three times the size of the walker. I shout, the town seems very close, but the sound is eaten up in the water.

'Remote' is better than 'wild', generally. 'Remote' has to be 'from' something whereas 'wild' can be invaded without changing status; the quality of 'wild' can be damaged while its status remains the same. But 'remote' means that other things have been successfully held away. That was what the birds required, the absence of even one witness; a lonely and desperate man could keep hundreds of birds from their shore, pilots without landing strips running low on fuel. Perhaps we should stop using 'wild' in the way that we have largely stopped using 'mad'.

I make my way back along the Warren. A light aircraft buzzes it, crazily low. The Shetland Ponies, one white and three black, are indifferent. The ponies are big.

I explain my mistake to the artists.

Beyond the now-redundant camp carriages, is the original cliff face, before the railway came, hundreds of metres back from what is now the shoreline. I feel slightly shocked, though it is a coast, that this is such a temporary, liminal and questionable un-place.

Under the Creep again and I turn past some holiday camps. I am too young to remember our holidays in places like this with my Ma and Dad. They grew out of such places and got a taste for ferries, *moules marinières* and Muscadet. I hated every minute of our holidays; I had nowhere on any continuum of pleasure to put the castles, restaurants and menhirs that seemed to fascinate them; each week was a baffling annual anxiety.

Out of curiosity I turn into one of the camps. Long roads of similar structures; mobile homes on skirts of brick are spaced at equal distance from each other. Given the regimented layout, it is less than sensitive that Vinyl Solutions is one of the firms chosen to provide materials for the camp; wordplay on the Holocaust is either intended to be provocative or spawned of an ignorance that is almost as bad. On the points of the roofs are diamonds, like on garden sheds.

There is something of the model village about it all.

At the end of one long road I find a large pond with a giant weeping willow. Large geese float. Red dragonfly. Green dragonfly. I stand under the trails of the willow. A leaf pokes me sharply in the eye. I jerk back and yet the leaf is still hovering in mid-air, malevolently, ready to strike again. It takes me quite a while to work out that it is hanging there by a single thread of spider silk. I thought Jane might have levitated it.

On my way out of the holiday park, I pass the camp's club, shop, pool, office and 'cantina'. Is this regimentation a comfortingly benign version of the structure of a certain kind of work? Of firm's parties and factory outings, mostly gone now? An echo of the rigorous disciplines of Butlins in its early days which in its turn was echoing the structures of mass production and National Service? Now those 'certainties' have disappeared and are replaced by very little, do these repetitive ground plans and collective provisions – the swimming pool with the sign to PLEASE USE POOL WITH OTHERS IN MIND – constitute a welcome and reassuring enforcement? No lifeguard will be in attendance, but the consumer can still enact the idea of one. Within the boundaries of holiday, this is a chance to live out a less chaotic life than in everyday precarity?

I follow the coastal path. A large white house, set back from the road in grounds dotted with huge rolls of hay has been broken up into holiday apartments: ordinariness behind a screen of luxury. The hips in the hedgerows are violently red. A poster advertises a burglary and loss of personal documents; identities are on the move. I keep passing balancing ponds. The information board lists the gales and storms that knock the Warren into different shapes each decade.

On one side, the railway line is at my eye level. On the other, a tall field wall. Between rough limestone sections are beautifully-worked, yellowy-grey sandstone blocks. I wonder what dissolved monastery has ended up here. An express service roars by a few feet from my head, bending into the curve of the shore. It sounds a warning. There's a footpath here, through a cast-iron kissing gate, directly across the tracks of the express. A train spotter is on guard, nursing a huge camera lens on his chest, and we chat. I ask if there is a footpath on the other side. Only when the mud is exposed, he says. "And if you've got wellington boots." I cross over anyway, checking in each direction four times. Directly in the water is the wreck of the 'South Coaster'. The spotter, who has visited the wreck, says it was a Cardiff-based steamer, built in the Netherlands. It had many names, but he cannot remember them all. Nothing about U-boats, either. It was just poor seamanship, then a storm that broke the ship. Salmon's story about the coal washing up on the beaches keeping the locals warm during the war – he has never heard. The wreck looks like a complete vessel, but the spotter explains that half of it broke up completely. One is inclined to misread a part for the whole.

Captain Peacock's 'Swan of the Exe' was usually anchored here, just off Starcross: a ten-berth sailing yacht shaped like a swan, with four smaller but identical boats (the 'cygnets') for tenders. This is seventy or more years before the South Coaster wrecked. One of the 'cygnets' ended up in Peacock's garden; another as HMS EX 359, an armed rowing boat operated by the local Home Guard. The sails of the 'Swan of the Exe' sprang from its neck and were strangely webbed, more like the fleshy 'wingspan' of a bat than the feathers of a bird.

This Peacock is another of the 'Devil's Footprints', the chain of 19th-century technologists strung out along this coast. As well as patenting methods for desalinating water and salving wrecks, designing a semi-submersible floating battery (Centrax might be interested) and an "unsinkable" bathing dress, his stand-out innovation, in 1822, was the screw propeller. As a good shipwreck modernist, Peacock thieved the idea after watching Archimedes screws raising water in Egypt.

Perhaps not surprisingly, given the coast at hand, the technologists of the route I am walking were mostly wet ones; even Babbage might be thought wet-brained. Inland they still seem to orientate to the deep; just as the earth and animal scientists oriented to the buried thing, to the cave and cavern to find the truth of biblical texts and evolution, so the technologists drew on fluidity and the dynamics of the ocean. Lethbridge in his orchard at Newton Abbot built a pool to dive in, Froude made tanks in his attic, and Forbes Julian (who went down with the Titanic) installed acid baths at his house in Shaldon. And there is something fluid too about the "bending of space" described by William Kingdon Clifford (born at Starcross, though brought up in Exeter) pre-empting Einstein's relativity, a rude grasping of how physical matter might be modelled as "a curved ripple on a generally flat plane". Just like mythogeography's characterisation of pleasure in walking: a wave of narrative around a layer of intensity.

At Cockwood (pronounced 'Cock'urd') I call in at the pub and eat a plate of mussels with a glass of cider. They are good mussels: an inoculation against the memory of bad holidays. Then take the stone bridge-like road across the harbour ('the Sod'). An egret of unreal whiteness is fishing in the waters streaming from a culvert. At the far end of the harbour, on the main road, there stands one of those houses of Georgian elegance, not a big house, which the next century's architects would denigrate; a pattern for the reactionary modernisms of Blomfield and Sharp. Unfussy, tall windows, simple lines, a cross-hatched balcony, a relaxed massing of flat surface.

Dead mouse by the road.

I try a route going inland, but retreat before the traffic. At Starcross a notice in a shop: "Have you lost/found or seen a ferret around Starcross/Cockwood area?" It seems rather too generalised an interest.

The Starcross Garage has shut for good and is up for sale. Just a couple of capped off tubes where the pumps had been; one of the few surviving independent petrol stations no longer surviving. Peering in through the window, a 'Marie Celeste': the tiny office, with a curved wall, a feel you get from 1920s' rural garages, out of place modernism, a new mass production making its first inroad into the old. It looks as if it was abandoned on a whim, or during an emergency; telephone numbers scribbled on the wall, the diary open and a biro laid across the page, a calculator on a scrap of paper, an oily cloth gaffer-taped to a stool, a wristwatch hung on a nail, opened post, an instruction manual fallen to the floor. Had illness come suddenly? A snapshot museum of a working life is fading in its frame.

At the side of the garage there is an old stone horse trough; so this might have been a farrier's yard before it turned to filling and fixing cars. This little stretch is a transport nexus. Just over the road a building with a breccia tower has a smart plaque:

ISAMBARD KINGDOM BRUNEL ATMOSPHERIC RAILWAY
PUMPING HOUSE

The first 'trains' to use the line I have been shadowing had no engines; they were just a procession of carriages pushed by air compressed into tubes between the rails by pumping houses like this one; its Italianate (more theft) top blown off (more composture) in a storm. A capsule inside the tube was connected through an opening-and-shutting flap of leather to the front carriage and that dragged the train. It made no sound. It pumped out no smoke. The energy production was centralised at the pumping houses. The common story for its demise as a system is that the crucial flap was problematical; it had to be kept greased and this attracted rats which gnawed away at the leather seals. Salmon is unconvinced, suspicious that the atmospheric system's dismantling was part of an ideological transition; the shifting of the power source to individual trains would eventually lead to the return of private train companies and the mass production of private motor vehicles.

Another redundant business: The Courtenay Arms. I grasp the irony later.

I had thought about taking the ferry from Starcross over to Exmouth. After my abortive attempt across the dunes, I remembered that one of the performance academics from Plymouth had been talking at Paignton about how their former outlying campus at Rolle, which is in Exmouth, was now being used for counterterrorism training. Gunfire, everything, scaring the locals. I was fascinated by the idea of a geography of fake cities, invented playgrounds for armies to test their tactics on dummies before loosing themselves on real people. I had read some of the work that Eyal Weizman had done on these as part of my research for the conference; how for a while the Israeli Defence Force were teaching the ideas of Deleuze and Debord to its officers, to inform their '*dérives*' through refugee camps. This was a punt that came to grief in South Lebanon in 2006 when the IDF sustained heavy casualties in ground fights with Hezbollah; an event of some significance, because the authoritarian Right has taken much from the left – postmodernism, anti-grand narrative, relativism, fragmentation of truth, the performance of everyday life, and so on – Russian oligarchs quoting Derrida and Lyotard. '*Dérive*', however, doesn't work for them.

From the ferry dock I can see the distinctive shape of A la Ronde, a late 18th-century, sixteen-sided house, originally the home of its possible designers, cousins Mary and Jane Parminter. It stands out, on the edge of suburban housing, an oddly shaped roof rising above the tree line; another of those Devon sentinels. It's a cabinet of curiosities, housing the collections and curios of the Parminters, decorated in sand, feathers, broken glass and china. Exactly who the Parminters were, even in the sense of what they thought of themselves, is fuzzy. Proto-feminist fundamentalist Christians set on converting the Jews as the unfinished business of the Coming Kingdom? End-times arty folk celebrating the end of civilisations in the arrangement of fragments collected on their Grand Tour?

The house takes its place among the sinister towers or 'points in view', along with the likes of Langstone Rock, Lawrence Tower, Starcross Pumping House, The Yannons, Matford Belvedere, Ashcombe Tower and the Powderham Folly.

I decide to turn away from the coast. I am finding no walkers this way. I have caught only one glimpse of a walker all day. Cutting inland, past Tower Cottage with its crenelated cast-iron gate and actual but unreal tower, past a poster for 'Meat Bingo', then through a play park, beyond which an archway takes me into an unexpected maze of new houses; built so close together that the way is cool and shadowy even on this sunny day. Finally, I am churned out onto a country road called Brickyard Lane and head away from the village. The lane takes me out among fields. I recall similar feelings to this as I left the suburbs of Torquay, but I am less anxious. I am more of a walker now. I relax into the pattern of the fields until I come to a junction. A small triangle of land in its elbow is roofed by trees and seems untended; I search for an entrance and, finding a gap, try to climb in over the rusted frame of a metal chair. Then, with an ankle becoming wrapped in a coil of thick wire, I am briefly in that scenario of 'the more I struggle the tighter it grips', but I shake it off in time to trip over a fallen branch. Within the wall of trees are the remnants of a long abandoned 'den', or maybe a homeless person's refuge: covered in leaves now, some corrugated sheeting, a couple of plastic containers, a branch arranged for a bench, and a pile of bedding that appears to be wrapped around something. I nervously nudge it with my toe; relieved that it has the light resistance of something fluffy and feather-based. There is a clear arched entrance in through the hedge; I had missed it, looking the other way at the thin, turquoise towers of the laboratories of the Animal and Plant Health Agency; inside they are anxious about the return of bird 'flu.

The lane begins to climb and to my left a five-bar gate reveals a long and broad strip of grass leading up to the woody hills, about 25 metres at its widest point; the remnant of a drovers' route?

At the top of the hill I turn into a large field. I can see the footpath sweeping around the hill. Walking so often in tall, hedged Devon lanes, it is a rare, liberating moment of seeing my way mapped out ahead of me. Further down the path I am walking in great waves of green, the fields folding and unfolding in long, soft sweeps of raw veg. And then a quite different kind of land; crossing, by right of way, the flat tracts of a country estate; smooth expanses of green giant trees dotted among trenches of brackish looking water.

A castle heaves into view. Solid, but not 'heavy'; a fortification, but a spectacle too. It seems a mass of thick towers.

This is the seat of the 19th Earl of Devon, a direct descendent (kind of) of the 13th-century Robert de Courtenay, not so long inherited from his father (who in 2008 refused a gay couple the right to marry on his property, relenting two years before his death). The 19th Earl was educated at Eton and Cambridge, admitted to the bar of Inner Temple in 1999, and continues to practise as a barrister. The present Countess is a former actress who, perhaps extraordinarily given her present status, appears in the 1991 Wes Craven horror 'The People Under the Stairs'; Hollywood's most trenchant assault on landlordism. The Countess plays Alice, the 'daughter' of psychotic landlords, who is rescued by abused African-American tenants. At various times the characters hide in crawlspaces within the landlords' house; eventually, by their own explosive means, the landlords are destroyed, the cannibal children they have created and imprisoned are released into the night, and their money is blown into the air to be gathered up by their exploited tenants. A couple of days later, I get to fast forward through this unpleasantness; it is striking to witness the future

Countess of Devon drop through a ceiling and beat a landlady's head against the floor.

The Countess suffers from fibromyalgia, which at its worst causes "excruciating pain almost everywhere". I look at the hard exterior of the castle and think of the vulnerability and sensitivity of a body in universal pain. It is easier to think of pain as a point, with a focus, but what of a pain which comes in sheets, or as a plane. What do you rub? Where do you go? How do you hide? That is suffering of an architectural kind.

The Courtenays arrived as immigrants from France during the reign of Henry ll; they gathered a fortune by marriage and Powderham came into their family's control as part of a dowry. For a while the family had four Devon castles and constituted a state within a state, but the late mediaeval period saw the family locked in a series of inter and intra-familial feuding; they featured on both sides in the War of the Roses and were variously dismembered, empowered and reconstituted under the pressure of a powerful independent Haccombe to the south and the rise of a chaotic Tudor patronage more generally. This reached fever pitch when Henry Courtenay was named as next in line to the throne by Henry VIII on leaving for the Field of the Cloth of Gold; insurance, perhaps, should he not make it back. Later though, Courtenay would be beheaded on the orders of the same monarch, and his son imprisoned until released to carry the Sword of State at the coronation of Bloody Mary; a doubtful honour.

Ubi lapsus, quid feci? (The ancient Courtenay motto: Where did I slip, what have I done?)

These were gangster aristocrats in gangster states. During the Civil War they shimmied via Forde House in Newton Abbot as Parliament laid siege to their last Castle. In the 18th and 19th centuries the Courtenays followed the trajectory of power and shifted their focus from intra-national politics to business and law and then to Parliament, standing and then sitting as Tories. William Courtenay, 10th Earl of Devon and son of a Bishop of Exeter was with Brunel on the board of the South Devon Atmospheric Broad Gauge Railway; the line running at the bottom of the grounds here.

Making my way along the wire fence, watching the herd of deer feeding on the other side, I run into a grove of old trees. It is like interrupting a meeting. The trees have the skins of old necks, their great boughs lie, exhausted, on the ground. A pile of broken branches has long dried up.

I sit in the gloomy shade and read the synopsis by Salmon of Devon-based John Trevena's novel *The Reign of the Saints,* a *Turner Diaries* for 1913, doing for extra-parliamentary conservative conspiracy what William Pierce/Andrew Macdonald did for the white supremacist militias of late-20th-century USA. The novel pre-empts, by some 60 years, the paranoid politics of Harold Wilson's Britain, when plans were mooted for a junta led by Lord Mountbatten and the chairman of the National Coal Board.

The central character of Trevena's novel is Hugh Courtenay: "they may hate a Courtenay according to orders, but this side of Exeter they would never lay hands on one. Parochialism is not quite dead". Hugh being the name of the first Courtenay to have the Manor of Powderham, a name that does not return into the family until 1998, though it was one Hugh of Haccombe who saved 'the line' on the accession of Henry VII. The surnames chosen by Trevena for his 'Blue' heroes are iconic: Cavendish, Manners, Howard, Cecil, Pelham, Montague, Talbot, Rodney and Fane, an eternal class that survives civil war, democracy and the severance of its own bloodlines: "all as resolute as their leaders, and pledged like them to a reactionary doctrine of work, self-sacrifice, and duty. No sign of giving way upon those faces, the only ones in England which revealed the lion's breed, and spoke of a connection with that race, hot-headed and piratical perhaps, but above all courageous, which had gone forth from peaceful homes at the clang of the danger tocsin, to make the coastline clear".

Pirates, like smugglers; a solution to the irritation of history.

Trevena's novel is bizarre, misanthropic and pessimistic, yet prescient. It depicts a future Britain where The Hedonists are the party in power, where football plays an inflated part in cultural life and has given rise to a rampant transfer market, with politicised and violent players "controlled by the cheque-book" and playing in stadia with sliding roofs. An information technology of 'wires' brings news and entertainments instantaneously to a people whose "history during the last two centuries" has been characterised by "the religion of agreeable sensations", marked by "less work, better food, more holidays, incessant spectacles and laxity of the marriage tie".

Later, I get a connection to a Gutenberg Project facsimile of the novel and skip-read it in an hour. "All roads lead to the Amphitheatre" in Trevena's Britain and the multi-racial crowds marching there chant "give us Commodities, we will have our Commodities" while on their banners is written LET US HAVE PLEASURES. This is the Society of the Spectacle as conceived by a Grub Street Oswald Spengler. The author writes in the voice of a pinched and mean ego, furious and offended at the pleasure of others; exaggerating and parodying the capacity of the 'other' to cultivate great appetite and its gratification, while never being satisfied. The poison in the prose is not so much in its slurs upon these others as in the creation of a space of auto-justified and privileged disgruntlement, transferable self-hatred and self-pity on the part of a slightly less dominant and slightly more guilt-ridden demi-elite.

The description of the social conditions of the working class – living in huge clubs "where each family had retiring rooms, meeting the others in the restaurant, the gambling-rooms, or the music and picture halls usually attached to such buildings" – sounds remarkably like the set up at the Dawlish Warren holiday camps. Trevena, in common with middle-class liberals, cannot bear collectively organised pleasures.

The cruder context of the fiction is a dystopian society where skilled artisans are played off against labourers, while their parasitic and/or incompetent leaders spend the economy into bankruptcy. As a new crisis approaches, the remnants of the business class and the aristocracy, the Blues, position themselves to gain most from a new revolution. Their leaders are pessimistic about the majority having the ruthlessness to change their circumstances: "a number of pale-faced youths, badly put together, toothless, rachitic, and impotent, threw back their pear-shaped heads, and squeaked like so many bats, 'Football and cheap food! Football and no work! To hell with the taxes!'" Trevena cannot hide his hatred for "a people which summed up life and duty in the one word Happiness"; their indolence entangled with his wish for action against the majority.

His enemy is not simply Socialism and collective action, but pleasure and democracy too. Initially he dresses this up as enmity to a "false democracy", but later that "false" somehow falls away; liberty and equality are next to go. He saves his special ire for golf and weekends. When a character accuses his Blue heroes of trying to bring back Puritanism, Trevena does not refute the suggestion. His feel for the apocalyptic is Jarmanesque; a Statue of Liberty that dare not show its face, a scene in which a court of children try one of their playfellows and then tie him to a railway track and watch him dismembered is as chilling as the burning pram in the 1978 'Jubilee'. Published in 1913, *The Reign of the Saints* has the feel of the 1970s (National Front demonstrations, ubiquitous football violence, economic crises) and it also has the feel of now.

The comparison with Pierce's racist manifesto is not an unfair one; Trevena, real name Ernest G. Henham, had been steeled as a writer during the 1885 Riel Rebellion in the Canadian North-West, when, according to him, "the loyal Archbishop Tache... crushed the rising spirit of independence in half-breeds and Indians and brought insurrection to a close". *The Reign of the Saints* is set in what for Trevena is a nightmare of miscegenation. Behind and within and in front of everything is the racial narrative – so explicit that it robs the book of any dynamic. In the USA the white minority are slaughtered by blacks. Wealthy Japanese consider buying Britain wholesale, and in the streets of London "the yellows [are] smiling contemptuously at the whites". This may be set in the future, but it is no fantasia; in his introduction, Trevena, who lived on the shifty Sticklepath Fault, asks the reader: "has it occurred to you during your walks about London that an entire change has taken place during the last two decades? The same outward show of prosperity, the same pride, but surely a great increase of swarthy faces. Has it struck you that the typical English face is none too common? That the well-known English character is liable to be forgotten during moments of excitement? Must not this admixture of foreign blood be changing to some extent the national character?"

The margin's fear of the corruption of the centre; of a metropolis becoming cosmopolitan.

In Trevena's future, white males have become feeble in body, and, horror of horror, white females, unable to contain their desires under a regime of pleasure, have turned to other races: "if the advanced women had been kept locked up, this country at least might have been able to resist the overwhelming advance of the Asiatic" (this was not a metaphor: as Trevena was writing it Oliver Heaviside had his sister-in-law's sister incarcerated in Torquay and sworn to racial purity); "many of a man's desires and thoughts must remain unintelligible to a woman; and it is the first aim of every woman to oppose and get rid of what she cannot understand. The triumph of woman had come: it meant the extinction of the race. It meant the loss of womanly softness and gentleness, of the graceful figure and beautiful face".

This theme of intelligibility is a key one for *The Reign of the Saints*; not only do women find men unintelligible, but English men find themselves similarly so: "the Englishman: he has never been articulate: ask him to explain his feelings, and he will only stare. He travels along the road of least resistance, accepting all the good he can get, but he cannot and will not explain his actions: he does not understand them himself." The "saints" of Trevena's reign are emotionally constipated supremacists, insecure and anxious to retain women as objects of private property. The psychologist Christopher Bollas describes such personalities as 'normotic', devoid of inner life, a kind of philosophical zombie, with the outward signs of sense and perception, but no actual qualia: these are the people – Trump, Putin, Assad, Erdoğan – who now rule the world.

Sweep aside the racist rubbish from *The Reign of Saints* and there is a far more substantial sub-plot of subjective death in an entertainment culture. Then push the racist rubbish back centre stage and what you have is a Devonian *Mein Kampf*, with the same contempt for "mad democracy" (in Putin's Russia the state-controlled media's word for the opposition is "demoshiza" – democratic schizophrenics), church ("disestablished, degraded, and reduced to a mere bogey of sticks and turnip-head covered with a surplice") and interiority ("the interior becomes darkened, a horrible mystery broods... a figure rises, an idol dark and fearful").

At the climax, economic crisis and political intrigue triggers an election and the ruling party narrowly hangs on to something like power, but the Blues win seats in the countryside – the ruling party can only hold the cities where they can outbid the opposition in bribes. A secret deal is done and the military defence of the country is contracted out to the Japanese government. The ruling party leader mobilises the Players (footballers) as death squads, organises "free meals for all... and in the afternoon a big game". Meanwhile, the Blues organise in an isolated cottage on the Devon moor, where a certain 'Edward Prince' is revealed as a king-in-waiting ready to form a new order of chivalry. The landscape of Devon is far from neutral in Trevena's construction of it; unchanging, it "reminds each knight that he was a son of the nature whose laws cannot be set aside for ever".

While Trevena's tale crudely favours the Blues and the authentic countryside over the corrupted city – "an endless stream of motors carried strangers, that is to say Englishmen, into the metropolis from every side. The horrible lingo of London became drowned by a flood of anglicisms" – his reflections on the operations of power are strangely contemporary. He is clear that on all sides the suppression of women is vital to reaction. On the one hand, The Players (contemporaneously iconic in their exploitation of young women) invade the chamber of the House of Commons: "'We will have no more women in Parliament... No more women-made laws'... It was passed in a rough-and-ready manner", while on the other side, to Hugh Courtenay, passing through small towns and villages on his way to Dartmoor, there is the heinous sight of "groups of women discussing the situation, and processions of other ladies marching solemnly to the end of a street with no other object than to march back, throwing stones at windows, so that they might feel they were advancing the cause of liberty". Trevena the narrator takes pleasure in the breakdown of rule under the thuggery of The Players when "[I]t almost seemed as if human nature had reasserted itself, as if man was still a fighting animal, and women were still wanting in good logic".

With the Players pointedly dressed in Red and Blue kits, the promised football game quickly develops into a violent confrontation between the two groups of supporters, and "as necks were stretched out, and the tiers became all mouths and teeth, and above them endless lines of squinting, half-shut eyes" the mechanics of the carnival are unveiled for all to see: "[T]hey, the spectators, were the spectacle, not the Players".

True to his pessimism, Trevena will not even allow his readers a feel-good Tory ending; the Hedonists are overthrown only for the Japanese contractors to invade.

I get up. The branches of the huge oaks are still dragging on the ground. As if they think, like yews, that they might root again. I pick my way over their fallen limbs.

At the gate I notice that blood is dribbling down the fingers of my left hand. I have no idea when or where I cut myself, but I guess it must have been climbing into the 'den'. I wipe it up with a tissue and lick the scratch; take away the iron taste by eating sweet blackberries growing along the side of the railway line.

Something is stirring in the herd of deer in the castle grounds. A stag with giant antlers – those ones that look unfeasible with huge pointed plates of bone, unbalancing the whole creature – is trotting around, and the rest of the herd are responding to him. Mostly shifting out of his way or briefly chased by him, smaller males emerging to stand before him and then folding back into the herd. All the time the male, his antlers like beams of frozen fire, incanting the same coughing howl over and over.

I pass a bed of rushes that are making mountains and vales.

The road bends around a graveyard full of Courtenays. By the roadside, lying in long grass, are three abandoned telegraph poles, according to their faded labels intended long ago for Torquay. Forgotten now, some part of the abject precarity teetering on disconnection. At Powderham Manor I take the footpath around the edge of a field and a view to a Folly opens up; triangular like the Eye of Sauron on Haldon, a model for it, maybe.

Part of me wants to climb up to it; to diminish it, to reduce it from a feeling to a fabrication. The tower is a dim and controlled ruin; nothing on the fiction that this place has provoked, by fury and rejection. Perhaps I should be bolder and trespass more? I hate humiliation. I feel it and I hide from it. I had surely inhibited the birdman at Torbryan. Without me he might have stolen in and found something extraordinary.

A pheasant takes off, with the sound of shaking metal tongs, a mad flapping of feathers and a trajectory of colours and line of body that are arrow straight; powder blue, sunset orange, Labrador brown. As I turn out of the field and up the curving lane, I am starting, for the first time, to suffer a little from my journey. Not that I am particularly exhausted. A little tired, maybe, but that part of me that has been sustained by the oceanic rush of intensity I have been experiencing for nearly a week... it was all too 'good' to be good for me! I am a creature of punishment and I have been baptised, with the zeal of the recent convert, in the "swimmer's poetics of feel, endurance, and mortal limits" (Mentz); a sailor who cannot resist another voyage, I am beginning to fear that I could not, would not stop, even if I wanted to.

> There is a tower that only stands in dreams
> And when you wake it falls
> And that is all you remember,
> That, the tangle of sheets and the tang of instability

I don't know, maybe it should be read back to front. The dream is the real tower and the real tower is folly. I lean on the wall at the roadside and stare up the bow of the field opposite. The Folly is somewhere above the field, but hidden by its brow which slopes abruptly on both sides, like cupped hands. I imagine myself, earlier on in the day, at the end of the spit of sand, cuttlefish bones, wooden pallets and salt.

I have had time to think. To imagine the waters of the estuary boiling as the incoming tide meets the outgoing flow from the hills. I have fallen for an old temptation. The comforting thought that all this is part of the same story. That when the walking groups moved, they did so in a kind of ballet across a cosmic ballroom; all moving to the same orchestra. Like that drama exercise where everyone in the room tries to start and stop at the same moment without a cue. But the real machine is more of a clanking engine, creaking like pheasants and howling like agitated male deer. With deep structural tensions. In the sand I had begun to redraw the movement as a map of conflicts: immersion against analysis, narrative against multiplicity, phenomenology against mindfulness.

A bus passes. One of the women passengers is wearing a hijab. Not such a common sight in this part of England, but hardly unique or remarkable. (Outside Starcross, where the erosion has turned a pedestrian figure in the pavement oddly green and white, I had met an interracial couple with their child. On the dunes at

Dawlish Warren an Asian man was walking with his tiny child and a white male friend, or his partner maybe.) That is not why I look again. Perhaps to those on board the pattern will not be so clear, but from outside the bus the chequerboard of empty spaces seems far thicker in the seats immediately around her.

The making of place and the ideas associated with it is always in the being there, the doing there, the feeling there. It is only when these makings escape into representation that the separation begins; criticism and theory (and politics) should be repeatedly set upon its feet and made to walk across new terrains; at the mercy of passers-by. That would be far less pleasant for professional opinion-formers, but much better for opinions.

I choke on a blackberry pip that has worked its way loose from my teeth and dropped onto the back of my throat. I hope no one on the bus sees me retching and spitting, bent over a wall.

The woman on the bus; I did not meet her among the walking artists and I have not met her on my path.

There is only a void there, a vacancy, a potential: "alternately invisible and too prominent". (Garnette Cadogan)

For my preparatory research for the conference I had read an essay by Andrea Gibbons on the Salvage website. It answered a question for me, though not in a very comfortable way; for if the travails of the Israeli Defence Force had suggested that 'dérive' doesn't work for them, but it might work for us, Gibbons suggests that it might be even worse for us. A lot of the stuff I'd been reading up on for the conference was connected in some way to this so-called dérive, this destination-less wander that had been practised, for a while, by these Parisian radicals called the International Lettristes some of whom became 'the situationists' and were influential in the student uprising in 1968; wasn't 'destination-less wander' pretty much what I was doing now?

Frustratingly – or maybe this is why it serves everyone so well! – there is very little documentation of those situationist wanders. And Gibbons has the reason. It's directly attributable to the failure of the situationists to defend their Algerian comrade Abdelhafid Khatib after his psychogeographic survey of Les Halles was cut short by arrest (in the context of the Algerian War this constituted an existential threat to Khatib); instead the situationists seem to have closed down the whole project.

The most significant casualties of this kind of silence are the people like Garnette Cadogan who walk in fear and then discover that "I was the one who would be considered a threat"; how easy is it for them to really *walk* with an agentive, hyper-alert state that can draw attention to the walker?

Gibbons's devastating thesis is that the tradition from which much walking arts and radical walking comes – and this is almost all the people I've been walking with in the last few days – is part of the rendering blank of the colonial subject "who can most fully realise the dérive". Not only is it racist, it's self-harming.

As part of her research for the paper, Gibbons recovers a set of abandoned theses on psychogeography written by Michèle Bernstein, who some think is the real brain hidden behind the glamorous bighead of Guy Debord, in which she acknowledges that "the geographical milieu conditions a situation differently for each of its players and has never acted equally upon the affective comportment of all individuals", specifically that "race and nationality... materially condition our experience of power and the city... our play, our movements, even our ability to fully carry out intellectual inquiry", and that these contingent processes are open to those who *dérive* "not [in] subordination to randomness but [in] complete insubordination to habitual influence". In the face of conformism (the conditions for which are created or exacerbated by colonialism) "[I]t is the colonial subject who can most fully realise the *dérive*, whose presence alone represents a complete insubordination, whose body tests the first binding upon the possible that must be smashed".

I walk on. Not at ease.

I see the hills in ways I have not seen hills before.

There are giant fields with few hedges. One vista unfolds from the bottom of the valleys to the base of a hill that then rises up as massive and smooth as the body of a gargantuan whale beached inland, a frill of forest on its nose.

I see the ruin of huge oaks, fallen and silver, and other trunks gone ferrous with the red soil under the slow sun, like ancient trees fossilised in iron. And one tree fallen across the road itself, its mass of roots and lower trunk ripped up on one side and its upper trunk and injured branches fallen on the other. In between, the trunk has been sawn through and cake-like slices hidden behind the hedge. I am feeling the whole terrain moving like a green wave and pushing me on.

The ache in my left ankle, which has been bothering me since Starcross, has shifted into a blister on my right little toe.

I laugh at a jellyfish shape, made of cattle tracks, on the green dome of a field.

A crushed plastic milk carton, its bottom ripped open, laughs back at me, making fun of my jellyfish thoughts under the late afternoon roof of blue.

A buzzard circles around me for a while.

From the garden of the only roadside house I pass I hear the laughter of children playing with their mother, their games hidden by a tall hedge. During all my walking I never see children at play in the woods or in the fields or even out on the roads, except in the towns and cities among the houses. And then an old lodge with a red sandstone coat of arms over the door; the three roundels of *tincture gules* (red balls) of the Courtenays; symbols from the very beginnings of heraldry. The googoogahgah of the aristocracy; that strange language in which the 'great families' once talked to each other and which almost no one else could understand; an inversion of the inclusive teaching symbolism of catholic churches.

A chaotic orchard with cartoon red apples; *pommes tincture gules*. A man parked up in a field flying a drone above the ploughed ridges, an antenna attached to his head, too engrossed to notice me pass by. I wonder what crime he is rehearsing. The lane passes through the hill it is climbing, walls of red sandstone slowly rising up on either side of me. I compute: the straightness of the road, with an MG sports car at one point doing that blurry heat thing in the distance, the lodge with the roundels, the expanse of the land, the orientation to the castle (passing below and with a good view of the folly) and now these cuttings through solid rock. I am on the Earl of Devon's personal coach path. No wonder I am feeling as if I am surging along in oceanic progress, raised up by the land around me despite the weariness in my body; it was cut exactly that way. And I want streams of people, massive crowds, marching like the Hedonists on their way to the Pleasure Game, to feel it too.

I imagine that I am walking in a procession headed by the Great Hedonist, William Beckford, retreating through the pages of his hyper-orientalist novel *Vathek*; a huge influence on Mallarmé and the Decadents. But instead of the "pavilions, palanquins, sofas, canopies, and litters", I imagine the Caliph Beckford held up by swaying crowds of football fans chanting "give us Commodities, we will have our Commodities!" and waving cotton banners with the slogan "Let us have pleasures!"

Beckford, accused by a reactionary relative while here at Powderham of conducting an affair with the male heir to the Courtenay empire, was forced to flee England; only to return years later, having married, but now a widower, and build himself a greater tower than any he might have been expelled from. The tower of his Fonthill Abbey, raised near Bath (and repeatedly collapsing until it fell with finality in 1825) was 300 feet tall; one part of a barely-feasible gargantuan gothic structure, its ruination built into its completion.

The young Courtenay heir eventually became the 9th Earl of Devon and did not hide his sexuality; yet despite his intense popularity among his tenants, he was forced to live abroad and, unlike Beckford, was never to marry and never to return. Despite their immense wealth (Beckford was the wealthiest commoner in Britain), neither man could buy their way back into 'society' (though, unlike Edward Brittain, they did not pay with their lives): such was the importance of heteronormativity to the ideological scaffolding of the empire's collapsible towers.

In *Vathek*, the Caliph (a parody of Beckford himself) builds a palace of the five senses and a huge tower – he built in words first, then in stone – "from the insolent curiosity of penetrating the secrets of Heaven" only to find at his tower's completion and on his climbing to the top that "he saw the stars as high above him as they appeared when he stood on the surface of the earth". Beckford, in exile, took pleasure in the 'lack' of that which, for others, denied him any being at all, but which for him was the very generator of his desires; he cut a figure which, though feared and maltreated, keeps returning even more pleasured and desirous than before.

Vathek's hubris leads him to turn from heaven and seek the abyss, its "slippery margin" and the spirit of the hollow hills; in grim pilgrimage he sets off with his immense entourage: "the great standard of the Califat was displayed; twenty thousand lances shone around it, and the Caliph, treading loyally on the cloth of gold which had been spread at his feet, ascended his litter... The expedition commenced with the utmost order, and so entire a silence, that even the locusts were heard from the thickets."

Lighting "ten thousand torches" to illuminate their path, the procession ignites a forest of cedar and the Caliph and his servants are forced to escape on foot: "Vathek, who vented on the occasion a thousand blasphemies, was himself compelled to touch with his sacred feet the earth. Never had such an incident happened before. Full of mortification, shame and despondence, and not knowing how to walk, the ladies fell into dirt. 'Must I go on foot?' said one. 'Must I wet my feet?' cried another. 'Must I soil my dress?' asked a third... 'Better were it to be eaten by tigers than to fall into our present condition!'"

That's a good lesson – the super-rich hate nothing more than walking!

I had no idea that such extraordinary people, nor such extraordinary ideas, could have emerged from these few miles – Peacock, Clifford, 'Alice', 'Vathek' – but I suspected that wherever I had walked the density would have been exactly the same. Yet, because they are separated from space – because education would rarely teach any of these fictions or their authors in any of the local schools I was passing on my way – these anomalies (screws, a curved ripple on a generally flat plane, beating a landlady's head upon the floor, hearts in ignition) have always been detached from the everyday and float free to be picked off only within the privileges of academe.

If we are too interested in a geography of foci, of named concepts, of points of contact, of trouble, of the edge of identity, then we miss the flatness; we miss the plane in which these anomalies can sit and spread. We miss the dynamic fields of everyday life; different from the pointed moment when power pivots around an issue in daily politics or a balance changes in a drawn-out war or a meme goes viral. Everyday life is not like them; it is not a war, nor a positioning, nor an escalation but a dispersal of pleasure and gentle just-being; it is a hovering of the fields and platforms where those without separate power live and have life. Not at the foci.

The genius of lay armies in the last twenty years has been to run away, to take off their uniforms and to 'be weak', un-engageable, unfindable, re-emerging in their own time, to their own timetable. That is what everyday life is: the protection of subjective life as a *modus vivendi*. As I walk what now feels to me like it should be my last few days, the news I overhear in bars and breakfast rooms is about how IS, having seized its own caliphate is now being surrounded and at least partially routed and destroyed; its 'principled' application of its own narrow authoritarianism has directly translated into the container of its own elimination. A brief period of compression yields a thick concentration of power and then its exposure and confrontation. Everything I have seen and learned from the walkers (except perhaps the unconvincing passage on 'cells' in *Mythogeography*, subsequently disowned by its author) is about diffusion and diffraction; about missing the point for as long as possible.

Being jelly. Float. Leave the assembling of flotillas to storms and tides.

I get it now.

Finally.

So, it is nothing to do with the history of the past in this part of England. It is not some awful burden being dragged about by its residents; the householders of Plantation Street beggared forever by the name, the tourists burnt and blistered by the aura from the plunders of Palk, Lawrence, the loveable Colonel Smith with his twin house in pink in Nice and the East India Company. No. They were making colonial space in the bus as it passed! They were, in that second, as it swayed by, making a body of lack right there!

And the whole map ripples.

Passing what looks like the start of a hollow lane, by a sign to Try Your Brakes, I pause to let a farmer load a couple of bullocks onto a trailer; driving away, leaving the rest of the herd to complain loudly to me. Then, at the top of the hill, beyond Crablake Farm, there is another golf course. As far as I can see there is no one playing on its extensive fairways. I am sure it is busy at other times, but given that golf courses cover about the same amount of land as houses (*sans* gardens) in the UK, and given the shortage of housing, two things strike me: maybe we would not be such a "crowded island" if there was no golf, and if there was no golf maybe there would be no homelessness. I wonder, if that happened, whether golfers would turn to terrorism, just as cat owners surely will when the predation on wild birds by domestic felines finally reaches the point of mass extinction and legislators are forced to act?

A line of hand-assembled Morgan 4/4 cars wait like soldiers under inspection.

Strange that so many different makes of car sport a brand logo with wings, when none of them fly!

Well, Supercar, I suppose? Chitty Chitty Bang Bang? AeroMobil 3.0?

OK....

On a road to my right a woman is wearing a gas mask in her garden. The government is poisoning the atmosphere.

The day after I pass through the village, communal bins are taped up and cordoned off; police search the property of a Royal Marine suspected of supplying arms to dissident Republican terrorists.

I pass through a jumble of cottages and modern houses, thatch and breccias, Victory Hall and Tesco Express. I am impressed that the clock on the garage (Independent Garage of the Year, 2000) is working accurately, and then something special. On one side of the road is a grand gothic portal with tall stone pillars and huge iron gates and two lodges, North and South; while on the other side is a modern estate, it looks just a few months old, with an equally epic portal made by the big side walls of two new houses, one of them three and a bit storeys high. I take the turning into the new estate, down a road closed to everyday traffic in the middle of an expanse of grass between two lines of houses. Behind each line are back streets accessible to traffic.

Unlike most of the 'new estates' I have walked through – recent or 1920s' – this one has a vista, a sense of its own landscape, a vision that looks outwards. The grass centre is broad enough to hold trestle-table parties. There is no uniformity to the houses; they have the same jumble as on the Main Road. I think I might have enjoyed growing up here.

The houses are on a slope down and then beyond the homes, the land rises again up to a newly planted, greenish hill with wide paths around it and ramparts and ditches. It is a fake fort, I think. The earthworks feel too precise, contrived. O, I hope it is a fake. That is the kind of luxury that everyone should be afforded.

After my little brother and I had left home, our folks moved into a little suburban house with a mediaeval moat across their back garden. Everyone should have these absurdities; and where they are missing, they should invent them. At the top of the 'fort' I can see to the ridge of Haldon Forest and the thickness of the big river as it approaches the estuary at Exmouth. I think I can just see the shape of the Folly over Powderham, but it might be a conflation of trees.

I smell sulphur. Maybe this is an old tip?

The play area on the hill is wonderful: writhing remains of dead trees and a climbing frame that looks like an explosion in a lumber yard.

Retracing my steps I walk up through the two lodges and their huge gates, along a nameless avenue lined with black trees, towards the palatial buildings of a former psychiatric hospital; Vathek's abbey. A clock on the large central tower, like Exminster Garage's, tells the correct time. Among all the threats of action against unsanctioned car parking, there is a map of the complex; it is almost identical to the illustration of a modern panoptic workhouse taken from Pugin's *Contrasts*, as described in Peter Blundell Jones's *Architecture and Ritual*: "[T]he relationship between space and activity is evidently neither a compelling certainty nor open and random, but complex and variable. What makes it so hard to pin down is that it is a two-way process involving a 'reading' as well as a 'doing', so that there must be some complicity between user and building".

Is the attraction for home-buyers to these buildings to be found in their ordering, their pseudo-collective structures, their now spectral disciplines and therapies providing a supporting net of spidery rules and etiquettes to their contemporary, well-heeled conservationists? Are these the better-off equivalents of the holiday camps?

I spend a moment reflecting in Bowling Green Park; pretty clear what this flat and square space once was. It is designated a REFLECTIVE/QUIET SPACE; judging by the litter blown by the winds into one corner, sugar drinks are an important part of contemplation here. What I reflect on is that there are still areas in the north of France, once under the occupation of the English, called "Le Bowling Green".

The road is bending back on itself towards the centre of the village again, so I take a sharp right turn up Farm House Rise. No farmhouse I can see, but I pass through a gate into some kind of nursery, between greenhouses and keep going straight on, following a black tarmac surface; I am not sure if it is a continuation of the street outside the nursery or just a path to the buildings; someone will tell me. I pass an enigmatic brick structure and some discarded machinery. Then I am in a massive field, with the black road still going straight across it.

The field is like a scene from a biblical plague.

Wreckage of maize plants lies smashed all around me and down across the long hill. I get the feeling I should not be here, yet under the shattered stalks and cobs there is still the road. I cross the field, keeping to the tarmac, and it runs out at the hedge on the far side. I was expecting some way through, but there is nothing. I look for some shadow of a trampled path. Nothing. I am uneasy now. I am waiting for one of the drivers in the huge maize-smashing machines far off in the field to come over and throw me out. I decide, against my nervousness, to follow the edge of the field. There is no visible path at all, but this almost immediately brings me to a break in the hedge and a set of soil steps in the bank down to a small road.

The road is Deepway Lane. (A cousin to Hollow Way, perhaps.) Wonderful name. I dither for a moment, tempted to take the steep turning immediately to my left down Coffins Lane. I go to satellite brain and I can match this lane to the black tarmac track I have just been following through the field and nursery and then by the old hospital across Main Road to the mediaeval red stone church in the middle of the village. Pretty obviously, which is often the most misleading state to be in, this is a corpse road for the people of the sparse valleys I can see beyond the fall of Coffins Lane. I resist and follow Deepway Lane with the prospect of a city and dinner in mind.

From the drive of Matford Belvedere I can make out the little white eye of the Lawrence Tower (Haldon Belvedere).

I find the corner of the giant maize field. There is an old iron gate fixed solid now by branches, but walkers have trodden a path around it. I watch the massive machine, with a device like a giant barber's clippers; it's tearing up the maize which is shredded and chugged into a bin, gristle spat out the back; it "has the bizarre outline of a prehistoric monster, and is perhaps in about the same stage of evolution". Across the waste of maize crop I can see down to a motorway, curving round a distant and huge flyover, cars and lorries shuttling over. It looks exactly like the opening to a kids' TV serial I would watch on UK Gold in the 1990s. We had a tape of it. The show was called 'The Changes' and it was all about how people suddenly turned against technology, smashing up all the devices in their homes, and began to build an agricultural economy. The machines that survived – like electricity pylons – spooked people out and made them sick. It all ends in a Hollow Hill where a talking stone reveals itself as the source of the chaos, "trying to make a better England" by returning things to pre-Industrial Revolution days. The young heroine puts it to rights. At least that is how I remember it.

I laugh. Because the road – this little lane – almost immediately takes me across an immensely high bridge (good thing I do not have vertigo!) over the motorway.

Someone has attached a very slow ticking bomb to the bridge: a steel padlock that will, one distant day, rust through and fall into the path of the cars.

Once off the bridge, the lane narrows and bends. Radio masts in a nearby field look like the tops of a grounded sailing ship. Down, far below, to one side is a quarry of startling blood-orange sand, piled into a perfect fifty-foot high cone; a secret facility for making giant Platonic Solids. The lane is travelling over the tops, with views to the approaching city and out to forests and river and hills whenever it is not cut too deep in the sandstone. I am a knife carving through the body of a county; but this is not as 'natural' as it always appears. What seems like a raw piece of sandstone, when I look more closely, is a piece of very old wall, red blocks piled at first one way and then another. There is always a play of fabrication around the organic. If there is such a place as "untouched" I have never found it.

At the bottom of the long winding lane I come, abruptly, to a large and busy roundabout. The beginnings of a commercial estate are just beyond the junction, and right on it is a hotel. In the failing light the elegant shape of a Georgian mansion is still detectable beneath the branding. I choose to press on into the city, until I see that there is a second and more extraordinary part to the hotel: a motel wing which, despite some recent makeover, cannot hide its gorgeous modernist origins. It looks like a machine too; an extendable clamp or an adjustable spanner fastening on the traveller. I book in impulsively. I hate horror movies, but this is as close as I will ever get to the Bates Motel and I love the new series with Vera Farmiga. She is my role model... as a mother, you understand.

I take dinner in the hotel's Carriages Bar & Brasserie: *gnocchi.*

The cars whirl and whirl. I have a window table. I spectate.

What is art?

Not what does it do, and why do people do it and watch it? But what is it? Like, existentially.

Isn't it discipline? Isn't that what those folk in the old asylum and in the holiday camp are after: an 'art' of living?

When I was 'kneehigh to a grasshopper', I just caught the last deathbed gasp of a certain kind of popular working class art: kazoo bands, majorettes, that sort of thing, the dust beneath the feet of choirs and brass bands. Mostly it was not actually happening, it was dead and in photos in frames on sills or up on club walls. Or memorialised in pennants. The last moment before the middle-class ideal of self-expression finally stubbed it out and swept it away under a carpet of egoism and disintegration.

All night, in my dreams, I am being waved over by a cop on a motorbike; hiding the notes for my conference report under a copy of Strindberg's *To Damascus* trilogy. When the officer finally comes to the window his face is that of the desperate man in the Paignton church.

Mount Pleasant Road, Beach Road, Dawlish Warren (to end of the spit and back, only at low tide), under the Creep, Beach Road, Dawlish Warren Road, at Cockwood bear right on road (Church Road) across the harbour, turn right onto A379, The Strand, Bonhay Road, play park, through gap in top right corner, Sercombes Gardens, wind through paths between houses, then Heywood Drive and right into Brickyard Lane, at the T-junction right into next lane and almost immediately left into next lane, at the next junction (with a 'den' on your left in the angle of junction) turn right until at the top of hill turn right onto a signed (with stile) public footpath, at the four directions signpost go straight on, cross over the busy road (Southtown) and walk left along the pavement, turn right onto footpath across grounds of Powderham Castle towards the River Exe, on the other side of the estate turn left onto the road running parallel with the railway line, Church Road, cross the field on the footpath starting opposite Powderham Manor, at the end of the field turn right onto the lane and follow this for about three miles to Exminster (crossing the A379), Main Road, right into new estate opposite gateway to Devington Park (former psychiatric hospital), Milbury Farm Meadow, take paths bearing left and walk around the hill with play area and back to Main Road, take road up to Devington Park, Reddaway Drive, Farm House Rise, follow tarmac road/path straight through greenhouses and straight across field, at top of the field move right along the edge of the field and look for steps on your left made in earth to climb down to the road, right along Deepway Lane, Old Matford Lane, Devon Hotel.

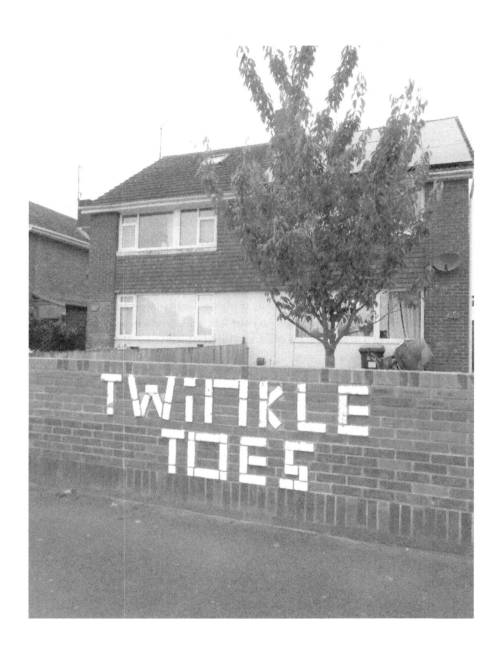

Chapter Twelve: Inner Exeter

I set off down Bad Homburg Way. With apologies to the Oberbürgermeister who opened it in 1987, I mentally re-name it 'That's Some Bad Hat, Harry Way'.

Cars. Hundreds and hundreds of cars. Not on the roads; these are stationary cars. 4x4s ramped up to look like they are climbing over rocks. A Mini hung with tyre marks to make it look as if it's flying up the side of its showroom. Supercar. The Ferrari logo is a horse, another symbol of spurious flight; it was the good luck symbol painted on the side of his aeroplane by an Italian First World War fighter pilot. I jump out of my skin as a prospective buyer guns his Ferrari out of the showroom, down a road of showrooms past the livestock market, where some kind of demolition has resolved itself into a huge accidental Dali, a whirling mass of bent steel grids with chunks of concrete suspended throughout; the spit of 'Head Exploding'.

Trans Plant Mastertrain. What the hell is that? I hope they supply surgeons with huge freight trains full of organs. They don't. They train general HGV drivers.

Back on Bad Homburg Way there is a jam of traffic backed up as far as the eye can see. I want the Ferrari buyer to be caught up in this. I check out the cars as I overtake them. Big cars, some of them. Expensive cars, most of them. A few works vans, but mostly highly polished trophy cars. The density of cars is very thick, with the huge showrooms packed one next to the other and the snail-pace of the bumper-to-bumper commuters. I see the whole horrific nightmare of oily dreams. The horrible graininess of work, grinding out painful years of labour and tedium in order to buy a better car to get more ostentatiously to further painful years of labour and tedium in the warm light of the jealousy of fellow commuters. I am becoming a bigoted ambulatory chauvinist. Fiona Wilkie would hate me. I turn off through a wooden gate and follow a fabricated curved rise that hugs a concreted brook. I rather like it. Then into Clapperbrook Lane: a narrow cul-de-sac with an odd raised pedestrian platform of packed earth on one side, its wooden rail now rotting away. Although an obscure little route today, I guess that the platform (which I avoid, it looks far more menacing than the road) was put there to separate walkers from its once considerable traffic; I have not noticed any similar efforts on far more unnerving roads than this.

I am rewarded with confirmation at an information board. It has been a while since I saw one of those; perhaps they have all been stolen and joined the metal forest off Long Lane. The name Clapperbrook refers to the type of bridge – they are common up our way in Yorkshire – by which the lane once crossed the watercourse when this was the main route down to Plymouth and Cornwall for travellers and their goods looking to avoid the distractions of the city. I find it odd to think of this little lane, so dark now and constricted, as the mediaeval equivalent of a Bad Homburg Way packed with horse and cart jams. There is some kind of centre; an inn, a cob wall, a St Michael's church (with the archangel busy spearing the mouth of the dragon) and a memorial with a restored wayside cross. The niche in the cross head is empty and I wonder what it would have held. An image or sculpture presumably. It's clear that the head is made of different, older stone than the shaft; the fracture is more evidence of the work of iconoclasts.

I am back to the jumble of old cottages, thatches, fake Dutch gables and 20th-century semis. I pass a group of schoolchildren and then a car passes me, driver winds down the window: "chaos, unnut?"

I realise how thin a line there is, for some folk, between normality and collapse.

The lane brings me to another large roundabout; I am weaving in and out of some bypass system. I run across to the centre of the roundabout and nervously push my way into the trees there. I am expecting that there is some kind of encampment of homeless people in the leafy haven within the whirling steel and aluminium, but there is no one here. I get caught in rose thorns, tearing my coat, and reverse down the hill until I can find an easier way through; finally the growth relaxes and I enter a small clearing in which, despite the heavy fall of leaves, I recognise a structure. A much easier way in; a set of wooden stairs. I trace them to the bottom and then back up to the top; hidden in the trees is yet another phone mast. I am disappointed; the curving leaf-carpeted staircase deserves better. I re-cross the road and scuttle through the underpass; cars racing beside me. I am tempted to explore the other half of the roundabout, but that feels like repeating myself, so I take the turning signed to Ide, partly because since that mediaeval centre back there with the niche that carved its emptiness into my brain I have been following Ide Lane and it feels like I should. The name is intriguing. Is it a place of omens? Only in March, maybe.

This is a good time to tell you about a meeting with experimental walkers that did not take place here, but somewhere similar to the hidden centre of the roundabout; close to busyness and yet secure and isolated. I am also not going to give too much away about the walkers themselves. I was never quite sure where they were drawing the line between intimacy and confidentiality, which is partly why I did not take them up on their offers. The long and the short of it, as my Dad would say, is that they invited me to join them in simultaneously pleasuring myself and a place; to engage erotically, to orgasm, with a vista and an object close at hand. They (and I will avoid specifying gender or genders) explained that they sought out places with strong textures (irrespective of design or natural materials) and an impressive view. They were not concerned with whether the landscape was natural or industrial or suburban or whatever, but they did specify some kind of instinctive sensual attraction to it. I had surprised them in their preparations – not quite foreplay – which appeared to me to be a kind of undressed archaeology.

I am embarrassed to admit that I did not accept their invitation, though I was tempted, which almost certainly means that I should have. Perhaps what put (turned?) me off was the idea of the sexual as magical, as somehow transforming the site more than any other kind of presence might have. If it had been a simple matter of taking pleasure I might have felt minded to join in; it was the prospect of sexual exchange that unnerved me; I'm being honest, now. I left them to their shooting, dribbling and squirting; the wind rose and a light rain began to fall for a minute or two, almost the only rain I saw on my journey. I did not feel disappointed in myself, but I think the terrain for a while was a little disappointed in me. It felt cooler for some time after.

It is further to Ide than I imagined. Either side of the road, in a cutting, are incredibly thick growths of shrubs and small trees. Except for a few spaces where a tree has poisoned a little of its own ground, the weave is impenetrable and forbidding. Nor had I expected such a fast road: cars at 70 mph. There is a pavement, but in the lanes I had grown unaccustomed to the proximity of such speed. Then suddenly, far up ahead, cars hammer to a halt, brake screeches, and a horse and a rider veer out into the road, the beast shying and stuttering across both lanes. Finally the rider brings the animal under control and they make their way, staccato, along the edge of the road. Horse and rider pass me on the opposite side of the road and I avoid looking at them, fearful of spooking them again.

I part with the fast road at the long, cream Pole House and take the quieter Old Ide Lane; I ignore another wayside cross for the seductively curly ramp of the steel bridge over the busy road. Strapped to its metal is a notice from Teignbridge Council (I have clearly re-crossed an administrative boundary) that the "Ide Rural Skip Service" will take place on the following Saturday. I hope that a "Hop Service" with much drinking and a "Jump Service" with much pleasuring will be observed, equally religiously. On the other side the bridge uncurls itself around a rich centre of dock leaves and other greenness, over an old bridge and past 'The Twisted Oak' pub and then past the Twisted Oak itself. 'Legend has it' that a troublesome imp is sealed up in its twisted trunk, put there by 'an Oxford-educated scholar'. Presumably in the days when scientists and alchemists were indistinguishable. The nature of the imp's mischief is intriguing: for it is blamed not only for the obstinacy of butter in the matter of churning and a tendency for cider to sour, but also for the sexual assault of women and the greater likelihood of neighbours arguing. And what if this scapegoating and transference were to be focused not on an imaginary force but on an Oxford scholar and his liberal arts?

I find the cross at the top of Little John's Cross Hill, in the garden of a modern house. It is a sister cross to the one at Alphington; I am contouring round the city, picking up its major arteries. I cross the main road to have a look at the freemasons' care home, but it is forbiddingly panoptic. Crossing back, the view to the city down

Dunsford Road is remarkable. From here, in 1877, Musopolus, a local poet, saw a "multiform'd being" forming over the maze of Exeter streets and heard from the station at St Thomas "the scream of the great Familiar, Steam".

The wide verge is a green carpet laid out to the centre of the city. Why do I not take it? I am not ready for a city, yet. And I have noted a little lane I want to explore. I am addicted to these things; after so many country footpaths, the smoothness of the metalled and stone surfaces of these lanes allows all my energy to go upwards and outwards without worries about footing. But I am mistaken; the tarmaced road quickly turns into a narrow and bumpy 'hollow way' under thick tree cover and, there, coming the other way, is the huge frisky horse that I saw charge into the busy road. On seeing me, it shies. I am only slightly less skittish and back up to a niche in the side of the lane. As they pass, I say to the rider "spooked by those cars earlier?" and she, surprisingly young, says to the horse, as he looks at me: "there, Mister, see, nothing to be scared of, you wuss".

For the rest of my time on the hollow lane I am alone in hobbit territory; gnarled and twisted roots and branches, and gates sculpted from broken lengths of corrugated iron seem to make it more mythic. Below in the valley are orchards, small cottages and columns of chimney smoke. I expect at any moment to meet more of the Black Riders, the remaining eight of the nine Nazgül under the sway of Haldon Belvedere. I turn down Roly Poly Hill and I am racing for the city now, emerging on a main road opposite a huge mediaeval farmhouse, Cowick Barton Inn, where Salmon says he first heard about *The Reign of the Saints* from the scholar Bob Mann at a meeting organised by the Centre for Fortean Zoology.

I keep pace with the backed-up commuter traffic, then cut through suburban streets and alleyways, past a group of girls nervously playing some game on an iPhone and a huge bricked sign on a front wall reading TWINKLE TOES, form fighting content, and emerge into a large and featureless playing field where one boy is playfully knocking about another. I am disoriented by the expanse, homing in on a huge flowerhead-like shape across the pitches. It turns out to be an immense seat, but empty now.

There is a park within the park. I walk through the gates: PINCES GARDENS 1912-2012. There is little more than a tree-lined path, and it does not get much more interesting when a set of dark wedges of topiary opens up on my left, but I go to look anyway and beyond it is something that appears at first glance to be a row of short entangled trees, but is far more: an extended arch of Wisteria, a tunnel of restless, thrashing and serpentine branches, a tornado twister of floral snakes attempting to crush itself to death in a purple storm. I wander within, bashing my head on the first of the low and unforgiving branches; the momentary giddiness only adds to my sense of being digested by flora. I don't know it yet, but I have entered the first of a sequence of equivalent spaces across the city of Exeter encountered over the next couple of days; the remnants of 18th- and 19th-century nurseries that for two hundred years – gardens with the life span of major factory processes – ran complementary to the politics and economics of the empire, ripped out its foreign flora and brought it here, and in the process transformed the ecology at both ends of the trade.

These dealers were inventing, filling and servicing the gardens of a generation of managers, bureaucrats and enforcers who were returning from working for the East India Company and its equivalents with immense fortunes to spend, settling discretely, but spectacularly, behind high walls in the Exeter hinterland. When contemporary horticulturalists rant on about migrant iniquities, Himalayan Balsam and Japanese Knotweed, 'we' invited them here in the first place.

This is where the Lucombe Oak was genetically and accidentally engineered; from Turkey Oak and Cork Oak parents. Their Dr Frankenstein, William Lucombe, saved planks cut from the original hybrid tree for his coffin; by the time he died, aged 102, the wood had rotted and new planks were sawn. The business became an empire in itself; with rock gardens, Italian garden, winter garden, bamboos and yuccas, a banana tree, even cottages around a fake village green.

The tree line that fringed the nursery is still mostly intact; the survivals are giant and exotic. Redwoods tower over the allotments. Without anthropomorphising these things, I want to acknowledge their abject lives; organisms that are not indifferent to their 'grounds' or their space. I have seen them in their enclaves, on lonely watch in gardens, penned in expansive grounds. I cannot help but draw the connection between these imported beings and the trade in human ones. The trees and plants were uprooted and cut, the seeds harvested and brought to do nothing but survive and display and die. There is an *arbor sacer* thing going on here; sacred trees that can be cut down by anyone. Their middle taken out when they fall on the highway; the rest left to rot.

Across the Croquet Lawn I get my first sight of the solid twin Norman towers of the Cathedral. Outside the gates the same girls I saw earlier playing with the phone are engaged in some version of Grandmother's Footsteps; testimony that digital and traditional cultures are not necessarily mutually exclusive.

I have reconnected to the artery running past the cross under St Michael's gaze. The jumbling of cottages and modern suburbia has become a mixture of severely faded pre-Victorian grandeur struggling to find a purpose and heavy Edwardian shells changing theirs, while small cottages have shrunk back like hermit crabs into stolen ground.

The garage with clunky iron gates that time has rendered down to an attractive starkness is one more card to a flush from Starcross through Exminster of longstanding independent garages that I will soon add to. The faceless corporatism of car sales, only baulked by the Morgan cars at Exminster, has not quite dominated maintenance with its diagnosis, improvisation, dependence and trust.

Passing a swimming baths opened by the chaste and chased and then "unchaste Diana" in 1985, I cross the hybrid bridge/roundabout. In the underpass are two fine graffiti jellies, one red and raw and goofy, the other melting, yellow and reminiscent of the ufological one in the ruins of SIMLA. Back at ground level, Fore Street is a street almost-happening, you can feel its straining at the profit margins, the precarity of its eccentric ventures and the energy of its designs. At the top, where it becomes the High Street, I cut through a gap in the buildings, the narrowest street in the world according to the plaque; its name – Parliament Street – was a snub to Westminster for failing to extend the franchise during the Reform Act conflicts of the 1830s. The author Phil Baker had once jumped the gap from roof to roof on a drunken night out; I mentally re-name it Baker's Leap.

I cut through the Guildhall shopping centre, amused at an abject clump of cobbles, rescued from a Roman Road, and these days mistaken, surely, for one of those uneven surfaces contrived to keep homeless people from finding a temporary home. On Queen Street I pass the Museum and four neo-classical heads above a beauty salon, possibly in Coade Stone. Later I meet a live artist enthusing about a spiral car park ramp behind St Sidwell's Church, her work a drag investigation of brutalism. What is it about female artists here and concrete?

I spot the Mercure Rougemont hotel and book in. Leaving my rucksack – I am getting used to staff hiding suspicion and disdain – I head back to the High Street.

Salmon mentions the collector C.V.A. Peel and upstairs in the award-winning museum I find a giraffe and an elephant (I cannot help flashing back on the bashful plastic elephant in the reeds around the koi carp pool) he shot – exercising "all the faculties which go to make a man most manly" – and then donated to the Royal Albert Memorial Museum on moving to a home near the city, in 1919, I am not sure exactly where.

> All at once we heard the crack of a branch, and knew we were up to the game. Scarce daring to breathe, with my heart pumping against my ribs, my rifle held ready before me, I advanced on tip-toe amongst the bamboos... One could hear the strange rumbling sound made by the animals' intestines... At last I saw a beast which was undoubtedly a male... I could not get a broadside shot at the bull, so fired a slanting shot for his heart. When the report rang out there was a tremendous commotion. All the elephants rushed together trumpeting like Sousa's band. The bamboos went off crack, like pistol shots, as the elephants tore through them down the bank. The earth literally quaked with the thunder of their feet as they moved off all round me... For two solid hours we tracked that bull, expecting every moment we should be charged. At last I got up within a few feet of him, and, taking careful aim at his head, I killed him instantaneously. He was a magnificent fellow, ten feet in height at the shoulder. His right tusk measured 6 feet 3 inches, and weighed 63 lb, and his left measured exactly 6 feet, and weighed 61 and a quarter lb... That night I had roasted elephant's heart for my Christmas dinner... This magnificent animal is now to be seen stuffed whole in the museum at Exeter.

When I look at that elephant now I think of Adam.

Adam was a butcher; for he changed his rib for a bit of skirt."

This was not his only butchery, however.

In 1927 Peel published a novel about a failed utopia, called *The Ideal Island*. It is an odd thing – an obvious autobiographical fantasy (just as much as Beckford's *Vathek*) in which Peel (in the guise of the hero) escapes from "vulgar newspapers which govern and order all our doings" and "the modern politician... [T]o him the Empire can go hang while he is plotting and planning to rob and plunder from the upper and middle classes in order to make the indolent working man of the present day still more indolent" to an "uninhabited" desert island with eleven single men and twelve single women; with the expectation of a smooth heterosexual pairing off. O my goodness, though, it turns out (as always) that there is an inconvenient indigenous population. That must be why Peel's expedition to an uninhabited island has packed a machine gun and a field gun. The natives are quickly exterminated:

> he gave orders that all the wounded were to be finished off on sight... the only safe way of dealing with such fanatical, frenzied people... The firing was so heavy that Frederick sent Queenie galloping up to us on pony-back to ascertain the cause and she returned saying that we were merely finishing off the wounded... Next morning we dragged the dead into the bush, dug a pit and put them into it.

Treated them no better than the theatre dead of the West Quarter.

> I cleaned the skull of a corpse for a museum specimen, much to the disgust of the rest of the company!

Ah no, that is different.

Peel died in 1931. In 1932 Peel's widow made a large donation of animal remains to the museum. In the 1930s the museum acquired three Melanesian human skulls; they still have them. The documentation for only two of them name a donor.

I found it difficult to be in this building; its adoption of a performative and participatory style left almost no space for contemplation. By animating their displays they had made them not only illuminating, but also blinding. It was only Joanna Southcott's ritual implements that saved me. And the fossilised burrow.

Salmon says that Southcott worked as a servant for the Taylors in nearby Gandy Street – one of many originals for J. K. Rowling's Diagon Alley – and I went there, to stand by the loading area behind Tesco's, by the dormant mesh-sided shelf trolleys, and the piles of cardboard, where the house of Southcott's employers had stood, and to channel Joanna, the woman clothed with the sun. In the last years of the 18th century, she dreamed visions every night, and every morning she translated them into doggerel. She was also an early surrealist, an exponent of automatic writing: "the

writing comes extremely fast, much faster than I could keep up by voluntary effort...
I need not look at the paper. I can talk on other subjects while writing".

Her publications of rhyming prophesies made her the first nationally read
female author since Aphra Benn. Rejected by the established church – believing she
might form a magical union with a Reverend Pomeroy (the apple king) – she realised
her own leadership: "Is it a new thing for a woman to deliver her people? Did not
Esther do it? And Judith? Was it not a woman who nailed Sisera to the floor?"

For some reason I remember Alice hitting the landlady's head on the boards of
the cellar.

The Strange Effects of Faith.

The thing about Joanna is that many of her prophesies came to be; from the
death of the Bishop of Exeter, through the failure of peace negotiations and the
Napoleonic forces' victory in Italy she demonstrated that the distracted intuition of
a woman servant was a better interpretation of her times than 'the experts'.

She gathered to her the followers of the Paddington Prophet and British
Israelite, Richard Brothers (whose ideas on the Jews were similar to those that
drove the Parminters' mission at A la Ronde), at that time working in an Islington
asylum on designs for the flags, costumes and architecture for a symmetrical New
Jerusalem. Seven of his wealthier followers – Joanna's Seven Stars – arrived at the
Guildhall on Exeter's High Street to collect a box of prophesies, bound with seven
seals, that would be argued over, advertised, hoaxed and faked, for the next two
hundred years. Rather pleasingly the 'authentic' box (one among many), when
finally opened, revealed numerous items, many rather 'everyday', including a bone
puzzle and a copy of Ovid's 'Metamorphoses' (I hope it was the wonderful Arthur
Golding translation).

Dying at 64 from a cancer she believed to be the foetus of the prophet Shiloh,
preamble to a messiah, howling crowds gathered outside her house in London. Her
followers kept watch over her reeking corpse in case of its revival, while others
proclaimed a spiritual and invisible re-birth: "and the dragon stood before the woman
which was ready to be delivered, for to devour her child as soon as it was born".

During the 1970s, odd little adverts would appear in British newspapers: "War,
disease, crime and banditry, distress and perplexity of nations will increase until the
Bishops open Joanna Southcott's box".

Joanna was a dangerous woman; embroidering treasonably the murder of the
king. She wanted a better place, a place to be "great again", to remake a scriptural
paradise now; she is the model of all those leaders of the inarticulate disgruntled (at
her death she had 100,000 'sealed' followers; her 'Seal of God' was in fact a seal that
she had found dropped in her employer's shop, which is why I am extra vigilant in
my attention to possible holy vessels and forgotten relics in Exeter's retail quarter),
communicating in approximations and complex non-complexities; the kind of ideas
that can be shouted across a noisy bar, the kind of Palin grammar that intellectuals
are contemptuous of and yet 'common folk' totally 'get'.

As the most important person between Richard Hooker and William Kingdon Clifford to tread these streets, she is, of course, almost completely absent. The ritual gifts for her son-cancer Shiloh were concealed for years in the RAMM's reserve collection, for fear that their display might compromise the institution by too close an association with the militant remnant of Southcottianism, the Panacea Society (last member dying in 2012). Now, the beakers and quilt – the things of Southcottianism, presents for Shiloh's baby shower – are keeping me going in the face of the unremitting racism and normativity of almost every other major figure I encounter. At least Joanna had the honesty to declare on her death bed, like a good Symbolist, of her writing: "it all appears delusion".

On my way out of the museum I see the fossilised burrow taken from the red sandstone cliff. The revenant of the work of some lizard-like creature from a Permian desert dune 300 million years ago; nothing of the lizard remains, this is not even the hole it made, this is the sand that later filled up the hole. There is nothing here to empathise with, not even a scaly animal; it is a representation of nothing. Wow, what a radical thing this is! Unseeable for what it is, 'it' isn't there at all, it has gone and yet it endures!

I want to form a gang with the ghosts of Southcott, Clifford, Lumley, Dumna and the burrow infill; the 'rebel rebels', the real rebels, and walk with them. I realise that, although I have walked with individuals, I have spent very little time with a 'drifting' group. The solo pilgrim, maybe, misrepresents the movement? The solo pilgrim most intensely excludes the other?

Out of Gandy Street, which becomes an alley, I slip into another: Martin's Lane, like the quiet passage of music before the symphonic finale. A pub promising much and delivering less, a sale of characterless pasties and a man begging; "as he walked down the alley, past the dairy and the old curiosity shop, it was of Hayward [a man condemned to hang that day in Exeter Gaol]" that the hero of Mary P. Willcocks's 1910 novel *The Way Up*:

> ...still thought. For Michael possessed the social sense, and every now
> and again, quick-winged like the lightning, there would come to him
> the perception of the unity of life. Such a thrill, once born in a man,
> never dies... Through the faint green tracery of the elm-avenue the
> stars hung in clusters like golden fruit; in front of the dark mass of the
> Cathedral sat the stone image of a great thinker. Clear for all men to
> see – the worn towers, the white figure of the old divine with a wise
> book on his knee and the golden galaxy of the sky. The visible universe
> was very good, but all that the wisdom of it could offer Richard
> Hayward was a broken neck.

The Cathedral Green is an orchard of the dead, a quarter million of them under the picnic grass. Springing from it I saw no king of apples, but the white statue of Hooker built over the old fountain. Salmon cannot quite disguise his gleeful hatred of this place. Its overriding of other cultures, Roman and maybe even before that; the cathedral church of St Peter, begun in Romanesque style and Gothicised halfway through its construction, its towers half converted, is a horrible mess of a rose-window surrounded by Romanesque arches. Car crash architecture, the feudal as rift. A split in the cosmos.

No wonder weird things happen here.

Was the cathedral originally a minster of early Saxon labyrinthine layout? The services were often held outdoors here and what could be more labyrinthine than that? Or was it always ordered and explicit; the place where Boniface was educated to cut down trees? Three hundred years later Canute was still issuing a statute forbidding "the barbarous worship of stones, trees, fountains, and of heavenly bodies". If this were not a cathedral and made in gorgeous stones from Ham Hill, Beer, Portland, Caen, Bath and Ketton it would have been up there with 'Britain's 10 most hated buildings' instead of the modernist Bobby's/Debenham's on the High Street, now a cosmetically re-veneered John Lewis, its gorgeous massing obscured; its role as a space quickly convertible to a hospital in the event of nuclear war long forgotten. The atomic blast is as scored into the centre (there are still enigmatic little huts on the university campus and doorways off Barnfield Road) just as it is rippled out into the suburbs, and ringed by Royal Observer Corps sites. In the noughties, walkers had followed urban explorers into the then derelict (now a 'paintball park') RAF Poltimore on the edge of the city, a semi-nuclear-blast-proof facility where they found an operations room with its control tables, and down dark corridors an office with a wooden chart on which were sliding shutters and against the names of each of the West Country communications bunkers a simple designation:

ACTIVE/INACTIVE

Chillingly binary.

I pop into the Royal Clarence Hotel, a creamy building, the first to be called a "hotel" in the UK, to ask them if I can see the skeleton in their cellar, but I have got the wrong building and they redirect me to the Well House Tavern next door. I drink a late lunchtime half of Otter and stumble-trip down the narrow, carpeted stairs to the cellar to pay my respects to the two-people-in-one; the bones of a young man and an older woman laid out as a single skeleton, echoing the local tradition of a joint suicide, nun and priest. Over the bones, a walker's epigram:

BIRTH IS THE FIRST STEP UNTO DEATH

Out on the Green again, I cannot decide which of the benches was the scene for the death of a homeless man, murdered by an assailant with the street name of Aslan, his defence that he was protecting an unborn child that the victim believed to be the Anti-Christ and sought to destroy. Father Christmas was called as a witness.

It was on these grounds that Bishop Phillpotts, whose Walk had spooked me in Torquay (that kind of anxiety seemed a long way back now, but I knew it could come close again very quickly), had been burned in effigy in 1831, a turnip for his head, a candle for his nose: inspiration perhaps for Trevena's "mere bogey of sticks and turnip-head". Bishop Phillpotts was a high churchman, which partly accounts for his infamy in 1831, but today it is more likely to be his executorship of a will compensating investors to the tune of £1 million (equivalent) for their 'loss' of 635 emancipated slaves. In response to his turnip-shaming, the Bishop called out the Seventh Yeomanry cavalry from Howell Road (named for the last 'British'/'Celtic' king) against the Exeter Party (the mob); a barracks complex built on the edge of the city specifically to keep the soldiers isolated from the revolutionary ideas growing among the civilian population. The resultant cavalry charge against the disenfranchised citizenry did nothing to improve Phillpotts's popularity.

Throughout the mid-19th century, Bonfire Night was the prelude to rioting on Cathedral Green occasionally spreading to the surrounding streets; this was the secular as well as the religious centre of the city. Sometimes burning tar barrels were carried and bowled through the streets, pursued by special constables, until they fell apart in hoops and cinders. The Green was a place of transformation and of rituals of danger. Preparations were elaborate. The 'guys' for the 1850 Bonfire Night included twelve Roman Catholic bishops, a number of Puseyite clergymen and former members of the Anglican Church now converted to Catholicism. These processions – almost as grand as Vathek's train – were flanked by "officers of the Inquisition with instruments of torture for Heretics". The "Renegade Members of the Church of England" each wore a Fool's Cap on their head, a bandage over their eyes, a padlock on their lips, while a band accompanied their shaming with the 'Rogues March'. Yet, despite this readiness to burn Tractarians, Puseyites, cardinals and Jesuits in effigy and chant annually...

Up with the ladder, down with the rope
Please give a penny to burn the old pope.

...there is no evidence of actual physical persecution or harassment of Catholics or of the 150 Irish families arrived in the West Quarter in flight from famine. Rather than a pogrom against a hated or feared minority – even in the very heady atmosphere of 1850 when a young woman, Miss Julia Munk, claimed to the mayor that she had been lured into an empty house "by an elderly gentlemen in black having the appearance of a clergyman... [and forced] to recant the doctrines of the Church of England" – the November Fifth demonstrators performed their resistance (often with much loss of their own blood) to a fake authority, their mummery threatening to agents of other authorities who each year were liable to become part of the Exeter Party's widening target. These accounts feel very contemporary: the raising of effigies, the hatred of fake authority, the language of intolerance to express a more structural distrust, revolutions can start in strange unrevolutionary ways.

Despite the oppressive drip drip of normative fictions and morbid theories of a fixed body, this 'rural' and 'provincial' city was the first to elect an openly gay MP, and has stuck with him through four subsequent elections.

Standing above the bodies I get a call on my mobile from the Crab Man. He is unwell, but would maybe see me in a couple of days. I am stuck here now, too slow to bargain with his health. I stand in front of the West Door of the Cathedral, a bank of statues. Step back to take it in; I am not sure why I am shocked to see the statue of St Peter, the building's consecrated saint, on its roof, stark stone bollocks and penis naked. How did *that* survive through all the Puritanical knocking off of noses?

> No doubt you've beheld us in passing this way,
> And wondered what caused this dejected display;
> Why our legs are so battered and bruised.
> Well... before we got old,
> We'd run around the yard, just to keep out the cold,
> And one or the other would often get tight
> At the 'Globe' or the 'Clarence' and stop out all night.

I find the uninjured martyr holding his own skin, and another round the side wall holding his own head; sculptural experiments with time. I know that Athelstan is in here somewhere; I ask one or two passers-by but they all fail to understand the question. I look for clues; I like the angel whose face has fallen off to reveal a fossilised mussel; as much a symbol of pilgrimage once as the pecten. I am tempted to pick at the little flecks of red paint that remain from mediaeval Catholic times in the grooves of the carved figures; before the Puritans' vandalism this display must have been better than television.

Saint/King Athelstan, somewhere up on this stone parade, collected over a thousand relics from all over Europe and brought them here, sending out his servants with bags full of silver; expelling from the city a surviving member of the Dumnonii for each relic. The relics include a portion of the burning bush (flames not included) and the spear of Longinus, used like a picador's lance to weaken the crucified Christ, a spectre of which the Torquay pseudo-author Trevor Ravenscroft turned into the *Spear of Destiny*, "the greatest one book occult hoax ever", according to Kevin McClure (who has seen a few); an alt-history (trash) at the heart of the after-the-fact myth of the Nazis and the occult.

What a charged space! And this is where Dracula's estate agent has his office...

I wonder about following the socialist novelist Mary P. Willcocks's Michael Strode, a disciple of Charles Fourier, into a time when "everyone has panaceas", back to a High Street where, just about the spot that Marks & Spencer is now, "between the granite pillars of the Market Hall a barrier of planks has been erected round a small moveable platform... a crowd of men in greenish coats and mud-bespattered trousers listening to a white-faced, heavily bearded man...'The wealth of the world is created by your labour and nothing else'".

I doubt, however, I will find such a "wayside Academy of economics" today, and I am sceptical that maybe Willcocks made it up even for 1910. But then perhaps I have been sold the same 'market town' myth as everyone else; for unlike the recognised mouthpieces of the authentic Devonshire farmhouse – Eden Phillpotts (born in Mount Abu, India) and John Trevena (born in Surrey) – Mary P. Willcocks was born and brought up in a Devon farmhouse.

Instead, I wander through to Bedford Circus and the new shopping centre. Not bad. Full of buyers. Clear logic and it frames what lies outside it. It has meaning. Only a copper plaque remains of the Georgian circus; a third of it survived the Luftwaffe bombing and yet the whole thing was pulled down. Salmon says:

> *they had a clear policy, partly on the advice of the town planner Thomas Sharp, of indifference to their heritage after the second world war, levelling whatever was even mildly damaged, clearing areas only partially bombed. They had inherited their attitude from those archaeologists in the 1930s who declared that 'the corpse of Roman Isca... has been crushed almost beyond recognition by successive monuments, medieval and modern, of militarism, piety and commercialism. But the loss is not a grievous one, certainly not so grievous that an excavator should spend precious resources in a laborious attempt to reconstruct the anatomy of the town from its torn and mutilated fragments'.*

If that was how they regarded their precious Romans, there was little hope for the remnant space of the colonised, for the Dumnonian enclave of Little Britayne and the great yew at Heavitree stuffed with concrete.

There was little sense to the demolitions. Sharp is clear in his book *Town Planning*, written while the bombs were still falling, that the architecture of a place like Bedford Circus represented an elegance traduced by the Victorians. Yet he applauded Haussmann's wrecking of Paris's "vast, squalid, insanitary huddle of narrow, crooked streets" (the streets whose imaginary reclamation inspired the first *dérives*); so in Exeter almost everything old that could go would go. As if they knew they were, in the name of a modernity they had never had, creating a gap, to bridge with nothingness, from the feudal to the postmodern. Look at the maps. The Luftwaffe destroyed about one third of the city centre buildings extant in 1890. With the exception of Cathedral Green and one or two isolated properties and a couple of ruins, peaceful forces of regeneration and modernisation destroyed everything else: Paul Street, half of Catherine Street, Southgate, Mary Arches Street, Goldsmith Street, Waterbeer Street and on and on. The gothic museum only just avoided Sharp's personal antipathy to its "smothering dough-lump of the Romantic Revival", he wanted it gone; the same for Northernhay Road and much of Victorian Queen Street. The fraud of the city's "historic" tag is staggering; if anything, it is anti-historic, toxic to history. There is a word for this: shame. The whole civic thing hangs by a tiny thread – like that leaf that poked me in the eye in the holiday camp.

But in Bedford Circus I witness a moment of restoration – the Irish artist Sean Lynch, working with the museum, is carrying a chunk of sculpted stone from the choir screen of the long-gone house of the Black Friars; he is making a video of its temporary and anomalous return from the RAMM to its long-trashed construction site. This was the site of a religious house of the Dominicans, converted in the 1550s into a grand secular townhouse for the Earl who replaced the unfortunate and dismembered Henry Courtenay. The next day the ambiguity, disconnection and idealism of the students here would strike me as I had to dodge and weave my way through waves of them, inured to the world by headphones and screens held to their faces. In a city with so much vacuum and flexibility it is scary to think that theirs is a detached knowledge, that while they may know *about* the world, they are not *in* it. That is a kind of *techne*-ism that could, in all innocence, be useful to evil machines.

Exeter is a dangerous place to educate so many young people. It is a city of spectres, the most haunted in England. It is a city without things. There is and has been no industry here since the mediaeval wool production that made the city the fourth biggest in the country. That is why I find Sean Lynch's carrying so moving; after all that was needlessly destroyed here, it is touching to see some 'thing', meaningless to almost everyone in the city, needlessly honoured; and there are the beakers and quilt of Joanna's. The students need things to hang onto or they will dutifully argue us to the obliteration of everything.

The pattern on the Dumnonian bowl dug up opposite the Guildhall in the High Street looks like the channelling of a prehistoric plant-jelly, its tentacles reaching out in front while its tendrils trail behind it. The piece of bowl, found when they dug the foundations for the now disappeared Woolworth store, from the period of the Nerva-Antonine Dynasty, is described in textbooks as of Neptune – but where is the trident? The head is missing too, no beard, and is that a chest or female breasts? What's for sure is that there is a double screw tail, like Starbuck's Melusine; twin serpentine. The patterns on the pottery of Dumna's people are just like the shapes you see if you close your eyes in a dark room; the white noise of the brain: this city, behind the rhetoric of "historic", is hallucinatory, ecstatic. On the Green it is delusion, the bonfires and riots of the Exeter Party, the vampire real estate, the most haunted part of the most haunted city in England (and as the most haunted building, that makes Pizza Express intense), bordered by 'Little Britayne', the last redoubt of the people of Dumna still mapped in the change of saints' names on the little churches, a cathedral built on a Roman bathhouse (an Exeter Mithraic Fellowship is nascent), a place where the invisible happens, where commandos from Lympstone covertly *parcours* the concrete brutalism in the night, where a chief economist working from a tiny office in his home near the clock tower can send the economy into a brief spiral, where they measure the prevailing winds of 300 million years ago in the sandbanks of red sandstone on one side of the Sowton Industrial Estate and predict briefly future ones at the Met Office (which until recently was part of the Ministry of Defence and still sends its Mobile Unit into battle).

It is a place where a miracle can be something that does not happen: "Unhurt one lies who from a tower falls...." (from '*In festo reliquiarum Exoniensis ecclesiae ad processiones*', 11th century).

The Giraffe Café in Blue Boy Square could so easily have become a memorial to mass murder; the bomber, a young man with learning difficulties, had intended to run into the customer area and detonate three glass bottles full of nails, kerosene and caustic soda. Instead, his large body became stuck in the toilet cubicle where he was priming his weapons and when one of the bottles exploded prematurely, it injured and debilitated him. His 'suicide note' cites the "disgusting" behaviour of others as one of his motives. He was reportedly manipulated online, but no one else was ever prosecuted for that.

What might have become a solemn space, twice bombed, a tarnished space, where the Roman wall has been pulled down for development, is the empty site of the missing East Gate where the roads come in, the Icknield Road from the east straight down the High Street, the Ridgeway arriving from the South East, weaving routes like the interweavings of the tributaries of the Great Bagshot River. The definition point between the Tory Trojans of the city and the outsider Whiggish Grecians (still the name of the football team) of the suburbs of James and Sidwella.

The incompetent bomber died in a Manchester prison while I was walking. At the same time the Prison Officers Association said that staff shortages had created the conditions for "bloodbaths" in prisons; riots broke out, suicides hit record levels.

I bend under St Stephen's Bow; walking under an altar. Here a mayor contrived to get a king to bow to him. A dangerous joke in fraught spaces, part of the contesting for the city between church and secular leaders which would leave a Chanter dead and his murderers (and their commissioners) either pleading 'benefit of clergy' or fleeing into exile. The cathedral built a wall around itself, and its gates, gone now, are still marked with names and small engraved stones. All this with the cross-hatching of sectarian divides and a 'ley line', identified by Alfred Watkins in *Ley Lines: Early British Trackways, Moats, Mounds, Camps and Sites'* (1922), as passing through the hall of Lloyds Bank, up the steps and through the library into Rougemont gardens, once the scene of outdoor Shakespeare productions where the gardens were obscured by artificial scenery, including, once, a representation of the gardens and city walls themselves, a few yards behind their stick and canvas copies, past the cherry tree, *Prunus glandulosa*, UNIQUE TO NAGASAKI AT THE TIME WHEN THE ATOM BOMB DESTROYED THE CITY ON AUGUST 9TH 1945, the ripples of the blast carrying seeds, and through a tower that is part mediaeval administration (with recycled Roman materials) and part a later Romantic ostentation – you can see the join where the hungry idealist gaze latches on to the older appropriation, where the necessity for defence (a watchtower become a gate) passes away.

Where the ley hunters got the whole thing mixed up, from John Michel and comrades onwards, is that having settled on the lines-as-energy-channels as their big metaphor ("as if they were great stone and earth pylons supporting invisible wires" [Joanne Parker]), they ignored the National Grid, much more a network of energy lines than churches and hills. They forgot that Watkins was not looking at a line of earthworks in 1921 when the landscape lit up for him; he was sitting in a car looking at a map! Ley hunting became a giant nostalgic obfuscation of what ancient energy lines had become: lines strung between pylons carrying high voltage currents. By seeking to be ancient again (how do you ever do that?), they had denied the reality of the ancient – "ley hunting held out the promise of adventure and genuine discovery at a time when the British Empire's cartographers seemed to have filled in all the seductive blanks on the map" – failing to see that the great social energies of the ritual routes that had brought folk from the highlands of Scotland down to the Stonehenge/Avebury nexus each year were the same kinds of meshwork powers as those of the pylons (and now the fibre-optics), distributing the subjective-Spectacle in just the same way as the ancient networks propagated the mysteries of the priests, until they would eventually fail along with the harvests they were tied to. It is not from what remains that things are learned, but from what is denied or reversed, from what choice is made to leave what after the orthodoxy is destroyed; legacy is always a negative.

Those Roman walls, they got knocked down, we build them up, keep Argyle out, wowowowoh! (Exeter City FC chant.)

Not far outside the city, in the "failed town" of Bow, a child of the vicarage became the commissioner of those electricity pylons. He is often inaccurately cited as their designer, but in fact he chose the model in 1927 from the catalogue of a defunct US firm. This was the fiercely anti-modernist polemicist Reginald Blomfield, a man who nailed his 1934 book *Modernismus* to the front door of the Bauhaus. So when it came to choosing a design for the National Grid he chose what was suggestive of the most ancient thing possible: an Egyptian pylon, gateways in the afterlife, conduits for the Ka of the dead: "as if men were putting a grid of reference over the landscape seeking to translate it to some new dimension and to keep their bearings in a strange land". Blomfield's morbid and anachronistic machine was quickly denounced as everything wrong with modern, though that was exactly what it was not, ancient in everything but its materials. Stephen Spender, like many, missed the point with his famous poem: "nude giant girls that have no secret".

Blomfield's *Modernismus*, to my amazement, is available from the stacks of Exeter Central Library and I sit, on Watkins' ley line, and read it in an afternoon in the airport lounge-like non-place of the refurbished library facility, the dimmed red book in my hand obstreperously real and weighty. It reveals a complex, and then disturbing, story; for here, the man who chooses the dominant icon of modernism in the countryside (until the recent arrival of wind farms, since when the pylons seem to have become invisible to sentimental reactionaries) rails first against the "bad Gothic churches" and "inconvenient houses" of the 19th century and then the functionalism and brutalist affectations of the New Architecture of Taut, Golosov, Le Corbusier and their English imitators. He finesses his opposition to constructivist and collectivist enthusiasms with an appreciation of New Architecture's "effort at simplification, its dismissal of meaningless ornament and contempt for prettiness, its anxiety to do everything with a purpose" as themselves admirable in principle. And then, patting himself on the back, he concedes "an accidental beauty" to certain machinic assemblages, especially citing "the thin lines of steel construction, such as... electric towers".

This subtle positioning is argued in detail in *Modernismus*. The source of architectural evil, an opinion he shares with Thomas Sharp, is Romanticism, and the dominance it brings to a literature of ideas over the arts of the visual and plastic. In its place Blomfield advocates an art that is not expressive of, but is informed by, "knowledge of antiquity". Not in order to create copies ("fakes") of old buildings, but to develop, by an intuitive empathy with the masterworks of the past, a subtle feel for forms, an intelligence for combining function and ornament. Such taste and standards are referenced to masterpieces and "what they mean and must always mean".

Apart from the questionable privileging of certain works as masterful, all this might be mistaken for common sense, but the Bow vicar's son goes deeper in to where practical ideals writhe in an arch hysteria within his deepest fears. Comparing a British sensibility – that which protects the British artist from extremism, collectivism and exhibitionism – to that of a Russian artist, or one from "those weird new European states", Blomfield invokes "the peculiar privilege of a thousand years or more of civilisation... that with many set-backs and failures has steadily advanced, and has implanted deep in our character ingrained instincts that will outlast any ephemeral fashion". What this precious thing that has been ingrained turns out to be is racism: Blomfield argues that Platonic idealism (in the form of modernist manifesto art) threatens traditionalist-empiricist-mediated-by-instincts mastery, but is as nothing – a "bright, particular star high in the spiritual firmament" – compared to the horrors of the "dull obscenities of negroid Art" or the prospect of corruption by "those primitive animal instincts to the expression of which such Art as that of negroes sullenly gropes its way".

That "sullenly" is telling. Here is the worm in the apple. Blomfield fears the rise and inversion of the repressed of the Empire, released by the Romantic and neo-gothic, both lustful for what it has no right to know and resentful without good reason. A shaky train of Hedonists, hearts cooking in flames, incapable of discerning anything in the eyes of their most beloved but "aversion and despair". Exactly the resentment that the liberal middle classes feel now about the politically alien disgruntlement of a working class voting against its own best interests as decided for them by the same said middle class. The chickens are coming home to roost; but all at the same time!!! It scrambles the white-privilege fear of the return journey of the slave ship (which once gave such apparent power and cultural authority to "those individual men of genius who from time to time have caught rare glimpses of eternal beauty") with blocks of poor working class animosity to just about everything except a *jouissant* bitterness.

If my feelings about the Passmore Edwards Library are right, then something of these fears courses down the pylon lines, down the landscapes of isolation with their hobgoblins in every lane, jumping from house to identical house in the former council estates. It makes me fear that the obvious thing is happening, and that there are no giant's shoulders to stand on any more, but rather that even to get a peep over the wall, let alone climb into the promised land, we will have to build any giant; not from scratch, but from the shattered pieces of *all* our fallen idols.

It is getting dark outside. I take a stroll through the Cathedral Green. Exeter is the holy city; Richard Brothers and Joanna Southcott did not need to imagine an abstraction. This is where astro-archaeology began, in the lecture room of the Devon & Exeter Institution over there, still going strong by the look of all the lights on, under its oval roof window, advertised by its globular lamp: as above so below. They must be holding some meeting. This is the city of the monad, where drinking water was piped in from the holy wells out in St James.

I eat at the Côte Brasserie. Mussels again, this time in a Breton sauce, for this pilgrim. Two bottles of Pelforth Blonde. Not obviously local, but I am almost next door to the Royal Clarence with its French connection; so, it sort of counts.

I turn in earlier than usual. Speak to my baby. Tomorrow, I want to explore the city's postmodernism, get away from the oppressively replaced history of the centre and find the present of the city's digital information industries. I know the Meteorological Office is somewhere on the margins, doing the old work of seers and shamans.

I fall asleep and in the morning forget my dreams.

Bad Homburg Way, Matford Park Road, Hennock Road, turn left through the gate onto the footpath parallel with Alphin Brook, left through the gate beyond a bench onto Clapperbrook Lane, Ide lane, across roundabout under flyover, take turning signed to Ide (continuation of Ide Lane), past Pole House up Old Ide Lane, right onto Fore Street, bridge over A30, past Twisted Oak pub, right onto Doctors Walk, left up Little St John's Cross, look down Dunford Road, take Hambeer Lane (footpath on right), at footpath sign turn left down Roly Poly Hill (footpath), turn right along Cowick Lane, left into Hatherleigh Road, left down footpath and left into Wellington Road, path on the right into Cowick Barton Playing Field, cross pitches to Pinces Gardens, Waterloo Road, Alphington Road, Alphington Street, Exe Bridges, New Bridge Street, Fore Street, High Street, Parliament Street, Guildhall Shopping Centre, Queen Street, Paul Street, Gandy Street, Martin's Lane, Cathedral Green, Catherine Street, Bedford Street, Bedford Circus, Princesshay, Blue Boy Square, East Gate, High Street, (through Lloyds Bank banking hall), Musgrave Row, Exeter Central Library, Rougemont Gardens, Northernhay Gardens, Queen Street, Gandy Street, Musgrave Row, Central Library, Musgrave Row, Gandy Street, Martin's Lane, Cathedral Green, Martin's Lane, Queen Street.

Chapter Thirteen: Outer Exeter

In the morning, at breakfast, I ask about the cells that Salmon mentions and I am led down to the kitchens and shown a part of the 18th-century prison the hotel is built on. My photos are dotted with dust orbs.

"There's something else, though, more interesting" and the waiters take me, at the same subterranean level, to the other end of the building, open a locked door and usher me into a dust-covered 1970s' disco, its fading cream and brown paint and its tarnished tinsel heightening the aching melancholy of its empty dance floor. It was once a favourite haunt of the commandos from Lympstone, downstream, but there had been, maybe a murder, or one too many fights, or the hotel had just lost patience with the bother and the nightclub was closed to gather amnesia.

I ask a few questions, just to stay here a little longer. I am listening but not to the answers, rather for what cannot be spoken here, for the anaesthetic dullness of the place, its colours washed out, the evil commonplace of sex with violence.

Salmon explains that the hotel is incomplete – like the monsters. It only has one wing, where it was planned for two, but the money ran out. If it were a bird or an Aero Mobil 3.0 it would fly in circles. It takes me back to the ruined chapel wing of the complex in Teignmouth cemetery; atmospheres overlap.

How did that happen?

I set off to walk Exeter. Not the centre though, I want to walk a doughnut shape around it, see what had been expelled outwards from its middle to its suburbs. It does not work out quite that way. Instead I spend a remarkable amount of time under tree cover. Mostly I am alone on my paths; if Exonians know of these paths, they do not use them. But there they are: a network of surviving hollow lanes along which one can circumambulate much of the city, in ancient footsteps, while sliding through the modern city, through council estates and industrial estates unobserved and observing. I find them by accident, so presumably there are far more, and the network far tighter, if one uses a map. They curl through enclaves of maize field and pasture and within the patchwork of suburbs and industrial estates.

But at first I think I have simply 'got lost' in an unhelpful way.

I pass the clock tower – a memorial to the author of *The Horse's Foot, and how to keep it sound*; it is decaying badly, knees falling from its sandstone horses, heads from its snakes, tails from its dolphins; the hybrid animals reducing down to approximate stumps. Through a cold tunnel of trees on the New North Road, away from the centre. Down around the railway lines there are grey mountains of ballast; the track up ahead at Cowley Bridge was swept away in the 2014 storm. These ballast Ararats are ready for future deluges. The plural is important; we will live in a neoliberal time not of Apocalypse but of many competing apocalypses. Above, a pair of buzzards are competing with herring gulls for layers of the sky.

I come to a portal with grey stone pillars. It looks like the entrance to something unusual. It turns out to be dull and oppressively fenced; a steep sloping path; a sign says that the fenced buildings are student accommodation. The door in the steel fence here is locked between 11pm and 7am. But the path is not part of the university and it keeps going up and up, between student buildings on my right and houses on my left, then leaves both behind. The fences have already fallen away; those fierce green prongs were just a display for lazy aggressors. The path itself changes from human-sized tarmac steps to high granite clambers and then to a pebble and brick base variously covered or not with trampled dirt.

I follow this upwards and then around, all the time in a tunnel of trees; it becomes almost tropical with the banks covered in wet, broad, waxy ferns. A couple of old signs to my left warn of the dangers of stepping into the University's Nature Reserve, which seems to have been sold off for housing. The same old bricks poke through the mud beneath my feet; not just on these paths but on a number of similar paths, as if an attempt was made around the same time, some hundred and fifty years ago or more, to secure them all. A brief digression through an adjacent field: a buzzard swoops across my path, followed by a jay. I can hear children playing on the opposite side of the valley. Through the mist I can just about make them out, tiny dots bouncing on a trampoline.

The paths are called Grafton Road and Belvidere Road; though they are not for motor vehicles and I saw no Belvidere. I briefly turn off through two concrete posts into suburbia, but it does not feel right, the first house is called THE END HOUSE and I have hardly begun, so I turn around and go back to the hollow way. A sign reveals that I have been walking on tracks, crossing private land, managed by a shadowy 19th-century trust. I sense that I am all the time crossing these invisible bounds, the vagueness and notions of which serve to keep any sense of who owns what obscure.

I come to a busy road and toss a coin to go left. At the next turning off there's a sidepath, so I take it, for no real reason but to avoid main roads. But why? I am getting romantic and bucolic; I seemingly don't want to commit to exploring citiness. The road-cum-path becomes a *bona fide* hollow way in its own funnel of trees. On and on it goes and I repeatedly consider turning back. Just when I have had enough of the dampness – with scampering squirrels repeatedly showering me with the condensed mist they knock from the leaves overhead – I come to a sharp turn in the path. Two gates; I peer over one and there is a stag silhouetted against the horizon.

This is why I have persisted.

I gently step back behind the hedge, lest I scare it off. I edge back so I can see it. It is still there. It is still still. And it stays still still for quite a while, its neck turned to display its headwear. It is too statuesque. I become suspicious and climb into the field. It stands stiffly. I walk the hundred metres to it. It is made of rusted metal, a sculpture artfully placed to catch the eye of the few walkers who ever make it down here; a mile or so from the edge of suburbia.

I stand by the iron and look at the hills.

I think about art and its aggression, how it barges into places, how it bullies for attention, and when it loses how it stoops to tricks and jokes; but I do not like iconoclasm either. That comes with too much dystopian baggage.

The hills are as unnatural as before. Poussin in sandstone and volcanic heaps, red soil, grass and oaks. There is no neutral base to work from; no touchstone. Nothing to draw the critical knife across and test its mettle. A mile further on down the green path, in what feels like isolation: a witch's mask, a stuffed Guantanamo Bay orange jump suit, a weird 'guy' on the balcony of an isolated house.

Later, back in the centre (although it was once part of the outside), I have arranged to meet a student at the football stadium. She is waiting for me outside the turnstiles. She explains that she is a postgraduate student looking at how performance explains communities to themselves. Her immediate subject turns out to be a visit made here – which is St James' Park, the 'ground' of Exeter City Football Club – by Michael Jackson!

For a concert? Bit of an odd venue?

No, it is stranger than that; it seems that Jackson was brought here by Uri Geller, who was then (dark days at the club, 'the circus years', apparently) an honorary director of Exeter City. Geller also brought David Blaine. Darth Vader (Dave Prowse) had been invited, but failed to show. MJ did not perform, but gave an address in which he spoke in the vaguest terms of "children with AIDS", bewailed living "in a state of fear" and drew the crowd into a hand-holding ritual, a kind of 'kiss of peace', at which point in the ceremony he abruptly begins to 'see' – "I see Israel, I see Spain, I see countries all over the world. I love you". Like a *darshana*, the idol makes things happen by seeing the supplicant back; the most watched person in the world turns the gaze back on the world.

MJ's visit was highly appropriate to the area, given its history as a place of pilgrimage and healing. Something to do with holy wells; people came to cure skin complaints here in the Middle Ages. MJ certainly had problems with his skin. Together, we study an old map which shows three wells: City Well, Cathedral Well and St Sidwell's Well. Once we get the map the right way up and start interpreting its symbols, we find the Cathedral Well quickly, marked by a small brick structure on the edge of the platform of St James Park Station, just below the football ground. According to the chart, the brick mini-'chapel' rests deep down under the ground on an oak platform. The actual spring is a little way to the side of the structure, and is capped off with a "lead disc 5 feet in diameter" sitting on a stone platform, a pipe through the middle feeds the well and then into another pipe which heads off to the Cathedral Yard in the middle of the town. Presumably the second pipe fed water to the Underground Passages. The hollow hills!

The entrance to the Underground Passages in Paris Street still shows a film with a very young 'Alice' and her school classmates. I go in; the entrance desk is closed, but there's a crowd of people: someone asks me if I have come to see the performance and I say: "yes". Always say "yes". I am always coming to see the performance. After putting on hard hats we are led down into a series of narrow vaulted passages, built in the 1400s to house pipes that took the water from the springs in St Sidwells into the city and to the cathedral; in operation up until the turn of the 1900s. There are no pipes there now, stolen around the time of the Second World War, but the performance maker, Signpost from the Wrights & Sites group, has brought water back to the passages in large glass urns, within which something organic seems to be turning, green and jellylike and alive.

Outside, in the warmer late afternoon sun, after the darkness below, I see colours cinematically; in reflections in the windows, in a triangle of grass, on steps to nowhere, in Speculation Place (with freemasonic compasses) and in the New Horizon café, (where I call in for *baba ghanouj*). The geometer William Kingdon Clifford lived on this street as a child; he would hurl himself at lamp posts and then swing to the ground in a spiral. Later as a student, for relaxation, he would hang by his feet from the roof of his college library.

I find the house where Clifford grew up – he was born at Starcross – and there is a kind of round tower with a tall conical roof on the side of the house. I keep noticing towers; not always massive things like Beckford's but I see them everywhere; the towers for wind generators that have lost their blades, towers for communications, follies and towers for drying fire hoses. They all connect heaven and earth, ideal and material, in some way.

Clifford appears in *The New Republic* as Saunders, but Mallock got his atheistic materialism all wrong, tying him to Progress: "the generation that travels sixty miles an hour is at least five times more civilised as the generation that travels only twelve". There is no hint in Mallock's book of Clifford's speculations about 'mind stuff', his first nod to the possibilities of a quantum biology pioneered by the likes of Jim Al-Khalili. As Professor Chisholm wonders: "since Clifford also thought that particles were some kind of convolution or warping of space itself... [d]oes this mean that space itself is also endowed with some basic quality of conscious?" Clifford believed in a cosmic emotion, subjective psychogeography on a grand scale. Wilde did the conflation even better, so collective provision forms the basis for individualism (and is its sole point), the collective supports the variegated subjectivities of all. That is something definitely never present in Froude and the other race theorists, but it is present in Clifford the materialist, who takes the irrational drive to the cave, to the hollow hill, to the hidden city beneath the waves and then translates it into a curved ripple around a generally flat plane.

William Clifford also wrote fairy tales, including one about a giant consisting of orthogonal axes, who gets stuck in a castle, like the big bomber stuck in the cubicle. In the tale, things change their shapes: a woman turns into a fork, a church steeple into a dagger, a meal of hay into a haircut. It was Clifford's partner, Lucy, however, who was the real transformer of bodies: her short story 'The New Mother', written after William was dead, is a terrifying play on Mallock's distortion of William's view of humans as "clockwork machines, wound up by meat and drink". In the tale, two naughty children are encouraged by a strange girl to torment their widowed mother for the reward of viewing a tiny dancing couple who are only ever visible to naughty children (there is something reminiscent of the Torbryan fiddler's story). In despair at her children's bad behaviour, the mother threatens them with their abandonment and her replacement by a new mother with glass eyes and a wooden tail. The children ignore the warning, no tiny dancers appear but the new mother does:

> a long bony arm carrying a black leather bag... beneath her bonnet flashed a strange bright light. The children escape from their house to the nearby forest, where they hide out with only bracken for their pillows... Now and then, when the darkness has fallen, they creep up near to the home in which they were once so happy, and, with beating hearts, they watch and listen; sometimes a blinding flash comes through the window, and they know that it is the light from the new mother's glass eyes, or they hear a strange muffled noise, and they know that it is the sound of her wooden tail as she drags it along the floor.

This is not a disenchanting of space. (If I didn't know better I would think Salmon was getting at me.)

The second well on the map, the City Well, is inside a house up by the turnstiles on Well Street (obviously), but there is no sign of anything watery on the exterior – why do we not knock at the door? – so we try for the St Sidwell's Well instead, at the other end of the street. According to the map it is also inside a property, but this turns out to be a workshop making and repairing Stained Glass. This time we do knock; a less private space perhaps? The young craftsman directs us next door to a café where the well, its mouth lined with large stones in an eight-sided shape (the combination of square and circle, the meeting place of finite and infinite worlds), has been decorated with a plastic frog, plastic duck and plastic ferns and backed by a mural of a giant rabbit and what the birdman calls "the standard bucolic scene"; a 'Nature' where nothing need die and nothing hunts.

The latte is OK.

We sit by the holy well and introduce ourselves; Beth describes her eclectic research which includes visiting the megalithic sites that inspired the Cornish surrealist Ithell Colquhoun: "walking became part of my practice by accident, I got a dog!" I tell her about my walk.

As we walk back to the football ground and say goodbye, I wonder whether, when people did come to visit here for healing, the holy well was really much different from how it is presented now; someone trying to sell items around it, maybe dressing the well with inappropriate ornaments. I even wonder whether it fell foul of the same authorities that destroyed those altars to "proud and disobedient Eve and unchaste Diana"? Did Sidwella (almost certainly a Saxonisation/Christianisation of an earlier 'Celtic' [ie. Dumnonian] water and regeneration myth) begin to attract an unwelcome kind of worship? Had Beth and I stumbled on an Old Grotto to Dumna?

Only very gradually are we (which 'we', though?) learning of the dynamic connections between place and affect. Sure, there is the common-sense thing (our use of a space makes it what it is) and, just as obviously, our feelings change the behaviour that partly determines that use that in turn determines that place; if we are scared of a space then we are likely to reproduce it as a place of fear. Recently, science is catching up, if slowly, with these intuitions and we are beginning to grasp the chemical (Tsing's fungi thinking) and sub-atomic (Barad's diffractive entanglements) meshings of space and consciousness, of the physical structures and energy networks of space's own agency and ambiences and production-by-affect. Despite the emergence of these sciences, there is little complementary emergence of a discussion about *how* to use them, in the absence of which they will be deployed for the same ol' control and exploitation of scaling and separation.

There is a chance though. That rather than the pseudo-science of functional applications (if I do this I cause this), there might be a "what if": what if there were a jelly-ish, intuitive, embodied, super-stranger-based knowledge making? What if the kind of geography of feelings and ambience such as I have been drawn into, produced by thrashing diffraction rather than cool reflection, can arm itself with these sciences and the critical theory that lives on their edges?

I worry that maybe very few people are really paying attention and that these opportunities are going to go for little.

Wandering through the suburbs, seeing the chunky brand new houses to the side of Apple Lane, and how reminiscent they are of the houses in Summerway on the other side of the town, a much earlier layer of suburbs built maybe eighty or so years before, I wonder if the 'death' of cities is so bad and that maybe it is time to slow their heartbeat down even more? That the concentrated city that 'everyone' loves, that film makers love, that writers love, that social planners love, is also the concentration of old war-making, that those bounded and walled urbanities are all about binding energy in, preparing us to burst out in aggression? Whereas the suburbs are about the avoidance of war; about spreading the people as widely and thinly as possible, getting as many people as possible away from the centre of the coming nuclear blasts, protecting and preparing a future generation; even before the atom bomb this had started (in 1940 the planner Thomas Sharp, responsible for the post-war regeneration of Exeter, wrote: "it is dispersal rather than concentration that gives security... the spreading suburb is more desirable than the town, and Neither-

Town-Nor-Country is more desirable than either"). They are not villages, they do not have the Saxon shape with the Devil in the north and the cross-shaped junction of roads, they are becoming much more like a kind of social organisation that existed prior to cities and villages.

So, as I walk up Apple Lane, tailing a young woman with a buggy and an elderly relative, half way through my day of geographical-walking of this city, I am hugely pleased to see that beyond where the new builds have been completed the land for the next phase of the development is being subjected to rescue-archaeology. A laminated information sheet explains that while no major finds are expected, given that intense ploughing over many centuries has pretty much broken everything up, there have already been finds of multiple examples of pottery and of field boundaries characteristic of what they called a "Romano-British" presence. Nothing to do with Romans, of course, these are the people who were invaded by the Romans, who lived, apparently peaceably, alongside their occupiers – as their descendants would do in Exeter with their Saxon invaders right through to the 10th century – like "oil and water" according to Thomas Kerslake, the 19th-century local historian (though he calls them Celts, as against the Saxon "Teutons") – before being driven out by King/Saint Athelstan, in the process of his founding something like modern 'Britain' (the name stolen from the people he displaced) by unifying most of a mono-Saxon area now called England. The double-defaming of the people of Dumna is significant given how little we know of them; in the sense of how little we recognise them. There are no temples, there are a few hill forts (I'd found one earlier today, beside the metal stag, its ramparts wrapped around with trees and its view to the valleys and the horizon immense, even in the vanishing mist), but mostly there is dispersal and diffusion. Athelstan did not drive them far; though the myth is that his forces exiled them across the Tamar, the evidence from the recent Welcome Trust-backed genetic survey is that outside Exeter (still Saxon) the old people are still there, all the way down to, but not across, the Tamar. And that landscape that the birdman and I had seen from the fields around the non-dedicated church at West Ogwell, Lovecraft territory, of isolated homesteads dotted through the land with equally isolated communal foci (the Church, Gaia House) is not the fruit of lost villages, but the survival of a diffuse and viable social and production system.

Peering through the gaps in the brambles and then through a gap made by the bridge over the railway, I can see a sheet of red clay-like soil and in it cut grave-size chunks and longer, shallower trenches.

Given what I had seen the day before of what happened in Exeter; how the hills did not fill up with factories and houses like Manchester, how the city missed out on most of the Industrial Revolution and thus slid from feudal ways directly into postmodernity, missing out industrial modernity (with the exception of a few technological adaptations); its own 'enlightenment' free from rationalism, hence the invention of astro-archaeology first presented in papers offered at the Institution that I had visited on Cathedral Green. Now, walking the industrial estate, circumambulating the Meteorological Office, there is still almost nothing that is recognisable as "industry"; it is all services, trading in information, retail. There is a kind of thinness to the whole place.

Even in the de-industrialised landscapes that I am familiar with from home up in Yorkshire, there are still pockets of manufacture and the long legacy of it, from the bits of metal splinters and shavings people still carry in their flesh to the languages they devised for communicating among themselves in loud factories. But here, the economy is faint. The history is fainter. And I slip right through it, down, first to that network of mediaeval (and much earlier) motorways, the hollow ways, the arterial retail system, and then I slip again, on Apple Lane, right through to the red planet of the people of Dumna.

I wonder if the model of diffusion, of dispersed foci supported on networks of greened communications, could work again? The diffusion is already there, but it would need accelerating and exaggerating by adding dispersed foci.

I cross out of the Moto Motorway Services and skirting Toys R Us there's a footpath, where no one has bothered to remove the previous security fencing, so it feels like the residents have simply ripped it down to get inside the old sandstone quarry with its massive wall of red and gold and orange, stupidly protected by another fence, not enough to spoil the splendour, though. Then up through the new housing, and there's Apple Lane's ancientness which takes you into the towering symmetry of the former Digby Lunatic Asylum, ('The Grange', euphemistically) with its grandiose ballroom building, its tiled clock glowing in a jigsaw sunlight, and its abject mortuaries boarded up, unconverted, nothing lighting the mournful patterns of its stained glass, and then up between KFC, Pizza Hut and Sports Direct is the most beautiful and fiercest symmetry of them all: the fabulous arches of a building standing alone and glowing, almost tangerine in the golden afternoon sun, attended by thirteen yellow sentry poplars.

Made from the local stone, this was the water tower for the asylum.

The suburbs could be organised around such anomalies and designed in homage to them. With the services and outlets woven in, not separated out in car-convenient strip malls and those dull council estate shopping blocks. Integrated, like in Lutyens's modern village: tiny cathedrals, one-person theatres, snugs. The economy of behaviour stood on its feet again; beginning with experience and then reconstructing it in subservience to intensity of affect. Stuff the country, we want our joy back.

I walk through the outer arches of the water tower, attempting to circum-ambulate it as I had the Meteorological Office – and as I will the thorn trees on the rise in Ludwell Park – but a tent blocks my way. I think of the tent in the Quarry at Cockington Lane and how failure to do a very simple thing, to collectively provide housing, something far poorer economies have done and are doing, is driving homeless people to functionalise ornaments, to turn wonders into shelters; lose lose.

The headlines I read, again and again on my walk, on the newsstands as I pass by, are always the same: migrants, migrants and, o, some mix-up that has benefitted migrants. Wars are mostly too far away; and too likely to cause the reader to make connections. Even crimes are now rarely addressed unless celebrities are involved.

On the industrial estate, the great blocks of granite, for keeping travellers (no more 'Romany Rye') from parking their homes on the verges, put me in mind of Oliver Heaviside's furniture.

The power has found its fear; the killer clowns emerge (which is surely partly about ordinary people taking back the power to scare?). No one needs to do anything about homelessness and its various junior relatives while the migrants ('refugee' seems to have temporarily slipped out of the language) can be blamed for everything. These are very old complaints; I am not old and yet I seem to have gone through wave after wave of these scares. These things accumulate in the soul. The identity of the villains slightly changes but each variation is always just to the side of 'us', just over the line of the 'other'; competitors for 'our' limited goods and pinched pleasures. These narratives turn the language of collectivism, of togetherness, of public life into a relation of exclusion and hatred; what 'we' are is not the collective force that becomes public by providing a network and a supportive scaffolding; instead, 'we' are a vigilante squad, machines for producing the very things that the machines fear. The media has turned everyday life into war; even for those who suffer nothing but the fear of things that have never even threatened, let alone hurt, them. Dupes of Badiou's zeroes, 'we' live in a permanent hallucination; while in the ornaments that should provide us with benign hallucinations the weakest and most frightened shelter in tents.

I walk through Exeter and I feel its ease and I feel the suffering of a minority and the intense anxiety and aggression of a much larger minority and I want to see the ease spread so we can be individuals in our own special, local spaces; so we can be individuals who can enjoy the precarity of the rim of the abyss (which is the base experience of all organisms) and make our own marks there.

There were times, earlier in the day, when I had worried for myself. The long footpath from the farm below the metal stag, along the edge of fields, emerges on a narrow, fast and sporadically busy road. I guess that the city is back to my right and go that way. The road twists and turns upwards and some of the cars race up. On the bends I cross to the 'wrong' side so oncoming drivers can see me.

Five Oaks. Rixlade. The Edge. The Eye of the World. The Cottage. Moongate.

It is a nervy climb, and when a path beckons I turn off under a large phone tower. There is a panorama of the city there, hazy, the Heavenly City sat in clouds. Vaporised. It strikes me how few tall buildings there are. The towers of the cathedral, after almost nine hundred years, still stand out.

Mile Lane is a mile of transformed hollow way. Once a way of skirting the city on the way to other places, it now burrows through, almost under, a council estate. Sunken below the expected, I am very close to homes and yet anonymous. When someone in their back garden speaks, I jump; they are so close and yet they do not see me and I do not see them. A dog grumbles, suspicious that I am here.

I surface.

A school with a Thinking Room.

Two girls pass by: "with another girl... still kissin' em..."

I walk through a short pedestrian tunnel beneath the railway. About as banal as a thing can be. It is magical and sinister and corporeal and bizarre. It takes me a long time, but I think I finally get it: the tunnel is circular, they must have used a giant pipe, then levelled off a walking surface by filling part of the bottom of the pipe with tarmac, so the walls curve and then disappear under the ground, suggesting the tunnel continues beneath the surface that the pedestrian walks on. The tunnel is a machine for evoking 'hollow hill'.

On my walk I have realised how I assume a neutral pessimism, a default 'realism'; but I have walked into optimism these past few days.

Later, as I weave my way between distracted pedestrians on their phones on the Heavitree Road, I enjoy their lack of presence and focus; they are those multi-sensory beings like David Bowie in 'The Man Who Fell to Earth' who can watch twenty TVs at the same time. The Moloch-Spectacle is being picked apart; even though it is the Moloch-Spectacle that is still doing the picking. I would not have understood the significance of Heavitree Road if I had not turned around in some despair in Meadow Way. There have been one or two moments like this today; I thought for a long time on the hollow ways out beyond Rollestone House that I should turn back, I wanted to pursue the actual (named-as-such) Hollow Lane, but lost confidence when it arrived at a main road, and off Heron Road I got into a cul-de-sac where Salmon had promised a huge ceramic mural on the wall of the local newspaper offices, decaying interestingly. But both newspaper and mural had gone. I do not want to give the impression that my walks were a series of smooth transitions between fascination and discovery. There were also long passages of disappointment and anxiety. Yes, they were all eventually relieved or alleviated, sometimes very quickly, but in the moment they did not feel like preludes, they felt like dead ends and failures of nerve.

It took me a while to find any upside at all to the missing stones. According to Salmon's guide there should be a section of the circumference of a stone circle in the play field by Willow Way (just beyond Kingsley Avenue); he provides an aerial map which shows the spectral completion of the circle through the back gardens and living rooms of nearby houses. Well, it is doubly spectral now. The actual stones have gone! I discover their disappearance just as a group of radical cartographers from the conference, with a poet who writes poems on rocks and carries them, inspired by the same story of this place, are arriving. They have come to complete the circle, but nothing's left for them to finish. Undeterred, indeed spurred on by their surprise, they set to work, and I briefly assist.

I ask a woman watching her children on the play equipment, but she has no memory of the stones. Maybe we have come to the wrong place; but I can make out a slight variation in the colour of the grass where the stones should be.

The map makers have brought along a 'model' stone to show to the householders in whose gardens and front rooms they intend, conceptually, to site the completion of the circle. I love the cheesiness and homemadeness of this *papier mâché* thing; a simulacrum of a simulacrum that is no longer there.

"They would have had to have been notional, anyway. We couldn't expect ordinary people to welcome an actual thing on their lawns..."

No one welcomes them, no one 'gets it', they might not have 'got it' if the stones had still been in place, anyway, but the idea of erecting a notional continuation of a thing that is no longer there has no pull at all. We live in a secular society. The cartographers have accidentally mapped faith and no one wants to climb into their chart. I feel as if we are in the middle of one of those anti-art moral panics; door after door is shut in our faces; amusement turns to suspicion as each resident grasps that this is not a joke, but a generous, philosophical offer. These maniacs actually want to give them the idea of these stones. They have some kind of grant, they can pay for the notional stone, notional transport, notional installation, notional insurance, they say. Until one door, where the stone's notional spot lies just inside the front window. A young woman appears and listens carefully. Then she says: "My husband died last week. I've been waiting for someone to come. Some sign. We visited Stonehenge together."

The poet coughs and explains that the stone circle was fake.

"Well everything starts like that, doesn't it? I suppose people thought Bethlehem was a fake to start with. I still think it's important that if you are going to do it, you should put it in the right spot. The spot that it says on your map. Can you bring the stone in so we can see?"

The *papier mâché* 'stone' is manoeuvred through the metal-framed door and levered from the trolley onto the yellow carpet. Wood splinters drop here and there.

It looks like a gravestone in the lounge.

"Someone might think it looks like a gravestone", says the unfeasibly young widow, "but I think it looks like a living being. I'd like it to be here. Do you mind leaving it?"

The poet explains that this is not "the real thing", but the woman refuses to believe that. "I think you are meant to bring this." It is real enough for her. She is the opposite, the shining sun to the dark spaces of those disgruntled ones who understand the garbled world and do not like it. There is some discussion about safety, fireproofing. I ask the poet if she has a poem for this stone. She says the stone is poetry enough. It is a thing in itself. But the widow will not accept that and the poet is invited to sit down and compose something for it in the moment. She improvises something between a prayer and a poem.

We all leave; without our fake stone the thing feels over.

Later, what will be missing in Meadow Way is Ford House, the home of Richard Ford, author of the 1845 *Handbook for Travellers in Spain* (some kind of proto-Salmon thing, I guess); gone are his house, garden and summerhouse made in a

Moorish style. His book *Andalusia, Ronda and Granada, Murcia, Valencia and Catalonia: the portions best suited for the invalid* must surely be one of the first travel guides for people with disabilities? I am so furious at this destruction of 'our' other architecture; I want it back, but no matter how much I stare at the stupid lozenge-shaped plaque, apologising for the absence of Ford House, it just gets further and further away.

I don't want Britain to be great again, I want it to be other again, even though I know that that otherness was thieved and not "ours", and I think it might really happen, because the Empire is coming to visit its origins and my pessimism has turned to optimism.

By turning around and back.

So I reverse out of Meadow Way and back up Church Street, but I don't like covering the same ground (stupid really, because that is exactly what Salmon has been doing repeatedly and exemplarily, and I am in a tick full of his feelings), so I turn away from the Conservative Club, Strawberry Hill houses and the Alma Place alleyway (black SKINHEAD OI! superimposed over white BOOT) through the graveyard of St Michael's and All Angels – it is Anglo-Catholic in worship like the other St Michael's in the north, which guards the city from the Demon's compass, standing across from the region of Hell below the Iron Bridge – even though it is getting dark and I do not feel invincible at all. I just feel reasoned and self-righteous.

Beside the tower, with its peculiar gothic points that I had seen so clearly from far off up beside the thorn trees on the rise of Ludwell Park, is a very old yew. Hundreds of years old; yet even it is but the regeneration of a much, much, much older tree (probably cut down when the tower of the church was rebuilt in 1541) and the remnants of that ancestor, including its roots, are still there in the ground around the present tree. Roots that are perhaps, in its turn, only one regeneration away from the great 'Heavi-Tree' itself, the tree that stood at the centre or in the circle of the meetings of the elders of Dumna's people.

I had stood in quite a few tree circles today: at Moto Motorway Services I had climbed up the 'picnic area' to a ring of trees around a thin metal tower that supported some light or camera or something; I had stayed and swayed with them for a while. Then on the top of Ludwell Park I had found a clump of thorn trees on top of a grassy hill: a hundred crows gathered for a parliamentary sitting. I had let the thorns rip me. I stood inside and I walked in a circle around it. I looked down on the tightly packed roads, eight identical layers of them. The Burnthouse Lane estate; where they moved the people of the West Quarter when they cleared and destroyed rather than renovated its slums (mediaeval merchants' houses) and its unique community: when the Theatre Royal, at the top of the street where Clifford turned his lamp post spirals, had burned down in 1887 with the worst ever loss of life in a British theatre, the 186 bodies of those laid out in the stables of the nearby inn were exclusively from the West Quarter. They had all come to see George Borrow's story of gipsy life, 'Romany Rye', in the days when there was still a popular culture of identification with 'outsiders'. They buried the dead in a mass grave. The people of the West Quarter were not afraid of collectivity, they did not turn on their Irish neighbours despite the annual November Fifth anti-Popish parades, bonfires and rioting on Cathedral Green. The uniformity of Burnthouse Lane, after the clutter and baroque poverty of the West Quarter, was a frigid 'Siberia' to them.

Coming off the old Ludwell Lane into the estate, a young teenager, maybe fourteen, is crouched around his mountain bike, sitting on the step at the garden gate. His mate, revving a smoking scooter, is speaking in long, low, slow curves of words. These young sentinels are not going to let me pass without acknowledgement. I nod, the cyclist grins through the frame of his bike. I choke on the scooter fumes; just as I had earlier on the fumes pumped out of the Meteorological Office's chimney.

What do you burn in a meteorological office?

That place was designed, enigmatically, to make you worry. The outside says nothing about the inside, anonymous and ungiving. "Knowledge Is Great Britain" said the slogan: what does that mean? The 'nature world' sculpted all around it, with blue tipped sticks for bee orchids (like the feathers poked in the Lovecraft Triangle grave), is a little unnerving too. Bee Orchids and Wasp Spiders; hinting at cross-lifeform mutation.

Fifteen minutes later and time loops as I bend around the streets and down Lethbridge Road. After viewing another of those foci/anomalies in the middle of an estate – this time the ruins of the mediaeval chapel of St Loye (who once shoed a troublesome horse by removing its leg, attaching the iron shoe, and then reattaching the leg) and a recovered wayside cross of granite with an inviting niche for a fetish, I am back on the ring of arteries; triangulating the city by its boundary crosses: St Michael, St John, St Loye. And there he is again! The same boy, same pose, on his own now, sat on another step, his mountain bike propped up on him, same grin, if sheepish now; he knows how weird this looks.

Emerging from the former council estate, I pass Chance Cottage, then Brookdale: Oratory of Our Lady Theotokos, from the door of which emerges a middle-aged man in a voluminous, bright red dressing gown and pyjamas (it is late afternoon by now) carrying a large red lily-like bloom: is such a plant possible? The dome of the church in Istanbul had opened up like a flower and the Virgin had descended like a bee.

Across the road, I follow a map that Salmon has provided, overprinting the roads here with a diagram (provided by Lois Olmstead, one of the many walkers who seek out the routes of hidden rivers and the creeks under cities) of the Great Bagshot River as it was 50 million year ago, with one of its tributary sources starting here, at the bottom of Birchy Barton Hill. I stand by the road sign for a while.

A group pass by, singing. I follow them. They are a choir called Sine Nomine. They process among the modest roads behind the main Honiton Road, a small audience following; residents appear from their homes to listen, some to follow. In Elgar Close they sing 'Weary Wind of the West', in Stanford Road 'Heraclitus', 'The

Evening Primrose' in Britten Drive and 'There Was a Pig Went Out to Dig' in Grainger Close. Similarly, they sing songs or choral adaptations from the composers named in Coates Road, Sullivan Road, Purcell Close, Walton Road and Delius Crescent. There is nothing in these small roads to connect them to their composers, the names are a convenience for the emergency services; there is a wonderful anti-logic in taking the streets 'at their word', rising to their best significance. There is some kind of model here.

I head for the city centre, assailed by various signs: a ghost CHEMIST sign, the letters of SOUTHWEST REPTILES stuck on with sellotape, the fiery temper of BROCK'S IREPLACES, four plaster gatepost lions named ASLAM, RA-RA, SIMBA and ALEX (Do they mean ASLAN?), a holy well full of leaves, a redundant Victorian post box painted black, a chip shop Neptune with no trident, the horseshoe and 'frog' (inner part of a hoof) symbol over the door of the Royal Oak (once a forge) that looks rather as though it might be a sign for the worship of "proud and disobedient Eve and unchaste Diana" and the texts, either side of the road, that were intended to have been bridged by a 'Heavitree Arch': a bizarre story that Salmon tells, of extensive public consultation for a new public artwork followed by one of those scare/panic/outrage things where there is an almost sexual excitement in rebel-cops and cop-rebels outraging themselves. I actually loved the graffiti that the over-excited protestors put up on the wall of the Gun Shop: a white elephant and a bureaucrat with hands over his ears watched by a little dog. I wish I had been one of the official artists; I would have tried to keep those 'rebel' images and work them into what I wanted. The protestors also wrote behind the arch (which, for various reasons, no longer bridges the road but stands against the wall [?]): NOW OPEN: 'THE DELHI NELLY'. The archway, they thought, looked like the entrance to an Indian restaurant; in fact, it is modelled on the archway portal into St Michael's and All Angels. The angry traditionalists were ignorant of their own exotic tradition.

Such a rich street of symbols, all buzzing around the *heafod treow* (head tree, heavi tree, Hefa's tree, you can pretty much bend these old names to get whatever you want) and its new Beacon of Intolerance, the recently repaired General Gordon Memorial Lamp Post on Livery Dole. Gordon, a virgin tortured by the repression of his sexuality and regularly seeking martyrdom, was another of those poisonous combinations of conformist and rebel. A devout believer, he was convinced that he had visited a fragment of the Garden of Eden in the Seychelles (the rest of it going down with the sunken continent of Lemuria [capital: R'lyeh]) and an advocate for the buttocks-shaped fruit of the Coco-de-Mer tree of the Seychelles, which he thought "represents the... true seat of carnal desires... [which] caused the plague of our forefathers in the Garden". A great choice, then, to evacuate Khartoum under threat from an insurgent 'radicalism' (ie. a 'conservatism' violently asserting the return of a fundamentalist Islam that it was inventing in response to people like Gordon). Predictably, Gordon disobeyed orders and independently decided to administrate the city, instead, legalising slavery and pledging to "smash up the

Mahdi", the conservatives' leader. The two fundamentalists were made for each other; Gordon died when the apocalyptic Mahdi's troops took the city.

Next to the Memorial Lamp Post, not long ago, was dug up the iron ring to which were tied burning Protestants, still loudly denouncing the Pope as Anti-Christ. In the abutting Chapel of St Clarus (built for prayers to be said for the executed; having your cake and eating it) – to which I was admitted by a friendly, elderly man, dressed in enormous slippers, from one of the almshouses – I find a document that describes the Heavitree Road as 'the Ridgeway'; part, then, of the ancient route linking the South West with East Anglia, calling in at the *heafod treow*.

At this moment, I prefer the company of trees.

Waitrose stands on the site of Exeter Maternity Hospital – where Crab Man told me 'Alice' had been born in the fruit and veg section. This in turn was built on the site of Exeter Workhouse, where, in 1854 a journalist found Dahlia Graham: "an old lady seated in a cane-wrought chair with considerable ease and dignity. She saluted us blandly, and we soon observed that she was of African blood. Around her head was tied a many-coloured kerchief, in the fantastical style that obtains in tropical climes." After being kidnapped while still a child and an adulthood spent in slavery, she was still working at the age of 90 as a servant for the Wardrobe family of Rose Cottage, Pennsylvania Road. Now 93, she was, according to the correspondent (the self-style 'White Slave'), "fortunate Dahlia... she has a mansion to live in, gardens to live in, and the lieges of the Queen of England to minister to her wants! How different an end to that which would, probably, have awaited her in her own country!"

That "probably" is stained with blood and poison.

After I had finished chasing after wells with Beth, I had cut up Devonshire Place to Union Road, for which Salmon has uncovered a bizarre press cutting from 1847:

> Union Road has been for many days, almost an impassable gulf – a sort of stagnant canal of slush – endeavouring to account for this strong manifestation of mudomania on the part of our worthy Commissioners, a notice reached us, which seemed to throw some light upon the matter: 'a remarkable invention for the formation of large figures has been made by Messrs. Moeser and Kriegk (two Prussian Artists), the material being nothing more than the scrapings of the public roads, which is cast and consolidated into a material like sandstone'. No doubt our Commissioners have had early intelligence of this precious discovery and are saving up road scrapings to be converted into public statues for the town.... we venture to suggest that 'Figures' of all our Commissioners be immediately done in mud and placed in some conspicuous spot, the grass plot in front of Devonshire–terrace would be handy.

Almost back at my hotel, I stop for my evening meal at the Dinosaur Café, next to the crumbling memorial to the man who cared for horse's feet: an extraordinary plate of Turkish home-cooked salads, a landscape all of its own with purples and rich yellows and moon-cratered courgette fritters. I chat with the equally extraordinarily friendly Aysha and Abdullah as I sip a thick, sweet Turkish coffee; I would pay for that later in my dreams.

I am staying in the big hotel opposite the Central Station. I have an expensive glass of Merlot in the bar there and ring home. The walls of the bar are lined with mostly hollow and fake 19th-century books; I imagine finding Mallarmé's *The Book* there; the collection of everything necessary to read, arranged for a single performance. There's the model for what every book should be. Totality.

I drop into the nearby arts centre, the Phoenix, in time to catch a shortish movie in the tiny cinema; 'Deadly Intent' is a locally made psychological post-traumatic-stress-disorder drama, lacking narrative originality – I recognise Teignmouth promenade – and afterwards they show a trailer for the same production team's 'Scary Crows', a comedy horror set in Dawlish with living scarecrows, men in suits with sack heads, featureless, half-formed like all the monsters here.

Back in the hotel bar, I can access the web and read up more on the leftist particle physicist Karen Barad's "aim to disrupt the widespread reliance on an existing optical metaphor – namely, reflection – that is set up to look for homologies and analogies between separate entities" with "diffraction [which] does not concern homologies but attends to specific material entanglements".

In my second glass of Merlot, white horses froth.

Imagining flames in the non-functional fireplace in the bar, I think of the waves at Dawlish, hitting the new concrete wall, and how even there they would bounce back not quite in line with the next oncoming wave; foam and fragmentation mixing, pulling and pushing, but somehow retaining the coherent flow of wave motion. Symbolists are wave-like, and waves are Symbolist-like; releasing images and reflections from their referents, then recombining these things on the loose on the basis of their entanglement with everything *but* what they are like.

There's nothing necessarily good about such patterns. They are the same as those that inform fiscal and economic deregulation. Their effects upon language and meaning are not entirely unrelated to the emergence of 'post truth'. They are what the activist and theorist Franco 'Bifo' Berardi reckons are the driving fabrications for our present-day neoliberal culture, in which "signs produce signs without any longer passing through the flesh".

In resistance to this Berardi proposes a new kind of poetry which also is "an excess of language... which enables us to shift from one paradigm to another", but in which "language cannot be reduced to information, and is not exchangeable". That's a powerful vision if you then see this poetry as incompatible with the whole society of information we live in; something that cannot (or should not) be exchanged, but which sits outside information channels. If you put that together with the way that Symbolism finds a connection in everything-but-the-reflection between any two images floated free, and then the way that waves that are separate and diffracted retain a common performative quality, then you have a wholly different kind of exchange. Not an economic one based on scalable and separated commodities, but a common poetic practice which refuses to put its work down in saleable bits and is more like the way that sculpture, as a representation of bodies, is restored as separate from the art market when it turns into walking, when it makes art "through the flesh".

And that includes the kind of performance that is "total", that is big enough to outflank the Spectacle, hanging over its edges, creating a margin for freedom, not fake-rebel, angry, let-the-authorities-do-their job 'freedom', but *real* on-your-own, subjective-guided freedom and too big and too organic to be chopped up into saleable parts.

That's why I can't go home yet. That's why I have to keep walking, until I have made a walk that is big enough to outflank all the lies I see.

I fall asleep and into the theatrical worlds of Maurice Maeterlinck and Auguste Villiers De L'Isle-Adam.

Queen Street, New North Road, Cowley Bridge Road along raised walkway on the right, turn right into footpath between two grey stone pillars, 'Grafton Road' (this is a footpath), keep bearing left on the footpath until you reach a hard T-junction (of footpaths) and take the one on the right going uphill, Belvidere Road (also a footpath), through gate on left into Belvidere Meadows (signed) and out next gate on the right, back onto and turning left along Belvidere Road, over Argyll Road and left up Pennsylvania Road, take the footpath parallel and to the left of Stoke Valley Road, at Rollestone House take the left path, and follow it for about half a mile or so under tree cover, at gates with view to hill fort and metal deer sculpture turn sharp right and follow path round to farm, follow footpath signs along the side of the farm, through the gate on the left, and then bend round to the right hugging the farm's garden and pond, then through the gate into the next field, and through metal gate along the path which turns to the right and then to the left, follow this mostly straight path for about a mile, at the road turn right onto Stoke Hill (caution required with oncoming traffic), after passing Moon Gate (house) turn left onto Mile Lane (a footpath) with broadcast mast at the top, at the end of Mile Lane turn left onto Beacon Lane and cross the road, opposite the lefthand turn to Lancelot Road, turn right into the footpath, at footpath T-junction turn left, at the end of the footpath turn right and through tunnel under bridge, then left into Summerway, Willow Way, cross the playing field, turn left onto Pinhoe Road, turn right onto Hillyfield Road and immediately take Hospital Lane on the left, bear right up footpath, cross Hill Barton Road and up Hollow Lane (caution required with traffic), turn right on Cumberland Way, Ambassador Way, Emperor Way, circumambulate the Meteorological Office, Coriolis Way North, Coriolis Way South, right into Fitzroy Road, cross over and right along Honiton

Road, take the footpath up steps on the left after Vospers Garage, Heron Road, left onto Bittern Road, right along Bittern Road (same name, different road!), left down Kestrel Way, right along Moor Lane, on left hand footpath, take the informal path just before lamp post through trees into car park of Moto Services (beware lorries!), cross car park to front entrance of Moto Services and turn right through the cafe and chairs and through gate to 'Picnic Area' and up grass hill to circle of trees at the top, down other side and exit the Services next to petrol station, skirt roundabout, onto Sidmouth Road, cross to the Toys R Us side and take the footpath on the left passing beside the red sandstone cliff, turn right and right again through the new houses, take Apple Lane Path (signed) on your left at the roundabout, end of Apple Lane go down the pavement on right and take Baxter Avenue/Close (signs vary) on the right (this becomes a footpath), almost at the end take the footpath on the left and across Clyst Heath, take footpath bearing left of the play area, South Grange, Clyst Heath, footpath to Etonhurst Close, turning left and up the steps on the right, at roundabout take Digby Road to next roundabout and turn right there up Digby Road, turn left at roundabout, left along front of stores and turn right onto footpath running alongside Currys, turn left alongside Rydon Lane, cross over at lights, and into Pynes Hill, turning left at T-junction (taking short cut across the grass mound), turn right into footpath signed Ludwell Valley Park, on entering the field head for the top left hand corner, through gate and then take the gate on the right hand side, and once through it turn left, along top of steep field, through two further gates and then turn right, past seat on the right and head for the cluster of thorn trees on the rise in front of you, circumambulate the thorns, facing the city, head for the far right corner of the field, at the corner ignore the path to the right and carry on through the gate in front of you, following the right hand edge of the field, take the gate on the right hand side towards the bottom, at the next gate turn left along Ludwell Lane (beware fast traffic!), right onto Rifford Road, St Loye's ruins, Hurst Avenue, Lethbridge Road, Rifford Road, Honiton Road, Sweetbriar Lane, Birchy Barton Hill, Sweetbriar Lane, Honiton Road, Rifford Road, Quarry Lane, Grainger Close, Coates Road, Stanford Road, Broadfields Road, Sullivan Road, Walton Road, Broadfields Road, Elgar Close, Purcell Close, Delius Crescent, Broadfields Road, Quarry Lane, Rifford Road, Honiton Road, Wonford Hill, Gordon's Place, alleyway (Alma Place), Church Street, Meadow Way, Church Street, through churchyard of St Michael's, footpath on right, crossing end of Sherwood Close, to Church Terrace, turning right up Church Terrace, cross over road to Livery Dole, left along Magdalen Road, right along Barrack Road, left down Heavitree Road, Paris Street, New North Road, Longbrook Street, York Road, Well Street, Devonshire Place, Union Road, Prince of Wales Road, New North Road, Queen Street.

Chapter Fourteen: To Stoke Canon and back

Today I go in search of a personal hero of mine. I am the latest in a long line of those who hunt for his remains. Mostly these people go to the Amazon jungle, but I go to Stoke Canon. If I can find it without a map. It can't be that difficult; just two villages along from the city. If I cannot find it conventionally then I can depend, in my hero's case at least, on telepathy, sympathetic mediumship or, in the last resort, necromancy.

I call in at the Dinosaur for another Turkish coffee to get me going.

"A righteous man regardeth the life of his beast": inscription on another defunct trough, this one has a stone dolphin half-mask.

I cut down a side road. In an upstairs window I can read (backwards) a note someone has written to themselves in red CAPITALS and stuck across their vista:

STOP PROCRASTINATING
STOP IMPULSIVE SPENDING
GET A JOB

At the end of the street there is a motor car graveyard. I find what looks to be the rusty wreck of Mike Mercury's Supercar. It is an anglicised (Austin) version of a 1957 Nash Metropolitan; which one is less likely to find in Exeter than Mike Mercury's puppet machine. Lost in admiration, I leap in the air as a scooter whizzes by. Not the last time today that I will be frightened by machines.

I am in the jungle very quickly. Stone gates with the words THOMAS HALL emerging from under the words THOMAS HALL. Inside I immediately detect the beginnings of the tropical. Avoiding a huge garbage lorry grinding up the driveway, unsure exactly how welcome I am, I edge a massive eruption of *Gunnera manicata*; immense specimens, leaves the size of African elephants' ears. There is something ghastly and obscene about them, as if the parts constitute a single reaching mouth; whenever I find them, any time of year, they seem to be in collapse or decay, combining magnificence in a decadent William Beckford way with Lovecraftian unspeakableness.

More impressive are the trees. If my meetings with the grove at the motorway services, with the thorns on top of Ludwell Park and with the latest issue of the Heavi

Tree have all inspired reverence in some measure, then this is my meeting with the Titans. They are impossibly immense; looming towers of bark.

Such weird tree landscapes in the city parks and on the private estates must be inextricably woven with the nurseries and through them to the activities of the men who worked the colonies to buy them. They feel even more systemically alien. Trees from American forests and Latin jungles glooming over neatly cut lawns and gravel paths.

Turning the corner, I find that a man is controlling a wooden gate for contractors. I turn around but he calls me back and asks me what my business is. I explain to him what I am doing – I describe it as a walking research – and he is courteous and informative; he is the caretaker here. And he does take care; he explains the renovation project in the big house to me: twelve million pounds spent on fighting dry rot. Hoteliers had wanted it, but they could not get around the 'change of use' restrictions and the Steiner school movement snapped it up. It does feel good. I hear the shouts from the kindergarten. When I mention the trees, he says: "Veitch".

Later, when I meet the Crab Man, he will describe an 'under the radar' tour of the house, when it was still owned by the university, performed by one of the leading radical walkers, and of disturbing events, fully sanctioned, when students filled the kitchens with dead octopi and subjected him, in a room the size of a cupboard, to still images of shotgun suicides.

Having squeezed across the first of the Cowley bridges, devoid of pavement, I enjoy a pause at Bernadot. The walking trio walkwalkwalk had come this way some years ago; they had emerged from a scary road from Exwick to find Bernadot's garden decked out in a tableau of costumed mannequins. Calling at the cottage, they met Dot who at that time was creating a different tableau almost every week, often on topical themes – sports, politics – and sometimes just something racy to "entertain the lorry drivers". All that remains of these costumed spectacles (some of which Dot would have to periodically rescue from the river after storms) is Indiana Jones, his high-crowned, wide-brimmed sable fedora incongruously replaced with a floppy straw hat.

This is the default coincidence of all hypersensitised walking, Oak's Law, because the hero I am in search of on this day is the real-life model for Indiana Jones. Someone I fell in love with a few years back, when I read his own account of his adventures: *Exploration Fawcett*.

During my literature review, I came across a dead Fawcett's description of his final expedition into the Amazon jungle told through a medium over a series of séances. Not as crazy as it sounds, given that since Fawcett disappeared in the jungle around a hundred people have died trying to get that story in the flesh. Sitting in a darkened lounge talking with the dead seems a far more sensible business than tramping around under trees that continuously drip ticks and flesh-burrowing maggots.

Percy Harrison Fawcett, a sailor who could not resist another voyage, never came back; lost with his eldest son Jack, and Jack's friend Raleigh. They had gone to find a lost golden city which they code-named 'Z'; they were living the Symbolist quest. As to what happened to them, theories range from their descendants still living happily in Z to their finding zilch and getting themselves clubbed to death as a result of Jack's improprieties with "a chief's daughter".

I cross the second of the pair of Cowley bridges, this one over the Creedy; William Froude devised the first of this particular form of helicoidal skew arch. Leaving the busy road I wander by one of many entrances to big old houses today; somewhere between mansions and palaces. The road is narrow, the cars fast. I take a public footpath, which had not been my intention; up to now thinking it might be safer for navigation purposes to stick to the signposted roads. Across a couple of fields and a railway track and I lose confidence that the path will bend back to the road (actually, it did) and so partially retrace my steps.

Another set of stately gates with alien giants on guard.

I wish a lady a good morning and her "hellurrgh" could have come from the Queen.

I wander deeper into the countryside; the fields get bigger and the cars fewer. Then, after a peculiarly eerie hundred metres of shadowy trees and shuffling in the hedgerows, a creepiness for which there is no visual explanation, the road eases, the hills relax and recede and the sun warms me and all that nibbles at the quietness is a gentle and distant 'weep weep'. I feel some inner part of me reach outwards and relax.

BANG BANG BANG BANG

I leap and then cower. A man I had mistaken for a farm worker standing chest-high in the crop field has just let fly with a shotgun. I thought he was mopping his brow, but he was shielding his eyes as he took aim. Pheasants wheel out of the field and into the trees.

I had assumed that the handpainted DWGC sign and car park full of 4x4s was some sort of Golf Club. No, it turns out to be the Duchy Working Gundog Club. I had even sneaked a look through the Club gates to see where its greens and fairways could possibly be.

And this is how it seems to work. The big houses I am passing are almost all divided up into comfortable not-quite-communal-but-interlaced mini-groupules of privilege, while the really big money has disappeared; the great villas snapped up by landlords or canny middle class buyers when the market for those big properties dipped two generations or more ago. Wealth no longer displays itself; the fantasies the rich tell about themselves are not Vathek's. In an age of spectacle, from what little I can see from the road, the rich and the privileged are disconnecting (with the exception of reality performers and businessmen-salesmen) from display; except maybe among themselves (how would I know?) The DWGC sign personifies this:

hand-painted, black only-just-about-even letters on a white background, raw wood peeping through along the edges, less than a metre high and stuck, gnomic, against a hedge; a little too modestly speaking the privilege of being a member, of knowing oneself to be a member and of reading the signs of membership.

Trying to photograph the sign I get in the way of one of the members' vehicles and there is an impatient suspicion in those eyes that I almost wish I had intended to cause.

Wherever real power lies it is not in representations of itself. Looking over newspaper readers' shoulders in pubs and at breakfast tables the healthy resentment of inequality is directed not against those who own and order, but against those who manage: immigration officials, middle-level bureaucrats, hospital boards, school governors, politicians, those who are flattered by status, but are never given enough resources to properly fill their roles.

While beyond display...

BANG BANG BANG BANG

Having uncurled myself, I notice the unmarked and unsigned track to where the shooting goes on. I feel something from it, but it will only speak fully to those who know what it signifies.

At the next turning I am reassured by the signpost for the first village on my route.

Then: CAUTION: PHEASANTS IN THE ROAD. There are. Many. All flat.

Did I mention Devon's bumpiness? I had thought the county would be a kind of East Anglia but less so. So much for that. On the up side (ha ha), these latest hills afford me views across new valleys to... more hills: land that according to the Devon landscape writer W.G. Hoskins has been uninterruptedly farmed for 4,000 years, through Dumnonian field systems and monastic estates, an area that he wanted to see developed as a "conservancy", kept free from further suburban incursion or industrial exploitation. It pretty much looks that way.

The notice board in Brampford Speke invites greater participation in the work of the Parish Council, advertises a Halloween party and the services of an "equispirit" healer who treats both humans and non-humans. I follow a footpath around the church – where the vicar was once banished from the living by Bishop Phillpotts for his belief in baptismal regeneration – and along one of those backs-of-the-gardens alleyways, feeling privileged to be allowed access, but variously hemmed in by old brick walls and latticed fences. After a series of right-angled turns, beginning to imagine myself a rat in an experiment, I reach a rather odd place; perhaps not improved by the cries from the playground of the local Church of England primary school – I hope I misheard "come here, you rapist!"

In the elbow of the field adjacent to the alley, there is an elegant, but rusted cage of thin bars. Beside it an armchair, a sofa and an occasional table made of breeze blocks and slates. I wander through the village, past a cottage with a large chimney called 'Chimney Cottage' and a chapel notice board asking:

"A welcome or Judgement; which will you give?"

I'm not sure if this is addressed to me or God.

Very quickly I seem to have walked through the village and out the other end, arriving at a steep dark lane to a junction with a footpath signed to the right. I take it, past a derelict building, half the shell remaining, bricks jumbled in melancholy confusion, and into twenty minutes of unexpected jungle.

The path, clearly rarely walked, brambles and nettles encroaching across it, bends around to the right and I am soon in a thicket of bamboos. I weave between tight clusters of the rattling stalks. It is a snaky path, but I do seem to be getting somewhere until the whole thing wrecks on a forbidding pile of greenish stones from another ruined structure. An old iron meter pokes up from the ground. There is no way through short of jumping in the river that has been policing the left hand of my worming.

I retrace my steps, this time tearing my arms on the brambles I had avoided on the way in, and now I take the leftwards path, and that brings me almost immediately into another mini-thicket. This one is of softer stalks and bright yellow leaves, plants about eight feet high, encompassing the walker. At first I think I have to trample it down, but once I have my head in the yellow canopy a maze of tracks, with multiple choices of direction at each turn, is revealed and I wind one way and then the other, until I end up exactly where I have come from: the entrance to the bamboo thicket.

Feeling that I am now in some banal but allegorical saga, shuffled from coloured room to coloured room of 'The Masque of the Red Death', trapped in what must be the overgrown garden of some lost villa, going round and round in circles of exotic plants, I fully retrace my steps – more stings and deeper cuts to my forearms – and climb back through the village, taking the alternative turning at the concrete furniture. I follow a snaky steel pipe-handrail down to the river, and cross the bridge there, a modern main structure with preserved Victorian twiddles. Then take a path I hope will bring me to Stoke Canon, the village where the Fawcett family were renting a property before Percy and Jack's departure for Brazil.

The path is just a little too straight, a little too level; I am on the raised line of an old railway, taking me all the way to the next village.

I canoodle with an iron kissing gate, cast in a forge in a nearby village.

At the level crossing, over tracks from Bristol and London, the 1876 signal box is comfortingly generic. The red lights begin to flash and I decide, on the spur, to wait rather than run the barriers.

After a bungalow with a traditional red telephone box decorating its lawn, I pass something older with a circular door in a tall perimeter wall; a 'Chinese moon gate'. I wonder whether this might have been the home of Percy and his wife 'Cheeky', both of them anti-conformists. I call in at the 'Stoke Canon' and, initially, forget to ask; this is a pub run by volunteers, but it is not serving food. We have a discussion about the possibility of food at The New Inn by Cowley Bridge – I had seen it on my way over the bridge earlier – and whether they still serve Chinese food. I remark on seeing quite a few Chinese students around; are they catering for them there?

"If it weren't for they Chinese weren't be no one 'n Exeter!"

He has the Devon way of saying the city's name; as if speaking with a mouth full of cream; "Exuurtuuuur".

When I laugh and say "something of an exaggeration, but no mind", he doesn't seem convinced. It is an obvious absurdity, but I begin to wonder whether it is a truth for him; a part of that landscape of resentment that is growing and growing every day, that the Brexit lies and the Trump miasma are generating as a global hallucination, an epidemic of not listening, a complete loss of empirical thinking; that the digital-spectacular has really now begun and we are back, as we were before there was writing and text, to a different kind of narrative-making, a different kind of testing of real and lies.

The man is incredibly helpful in directing me to possible eating places; but I think he thinks I have come by car. He wears a poppy. His son, propping up the bar – maybe the 'dad' is a nickname, though – seems mildly embarrassed. Why do I not stay and have a half, at least? But I fear these new and slippery landscapes of resentment; of old men who can barely move now for their bellies, of young men and women who work in dead end, zero-hour jobs. They have their own Amazonias of humiliation and retributive fantasises. And there is a Great White Brotherhood living in the media jungle, obscurely, waiting to replace their souls with their own, waiting just the other side of the Chinese moon gate.

"Do you happen to know where Percy Fawcett the explorer lived?"

"I do."

A voice from the back of the room.

I join her and she lets me buy her a half of Avocet.

She speaks in a considered and mannered, if resentful way. Some of her sentences would run into ruins, like my own encounter with the green stones among the bamboos. When she speaks she seems to be composing notes out loud for a poem she will never get around to writing. She even forgets to tell me where the Fawcetts lived.

"What do you know of PHF and Z?"

I describe my infatuation as calmly as I can; of my admiration for Fawcett's anti-racism, his hatred of the colonial system, his independent thinking and questing after the lost city of Z.

She assures me that I am wrong in almost every detail, but that she will happily educate me about PHF's great Scheme.

"I'm shocked."

"Continue to be. Continue to be."

I cannot help myself from wondering by which roadside the paper mill strikers had camped in 1918; expelled from their tied cottages by the mill bosses, for striking during a world war. That would not have been easy. Were they still here when Fawcett and his family arrived and, if so, what would he have made of them? Would he hate them as that other 'explorer' Peel hated them? I swallow a little of my Exeter Brewery bitter. To sharpen my thoughts, I focus on a sting inside my boot.

"As a child, born in Torquay, Percey Fawcett went exploring the Devon wilderness with his sister, remember that he had a loveless childhood, father was a swine, mother little better, endless canings at his Newton Abbot school, and they found 'Roman treasures'..."

"The parents?"

"His sister and him, in the Devon wilderness, including 'hoofed gods'... you've read *Exploration Fawcett*, obviously? Not written by Percy! Not him at all! A confabulation by his second and less-favoured son, Brian. Says 'editor', means 'ghost writer'... appropriately, eh?"

She laughs long and sips.

"In Brian's book, 'Daddy' is Indiana Jones, but in the Secret Papers that Brian kept hidden for years, PHF comes over as a socialistic, ultra-democratistic, pacifistical, vegetarian ascetic, he's an anti-establishmentarian and a visionary of the esoteric!"

She looks around the bar and lowers her voice.

"Amazonia might have been as physically gruelling as hell, but for 'Daddy' it was 'preferable to so-called civilised life in Devon', those were his own words, and they were not lightly used. His idea, for his journey to so-called Z, was to set off into the Amazonian jungle in the full and confident expectation of not only finding the ruins of a lost city of 'Atlantian' origins, his words again, but of meeting there a full chapter of the Great White Brotherhood!"

"Bloody hell."

"'Daddy's 'Grand Scheme' was built on imagination and romantic notions and their psychic confirmation by a bunch of globally-organised self-styled 'seers'; if you think the Internet has uniquely skewed things, you have no idea what the postal service could do in those days, my darling! The pamphlets! Let me spell it out for you: the whole purpose of the expedition to Z was to fulfil a politico-spiritual objective, and the manner of its reaching was to serve as a religious allegory. PHF believed that the union of a person with the gods comes only through the individual and with great difficulty. Turning up *en masse*, so to speak, at a particular building every Sunday is not that journey. Understand? Percy Fawcett was looking to create a colony of spiritually inclined settlers, and his son, Jack, born 'miraculously' on the Buddha's birthday and in fulfilment of prophesies by Ceylonese mystics, was to be their global leader. The real 'Great Scheme' was not an expedition to a treasure city: Z means the creation of colonies of super-people who will provide the next new leaders of the world, taking over from the governments and bringing into being a wholly new race. To achieve his overseeing mastery, Jack's body was to be taken over by one of the Great Adepts his 'Daddy' believed to be living in the ruins of a once superior civilisation in Brazil."

"Where did you get all this?"

"From the hidden writings of Percy's son Brian, who covered it all up under the influence of M."

"Who's M?"

"I haven't seen those particular papers, but they apparently reveal a 'beguiling and ageless 'sith''"...

"A Sith... like Darth Vader?"

She shrugs. "I don't remember the papers mentioning anyone of that name. I can tell that you are laughing at me, but you look like the kind of person who believes what they read in the Guardian newspaper?"

What can I say?

"According to the Guardian, M 'appears only to the Fawcett family and those who try to track the expedition's path'. She is that 'erotic siren who draws white men into the jungle'."

And with that she bangs the table and is gone.

The men at the bar do not know who she is.

Is this a grossly distorted Dumna? 'M', not the woman. Or maybe both?

The real Fawcett, who has been my hero ever since I read beyond the fanciful séance readings, is also an invention it seems! Maybe that is *exactly* what a hero is! Fawcett could only have inspired the inventions of H.G. Wells's Professor Challenger and Stephen Spielberg's Indiana Jones by co-inventing himself. There is no absurdity or criminality. This is the *modus vivendi* of the mythic: a decent, internationalist, universalistic anti-colonialist adventurer and pilgrim could *only* be manifest by hoax, when in reality, in the words of David Grann, another of those who have disappeared into jungles looking for him, he "could not rid himself of the pernicious disease of race".

The PHF of *Exploration Fawcett* is a rebel, a non-conformist; he calls the European slave traders "scum", he never raises a gun to an Amazonian Indian; he learns their languages, their rituals, he communicates in accordion music and the rain of natives' arrows dies away. He despises the colonialist abroad just as he despises the 'civilised' at home, and he believes in a connection to something basic, fundamental and intuitively instinctive, so when he leaps to avoid the strike of a pit viper *before* he sees the beast, he is like me leaping out of the way of the buzzing scooter. Yet even he "could not rid himself of the pernicious disease of race".

I leave the village quickly, stupidly, I had come to ask about where the Fawcetts lived, but I became frightened of... what? People?

A few minutes later I am walking over the village's 13th-century bridges back towards the city and, just the same as on that narrow little Cockington Road, a young male in a car comes straight at me at speed, sheering down the weeds in the angle of the surface of the road and the wall of the bridge; I wave to him and he must see me but he does not slow, his face is expressionless.

"What are y..."

And somehow I manage, in a blank flash of darkness and bladed existential fear, to turn, balance and then pirouette in the few centimetres between the metal of the racing saloon's body panel and the low mediaeval breccias of the bridge without falling into the muddy Culm (and whatever it conceals): "psychometry... the theory that every material object preserves in itself the record of its physical vicissitudes, and that this record is available to a person sensitive enough to tune in". It is not me that saves me, but the unholy alliance of breccias, panel and a supra-me sensitivity.

I don't believe PHF would ever do something like that driver did.

At the next junction, I choose not to pursue the prospect of hot pot at The New Inn and take the left fork up the hill.

Almost immediately to the right is a driveway and a house name: The Round House. I remember the Round House at the end of Long Lane that is no longer round. But this one still is; it was designed by the architect Peter Blundell Jones. Oak's Law of Ambulatory Coincidence: Blundell Jones's daughter, Claire, created one of the most iconic walking performances of the first wave of walking's 'new movement'. Called 'Tumbleweed', Claire walks with an ordinary commercial leaf-blower pushing a tumbleweed purchased off the web. Given its ghost-town connotations, she instantaneously transforms a bustling financial centre into its future decline, a busy road into a racetrack for winds...

For the next hour or so I climb, almost crawl, from the bottom of the valley to the heights above the city. Much of the time I am under tree cover; occasionally it opens up for huge, aching, rib-easing vistas to giant fields.

I trespass, despite stern warnings, onto a trenched, dell-pocked zone between the road and the fields; dark under mature trees, and deeply carpeted with thick layers of leaves that sink as if no one has been here in years. There is something enigmatic about the space. The land is shaped in curves, but not clearly. I find two stone bases, but I'm not sure what of? I cannot read the place and get back to the road.

The Eye of the World is up for sale.

Car after car passes; I wave and all of them draw out and slow down to let me pass safely. I think maybe upwards of a hundred cars pass me like this, but not a single pedestrian (of the two people I did speak to earlier, one was the "hellurrgh" lady loading her dachshund into her car and the other a man working from a van clearing leaves from drains); I wonder what a different kind of wealth I would have gathered with a hundred pedestrian encounters.

The sign for the ST REGIS PAPER CO LTD has a little logo of St Constant to remind me of the militancy and holiness of my quest. There is a second logo: of someone juggling clouds, or maybe being eaten by Langoliers. Outside a farmhouse a broken cupboard displays what appears to be a set of poorly realised Platonic Solids.

I am tempted by the sign to Poltimore (and a chance to trespass in the bunker), just 2 miles away. But plough on.

Something happens then. Perhaps planned. Or maybe just one of those Oak's Law coincidences. For not long after passing the gap where the footpath from the farm by the hill fort meets the road, (which means that I am now re-walking this part of my route from yesterday), I pass a gate that I stopped at; I had leaned over it yesterday and examined the fly tipping, black bin liners full of something mulch-like, some piles of magazines. I pause again today, I have been thinking for the past few hundred metres about maybe being able to see the hill fort across the fields, about two miles off. I take the chance afforded by the gate's clear view. I trace the line of trees where I think yesterday's footpath must be, then I follow that line along and up towards where the farm is, looking for the sharp crook in the path with the two gates. Eventually, yes, there, pleasingly, is the camber of the fort top, and right beside it, precisely framed by the trees that grow along its rampart, a tiny but o so sharp black punctuation mark against the ashen blue of the sky, is the metal stag.

I had not expected this dark nick in the fabric of the universe.

Did I find union with the gods? Yes, of course I did. Even the 'hoofed gods'? Yes, yes, with them especially...

I stride on, levering off from this notch in things.

At a farm double-gate, where bouquets had yesterday been tied in memorial, a few rose heads lie on the ground, the bouquets are tossed into the hedge.

I lower my eyes in respect as I pass a hearse pulled up beside a cottage, from whose lollipop tree yesterday I scared away a hundred tiny birds. The back door of the hearse is open and elderly folk gather around the bright shining box. There is weeping.

There is a lot of death on this road today.

Yes, yes, of course, I did.

I pass the end of Mile Lane, and take another look at the holy city from under the phone tower. There is a small trace of smoke from the centre, like a signal for a change of order.

A hub cap rotates on a branch.

I re-enter the city proper at a red breccia bridge, over the North Brook, which passes the source of the Great Bagshot River at Birchy Barton Hill. I take an agonising footpath up alpine steps. Then I cut through an estate of houses on stilts, ready for postdiluvian times. In its gardens basks another alien slave monster; a titanic fallen tentacle resting on the green, trying to raise itself up on its elbow. I briefly explore an enclave of tree cover between two roads; there are stone pillars at the entrance, but whatever its function, and ownership, it appears forgotten and abandoned. An odd waste so deep inside the city; it is not welcoming.

At the roundabout that marks the end of the road, the 'Hill' I have been climbing and descending for the past hour or so, there is a scored boundary stone marked with the names of the abutting parishes: HEAVITREE and ST SIDWELLS. Beyond the cast iron dragons on Zanzibar Cottage, there is a face-off between Georgian and Victorian terraces – striking dolphin plaster mouldings from the latter, elegant restraint from the former. I pass the house where the postmodern performance-maker Tim Etchells, founder of Forced Entertainment, slept one night with a heart monitor and awoke to find from the readings that his heart had stopped in the middle of the night and been re-started by a dream. I wander around in the back streets behind Albion Place.

Extricating myself from a dead end, I re-emerge onto the street I had strayed from, and wind around the yard of an orthodox chapel of the Ecumenical Patriarchate of the parish of St Elias, trespassing for a moment inside its walls under the pretence of reading the service times on the chapel door: I WAS A STRANGER AND YOU WELCOMED ME. The site of a mediaeval hermitage, a John Wygwer (ancestor of the later Widger?) collected money, including from the Earl of Devon, to build this chapel of breccias in the early 1400s; it has been rented by the Orthodox Church since the 1980s. In the alley at its back is an old (as in 1930s old), empty, discarded suitcase; similarly, another of identical age in the water of the adjacent horse trough. Props for a script I cannot even guess at.

I run onto the roundabout and find a quiet place in the dip of it; but when I squeeze through the connections box beneath the phone tower, I am almost burned by all the chatter.

Sidwell Street is the first street I walk that feels like England.

My England.

And then I realise why this walk is wonderful; because it makes me an alien in my own country and that is how it should always be. We all need to be embraced as strangers close to home. All the hermit-syndrome fallen-to-Earth children in their bedrooms, connected to clouds; they have it right. They are protecting their inner darkness, the thing that makes them them, that even they should not know and cannot see. But there is a brighter way to that darkness; by being a stranger under your own sun, by being pilgrim across the ordinary world and making it strange. That is what I have been lured, or lured myself, into doing.

I hear chatter in Polish. Women wear headscarves. Someone is on their way to prayers. Someone else is picking at popcorn chicken from KFC. Dumna is in her heaven and all is well.

A group of young people are carrying a door in a frame. I assume they are helping a friend with a new home... but they stop, put down the frame and invite passers-by to step through their doorway. I do it. They say that I am welcome; wherever I have come from and wherever I am going to I am welcome. It is a portal to civility. They demonstrate the door to the small crowd that has gathered; the whole structure stands when the door is open, and when closed, it falls.

At the junction – under two terracotta 'Green Men', one with a jungle moustache, the other too strange to characterise, and between them, perhaps Sidwella? Or Dumna? – I turn down past the Spiritualist Church and then the mosque, and then along Blackall Road where there is a plaque in the wall which announces:

I DON'T LIKE TEXT IN ART
BUT WALKING ALONG
THIS ROAD HOLDING THE
HAND OF A GIRL I LOVED
WAS THE HAPPIEST I'VE
EVER BEEN.

Cruelly, behind the wall, are the remains of Gergana Prodanova, a Bulgarian woman; it will be a few days before they find her. I have had enough of murder.

I decide to have my dinner at the Dinosaur. I have got a bit obsessed and dropped my rules about seeking new eating experiences.

But when I get to the decaying dolphins-horses-snakes of the clock tower, I can see that at the other end of Queen Street black smoke is pouring upwards in thick spiralling columns above the winking lights of emergency vehicles. I jog quickly towards the flames, a vampire afraid to miss a drop of blood. I race past the entrance to Northernhay gardens, the oldest public recreational space in the UK, where Bram Stoker observed his boss, the gaunt and chiselled Sir Henry Irving, perambulating in the mist, cloak and all.

I crab around the Cathedral Green, cut off at every turn by blue incident tape. Behind Wagamama I am shouted at by a Princesshay security man and scuttle back behind the tape. Finally, by walking up beside the Bishop's Palace I am able to squeeze along the side of a fire tender and get a view of what is going on.

The Royal Clarence Hotel is burning down, and has been almost all day. From a crane, fire fighters are pouring foam down onto its gutted facade. Somehow, in my anxiety to get to Stoke Canon I had missed the early morning drama in the High Street, racing off in the opposite direction. A fire in a Cathedral Green gallery, being converted to luxury flats, spread through the Well House Tavern (O no!) to the Clarence. Even as I watch, the fire finds new materials and darkening smoke boils upwards in thick serpents of vaporised gunk. Spiritualising old Exeter.

No one knows how far it will spread. Maybe into the High Street: there is a mediaeval merchant's hall concealed behind the facade of Costa. That sort of thing. People want to talk to each other at the blue tapes. I begin a conversation with a young student and three other people join in. I am surprised in how many languages melancholy is expressed.

"Why did we not know about the places inside these buildings? Who knew that Costa was mediaeval? Only now we are told as it is all being destroyed..."

We are all held back behind flimsy plastic tapes. A few of the privileged – media, politicians – are allowed through. The Tory Police and Crime Commissioner is observed, behind the tapes, taking a crass selfie with a fire fighter. But for the rest of us, long term residents, recent arrivals in headscarves, language students speaking in excited Spanish, an American historian, and me – a Tyke interloper – all take our place in the exclusion zone. When the theatre burned down in Longbrook Street the people of the West Quarter flooded up Fore Street; there was no tape. The people carried out the dead, dampened down the flames.

Tape is the means by which the insurers and the bureaucrats ensure that, except in the most extreme of catastrophes, the ordinary person is allowed to play no part other than spectator or consumer in the spectacle of their own catastrophe. Shock, accident, attack and disaster – to which once ordinary people rushed to help – are increasingly the province of private ownership and state control. Shock and disaster are investments made by powerful others; they have ownership of them, they are no longer fallen within the democratic domain but are processed through the discourses of investment and redevelopment. Just as the suburbs and their ripple structures have been formed by nuclear blast, so the centres of cities are in a soft lockdown in response to the home-made terrors of the media's and authorities' authorship. They take the uranium of the unpredictable and lonely hatred, the poison of internet hermits, and they process it into rings of steel, lines of bollards, loops and shivering lines of tape.

The way that each step of terror has proceeded is to place bollards and barricades between power and the most exploited; at the very moment that the empire is coming home they have intensified the principle of separation to pixel level. The combination is strategic; the deprivation from its own public lives of a public that is losing what little privilege it had as a public; this spastic welding of exclusion and inclusion, cultural definition and a Super Other is like making a social IED and then planting it in everyone's way.

I now 'get' why some walkers want an extreme extension of the Right to Roam to dangerous places and sensitive sites. The logic of public protection is like that of an abusive husband.

The flames rear up again within the emptying facade.

That night I dream of a landscape made up of university buildings and mediaeval ruins. There is a certain smoothness to it. I am with my daughter, who is in a hyper-modern wheel chair. In real life she is not a wheelchair user. All is fine until we try to return to wherever we have come from, and then she disappears, the machine whisking her off, while every turn and staircase and boulevard I chase her down seems less possible than the last until all I have is my useless forward momentum into less and less recognisable baroque twists and turns, each of them beautifully detailed and terrifyingly incoherent.

Queen Street, New North Road, Hele Road, St David's Hill, Red Cow Village, Cowley Bridge Road, King Edward Street, Cowley Bridge Road, Crediton Road, Upton Pyne Hill, immediately after the bridge take the footpath on left, follow around left edge of the field, across railway line (take care), bear left and through gates into field, then turn around, back through gates, cross railway line (carefully) and bear left along top of field, through gate and left onto Upton

Pyne Hill (take care with cars), turn right onto Burridge Road at the signpost for Brampford Speke, at Brampford Speke turn right into Church Drive, take footpath through the churchyard and into alley, at the end of the alley straight on and down Chapel Road, at junction take footpath to the right – explore the 'jungles' – then back up Chapel Road, bear left at entrance to the alley and almost immediately bear left down footpath with handrail, cross bridge over river and turn right along footpath, follow footpath to Stoke Canon, cross the railway at the unmanned level crossing on Green Lane, bear left along Chestnut Crescent, at T-junction turn right onto High Street and Stoke Hill (take care on the bridges), once across the bridges bear left and up the hill (still Stoke Hill, take care for the two miles of this road, there are some narrow verges, but often not, take extreme care on any corner or stretches without verge), at junction with Collins Road take signed Widecombe Way footpath, top of steps bear left past school and down ramp turning right onto Stoke Hill, at lamp post and metal barrier turn right up steps, along alley into Monterey Gardens, past enormous tree on your right and take the pavement to your left, down Rosebarn Lane, at wooded area turn left and then immediately right onto Stoke Hill, turn right up steps into wooded area, turn around, back down steps and turn right along Stoke Hill, over roundabout and down Old Tiverton Road, Albion Place, right though gap in wall into Toronto Road, bearing left to the end of the street, take alley at the end on the left, then take alley on the right, at the end of this alley turn left along Old Tiverton Road, after Chinese takeaway turn left down alley, right onto Blackboy Road, onto roundabout (take care), Sidwell Street, York Road, Longbrook Street, Blackall Road, Howell Road, Elm Grove Road, Queen Street, High Street, Bedford Street, Bedford Circus, Southernhay, along Roman wall, South Street, Palace Gate, South Street, High Street, Guildhall Shopping Centre, Queen Street.

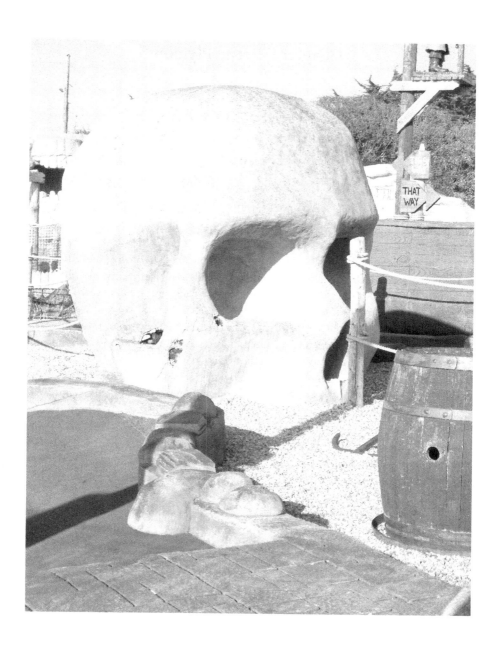

Chapter Fifteen: Plymouth

Crab Man has cancelled. His illness goes up and down, and he is down and immobilised. "Allow me two days' grace". I suddenly have a deadline, a target for ending my walk.

Well, I have other options today. After the split at the Paignton conference more walkers went west than east; my cosmopolitan, urban and Northernist prejudices are uncovered. I catch a train to Plymouth. I intend to doze, but quickly realise that, at least for a while, my walk has repeatedly hugged, crossed and woven itself around this line, itself a slow snake; it runs so close to the sea, corners around the hills. The train never gets up much speed and I can pick out landmarks from my walking, and others that Salmon fixes on and I ignored or missed.

As we set off, the city is dominated by the anomalous twin towers of the cathedral. There is still more than a wisp of grey smoke from the burning Close.

On the other side the skyline is patrolled by Haldon Belvedere sat on its pile of hills. Closer is the tower of St Thomas, from which a pro-Pope vicar had been hung "in full canonicals" along with his "holy-water bucket and sprinkle, a sacring bell, a pair of beads and such other like Popish trash". Trash, rubbish, waste, bloody flux. The body was only taken down, as a Courtenay was simultaneously released, when Queen Mary, bloodiness herself, was crowned.

We race parallel with the ship canal for a while. An unusual one, this. Canals are generally symbols of the Industrial Revolution, but Exeter's canal was built in the 1560s, long before the cotton gins and carding frames. I try to imagine the two-metre-long pike living in its waters, narrative revenants of the Cold War midget submarines – X Craft – that were tested here. Salmon quotes an oblique, but jolly online account of a social call paid in 1956 by Sprat and Minnow, two Stickleback Class submarines, negotiating the locks into the Exeter Canal Basin, close to the city centre. There is talk of cider, the crew emerging from their claustrophobic craft as the "great unwashed" and cricket played in a haze. But the visit may have been far from social, a covert part of Operation Cudgel, the project to secretly lay Red Beard nuclear devices inside Soviet harbours. Given that Red Beard was designed to explode up to a week after priming, it was clearly not a weapon of response; what was being rehearsed on the 16th-century waterway was a nuclear first strike.

They would not have used a live warhead in rehearsal. Of course not.

On the landward side of the tracks, I recognise the folly and then the grounds of Powderham Castle, where great oaks and conifers have fallen on their sides, their roots up in the air, like giant insects fallen on their backs. The herd of deer move complacently as an old forest moves through them. On the other side, on the far bank of the estuary and just above the town, I can just about make out the sixteen-sided home of those mad, anti-semitic, apocalyptic biddies (sorry, I mean proto-feminist architects and arts and crafters), its frozen carousel stuck forever between *ferme ornée* and a torture wheel from the 'Triumph of Death'.

Looking at the castle, I cannot help seeing Beckford's tower at Fonthill falling down and the landlords' house at the end of the horror movie blowing up.

THE AT OSPHERIC RAILWAY – the pub sign at Starcross.

The wrecks in the mud of the river, one a ruin, the other an elegant black skeleton, are topped off with cormorants, wings open like coats of arms. Then the larger body of half of the 'South Coaster', only the last of its many names: 'Oostvorne', 'Cwea', 'Martin'... like Mentz's descriptions in *Shipwreck Modernity*, there are no simple narratives for these wrecks; they do not clarify but make complex, they have multiple identities, cargoes, sources, suppliers and owners, and multiple and unreliable accounts of their demises. They do not explain but implicate; discovery, like mobility, is an ecological and human catastrophe. Eight days after going aground, eight days of efforts to refloat the 'South Coaster', the captain and crew were rescued by the local lifeboat. The boat, too damaged by the storm to repair, was towed and beached where it lies now and cut up for scrap – its guns lifted out and taken away. Its load of coal spilled out and rolled up on the shore at each high tide, a few pieces at a time; fuel thieved for the locals. What I had assumed was its mast – in fact a loading boom lashed to the deck at the time of its salvages – has now fallen across its bow, brought down after seventy plus years by the high winds that blew me about a few days ago and dropped boughs around me. The silhouette is skin and a few bones.

The train passes by The Sod and over The Creep.

The giant, anatomically absurd skull on the crazy-golf course, the sad carriages. The route out over the sea. On the other side, the red desert in the cliffs.

Just before we enter the tunnel at Coryton Cove we pass the terrace of four-storey houses, where the anti-hero of *A Perfect Spy* is hiding out; the modern flats where the police cars are hidden during their siege, and the top floor where the double-agent shoots himself in the face.

We have picked up the Devil's Footprints by now; then through the tunnels, under the former garden of the fugueuse's sculptor lover, by the Parson and the Clerk; more Devil. Shag Rock looks distinctly *lingam*.

The tide is out, but there are no signs of the wreck off the beach just before Teignmouth. There has been a desperate wish to make this an Armada wreck, to distil history down to a few improving stories, but the seals and insignia raised suggest that this ruin was a trader, probably Venetian, and almost certainly a galley, which means its oars were manned by slaves. For all the thrill of the recovery of cannon, there is no complementary concern for the dehumanised, no designation as a grave. No scallops to save their torsos. The dull thud of the Homogenocene, jelly-thinking, bites off the head of the saintly human race, yet still the body thrashes about demanding that all is fine, complete, whole. Slavery is where totality, mortally wounded, its mast blow down, becomes totalitarian. Some three miles further out, the SS Galicia blooms with anemones and corals and odd white lumpy growths; a multiplicity grown from the sharp point of a 1917 explosion.

This is where Norman Wisdom walks down to a train station that does not exist in 'Press for Time' (1966). Its sign says: TINMOUTH. We curl past the end of the Promenade, two women in deckchairs, backs to the sea, staring at a concrete wall. There was once a double arch here, made of whale jawbones, by the start of 'The Old Maids' Walk', symbols of the mystery we spend our whole lives seeking and that then eats us at the end; our way to a deep cosmos. But the bones are missing, like the ufo parts in an Exeter attic or the plaster statue of Drake on its back, a fallen pylon on the Haldon Hills waiting to confuse future archaeologists until it was recovered; just what the area needs, further distillation. The bone arches had been put up by Pike Ward, a local fish trader, insurer and all round marine entrepreneur – a Pike Ward company, Shipbrokers, still operates from the town – one of Ward's less successful ventures was 'Utopia', a trawler whose crew did more drinking than fishing.

We turn alongside the Teign, picking up speed; the tide is out and I try to spot the little chapel with its magickal parking space. Mussel cages are exposed on the tops of a sand bank. And there are thousands of wooden stakes in the mud; with rubber boot prints like join-the-dots. I watch as a man lifts one stake at a time, picking out pea-crabs, parasites that grow in mussels, bait that fetches a good price. He farms on land that no one owns; Salmon says that property disputes have been settled with fists in the past, but now the Environment Agency, without any authority except good sense, mediates. The boots of the outlaw-picker sink deeper into the rich brown dirty life.

A woman with a red rucksack is doing restrained tai chi on the New Quay.

Just before the unhappy Dream Church is the supermarket car park where The Newton Abbot and District Model Engineering Society's miniature locomotives, pressuring up in their steaming bays, were once tooted at by passing trains, saluting from one scale to another; a god to its fetish. This piece of line has a thing for throwing off its own simulacra. Inside the miniature railway track, round-the-pole tethered racing cars had circled worthlessly.

Then, something else: after Newton Abbot, just the slightest tip of a priory tower above the brow of the hill, and maybe only me on this train knows the secret of the "Chapel in the Woods", in a field full of downed trees, their kicking legs stopped mid-tantrum, is a fallen pylon, abandoned beside a working one. By its discolouration, it must have lain there for years, grass has grown up inside it, cows scratch their sides against it. Levelled like this, it is clearer that it is a hybrid portal, the two pylon shapes combined are closer to an obelisk; a frozen ray of sunlight.

Steep fields.

A pheasant on a concrete bridge. Gold and grey.

On top of the bridge is a white van, with a Pilsbury Doughboy, or maybe it is a Michelin Man, puffy and perished in the sun, stuck to the roof of the cab, waving yet another pirate flag. The romance of the bully-rebel is strong here; men (I think mostly) refiguring themselves as the disenchanted rogue, the disgruntled maverick; a glint in their eyes as if prejudice is some kind of originality. The 'reb' of the US Confederacy and the Prayer Book Rebellion; bad losers, defenders of reaction, Jesse James and Harry Callahan dissidents, Royalist rebels under Hopton, bushwhackers romancing murderous family disputes into principles, Robin Hoods dropping their knee to the Pope, betraying their language to a worse establishment, their heads full of trade winds and slavery, tasers hanging in their belts, an entrepreneur with sun-dried skin and salty accent, a strain of authoritarian populism, a kind of fascism, in the vacuum left by the dwindling collapse of independent working class education and culture: trade unions, non-conformist chapels, Antediluvian Buffalo lodges, WEA branches, co-ops, charities, Socialist Sunday Schools.

The field for 'independent' thought is left open to a populist Right, drawing on rich seams of prejudice and fear in sophisticated forms – Mallock, Trevena, Bulwer-Lytton, James Anthony Froude – ready for new demagogues. The majority (just) voted for cosmopolitanism in Exeter, but that is true of nowhere else I walked; the 63% in Torbay for leaving Europe were an alliance of big house Tories and the 'just about managing' poor.

Ruinous woodland.

Quarry buildings up against the track; hi-viz and rust.

More thick, dank, ivy-clad, rotting woodland.

In a surprising number of fields there are isolated caravans tucked into the elbow of a hedge for protection; lonely or cosy, I cannot tell. After the dark of a tunnel, the shock of apples unpicked on the floor of an orchard. Land rippled and folded, pylons marching to a strange knot as one power line passes under another, by a trapezoidal frame, exotic trees on private grounds, horses and the cluster of trees on hill tops. A huge barn. Mist above the marsh outside Totnes. On the other side of the tracks a steam locomotive is harrumphing its way out of a tiny station. A derelict hospital-green factory, a café in a signal box, slowing down; the weird hill is a Saxon construct not the ancient *gorsedd* of Mrs E.O. Gordon's British-Israelite imagination, cemetery, streams, HOWARD HARVESTORE, huge silos, fields like nitrate waves, and the trace of an old path curling around a hill, disappearing into nothing any more.

A line of washing, chickens, sheep, a church with a needle spire, "R&D" machines steaming, cable maintenance men in a field, more pylons, radio mast, wind turbine, an overgrown garden and a moto-cross racetrack cut into the side of a hill (a mark of Cthulhu according to the birdman!), sheep with turquoise dots, and then the land rolls out and up to the tops of tors on the moor. The train bends to skirt the moor and the land turns scrubby, we pass over three viaducts across deep valleys and an industrial estate far from anywhere, then a huge 18th-century house, probably with hidden older parts; although there are few dwellings, there is very little sense of wilderness. Instead there is land-in-between: private woodland, hedged green fields; I see no one walking. At Ivybridge there are bamboos growing over the platform from a large private garden. Monohousing; suburbia without a city.

Unlike the first half of the journey where my walk has sometimes been visible from the train, and things and shapes are soaked in stories and stuck in webs of connections, since somewhere this side of Newton Abbot I have been looking generically, seeing a Ladybird Book of landscape, a place defined by collective nouns. Maybe this train journey is not such a good idea.

Then afar off, and again remarkably close up, is the huge blank tower of Centrica Langage Power Station, a fossil-fuel burning state of the art operation; it has been up for sale, but no one will pay the asking price; the company is trying to raise capital to cover costs caused by – (drum roll) – extreme weather conditions caused by climate change.

Two massive troop transporters pass a few feet over us, swooping down into the valley to the south then tipping over the tops of the hills, full of grace and murder. I suck in a lungful of the stale carriage air, involuntarily, at these circus elephants.

Beyond the sprawling edge of Plymouth, the lunar landscape of white clay quarries, then a hollow building where the fire brigade rehearse their fire rituals, an abstraction of a building, shadowy as the ghost house at Dawlish in the photo in Salmon's pamphlet. Stained warehouses and stumpy 1960s' office blocks, and the white PVC-coated polyester sails of the Navy-inspired Sainsbury's, the wreck in the river mud. The tide is out and there is an intriguing river in the bed of the river; tiny dimensions curled up inside the bigger dimension. A giant school, 1960s' monohousing beside Victorian monohousing.

I have arrived at Plymouth.

I'd been expecting to be met. Two minutes of feeling foolish and a man in a thick tweedy suit enters, breathlessly, through the swoosh of automatic doors. As we walk towards the town he tells me he is a kind of tour guide.

"Like a mis-guide? Like a counter-tourism thing?"

"No, I know those things, but no..."

He collapses conventional guided tours together, exaggerating their existing qualities.

"I'm not interested in myths or fancies. History is quite strange and entertaining enough..."

"Entertaining?"

"In the sense of being a history of entertainment."

To demonstrate he takes me to an ornamental pond to talk about 'Behemoth the Sea Monster', partly set in the sea just off Plymouth; we don't have time to go to the Sound. On the way we pass through the university campus, a strange mixture of cobbled lanes and tall glassy unremarkable buildings, with large 'Big Brother' portraits of young alumni. A curled silvery snake discarded, temporarily, from a laboratory.

I recognise the green dome and we go to look. It's the Immersive Vision Theatre where Percy Seymour, the cosmic magnetism man, had once been director. My guide is not an academic, but we sneak inside. All is gloomy and locked, no one is about, but on the floor of the lobby is a sun symbol, not entirely straightforward: a twenty-headed corona around a black disc, an eclipse. Outside, due to the curve of the building, the decorative wooden panels have been sawn in pieces; a fish swims in two halves, its head angrily berates a shipwreck on the sea floor. Above the wreck a jelly attacks a knot in the wood. A vertical panel measuring oceanic depths – Abyssalpelagic six kilometres down, Hadalpelagic a full ten – has a submarine floating above an angler fish. My guide explains that male angler fish only live to find a female, biting into the female's body and fusing completely with them, dissolving their eyes and internal organs (apart from their testes) until they become a small, fertile fin-like addendum. I wonder if this is a very obtuse proposition, batting it back to the guide with a suggestion that he fuse with the submarine.

Seymour's grand theory begins with what sounds like a solid piece of science: Ernst Mach's famous principle that the mass of any body is a product of all the matter in the universe, hence its conservatism and its resistance to changes in its position or motion. His mistake is then to anthropomorphise it: "in other words, the universe exerts a form of social pressure on the particle to maintain the status quo". This quickly leads to a swampy recruiting of "palmistry, graphology and physiognomy" as "a natural consequence of my theory" and then he nose-dives into the sophistry of the pseudo-researcher: "investigations showed that outstanding politicians also tended to be born with the Moon in these positions". "Outstanding" by what criteria, standing out from what?

The whirl of symbols at the Ringmore parking space is mirrored at the centre of Seymour's theory, where the magnetic fields of the planets tweak the movement of the Sun about the centre of the solar system: "squares between Mercury and Venus will be important... If the tuning of a magnetic canal lies between the angular speed of any two planets, then the squares between those two will be important... This tuning will gradually shift from the inner planets to the outer planets", and as it shifts it "re-tunes" people. The plethora of signs in the parking space is marshalled to the conservative behavioural psychology of (tobacco-sponsored) Hans Eysenck, at the time of his death the contemporary psychologist cited most often in peer-reviewed literature. The black sun makes more sense.

Trying to make his case, Seymour repeatedly resorts to mechanistic analogies: a telephone exchange, a television set, but most strikingly, an explosive mine: "detonated by a device triggered by the magnetic field of a passing ship... If we consider birth as the explosion... the nervous system is the magnetic aerial and trigger".

The degradation of Seymour's science leads him from an intuition that, if he had stayed within the disciplines of electro-magnetism and gravitation-studies, might now be curling round to meet the advances of quantum biology coming the other way. Instead, he spirals off to the entrepreneurial margins of esoteric publishing, then curls back to the surprisingly close entanglement of New Age esotericism and right-wing Big Science.

The architecture changes for the better. A giant canyon and two sides of semi-iconic building, lovely brown materials, a huge screen, and three wonderful giant blobby sculptures, shifting gears through fruit to geometry, that no one seems to be noticing. It only needs a few market stalls to feel quite 'Bladerunner'. And we find the stalls! In the vacuous ground floor of the Roland Levinsky Building. I think this is the first time a very recent building has excited me in all my walking; Exeter's Princesshay was OK, elegant and inoffensive, but this is such an invitation. I ask my guide who Levinsky was?

"Hmm, 'was' is right, and he leads me over to an empty space by the revolving doors.

"Well, there was a portrait here..."

He speaks to one of the staff on a reception desk.

"Apparently his widow objected to the rubbish one they had here and another one is being painted. Roland Levinsky was the son of communist parents; his father had emigrated to South Africa from the Polish-Lithuanian border to escape the pogroms only to find his family the subject of repeated police raids by the apartheid regime. Roland came to the UK and worked as a top paediatrician at Great Ormond Street, then shifted into management and became the vice-chancellor here, turning the whole place upside down. In those days, the university was spread around with different schools in different towns and he brought them all together, here, and put up new buildings. I remember how everyone complained, these little outposts were losing their independent identities, but by putting them in a city centre and in touch with each other, the different disciplines rubbing along side by side, he helped, just a little, to counter the general homogenising rush of universities; but, yes, maybe he made this place vulnerable to that too, made the target too big, I don't know whether they still use the title but not long after Levinsky was killed the university started calling itself 'The Enterprise University'..."

"'Was killed'?"

"Yes, one Christmas, he was out walking..."

"Knocked down?"

"No, it was stormy, power cables had been blown down, the current from a broken cable jumped to his body and killed him. It was very unlucky; apparently it was unknown for a cable to break like that and not short out the whole system..."

Electro-magnetism.

"...he was just about to make a bid to bring Dartington here..."

"The college?"

Before I get to hear that part of the story, I am kidnapped. I am supposed to be meeting a dancer after the guide has finished with me – an apologetic Crab Man has recruited contacts in Plymouth to help me out with finding delegates from the conference – but she has spotted us on our way from the former planetarium and laid ambush. She marches me away.

"Quick or we'll miss it! You don't mind, do you? Why don't you come too? I'm sure it will be fine."

The guide is unsure.

"What is it?"

"Live art."

"Will there be blood?"

"O, I think so..."

"I'll wait here, if you don't mind?"

In a dark black box studio; it does indeed begin with a flow of blood, as needles are removed from forehead. It splashes down her face and chest, and she moves with a long sheet of muslin (I think), her nakedness is not about exposure, but her relation to what becomes a Möbius Strip, held in her hands and escaping her hands, movement about an eternal or giant exterior. She is vulnerable in the embrace of the Great Indifference of distance and closeness, powerful in her casting of herself outwards into a place where there are few gaps, where there may be no gaps at all. In this sudden dark space I see the church paintings to which the birdman led me come alive. She completes the three: Dumna, Mary/Sidwella and herself.

The dancer leads me outside.

"What did you think?"

"That it should be available on the NHS. *That* it is the ritual I have been missing in all the wonderful places I have been..."

She hands me back to the guide. "I'll see you in a few minutes."

The shopping centre is a car wreck; I can only imagine they gave a different bit to each junior in the office to design: a wave ceiling here, a forest car park there. It is almost as big a mess as Exeter Cathedral. I am gobsmacked when my guide tells me that the same architects designed this and the Princesshay shopping centre in Exeter. I think there was some politics of status involved.

We dodge the traffic and sit on the edge of the Gdynia Fountain in the middle of the busy roundabout. The guide is excited to show me the heraldic shield of the Polish port under the waters of the pool. He produces a plastic brontosaurus, although I think we have to call it something else now.

"They had wanted the monster to be something like a radioactive blob, more like the monster in 'X the Unknown', but..."

He looks up at the clock on the empty, impressive Royal Bank of Scotland Building, its blue mosaic tiles glittering between the shadows of its pillars.

"Now you'll hear the behemoth," he says.

And a wailing begins to snake up from the other end of the Royal Parade.

"If you hear that at any time other than 11.30am on a Monday, reach for your potassium iodate tables."

Stephen Barber writes that "[T]he presence of the tenacious film image... collides harshly with, and reveals the visual structure of, the city".

Not just the visual structure, Stephen, but its aural and atomic ones, too.

We cross back, perilously, from the fountain pool in the centre of the St Andrews roundabout, gold crab insignia winking behind the pillars. My host climbs up the churchyard wall and rolls onto his feet; leaves have stuck to the back of his jacket. He takes from his pocket a large length of chain and lays it on top of a stone plaque.

"They put it in just a few years ago, unbelievable, how can they do that? Memorialise Sir John Hawkins!"

He reads from the plate:

"He helped the poor of Plymouth... a highly-respected citizen of Plymouth, a parishioner of this church of St Andrew".

He kicks the chain and climbs down to the pavement. No one has noticed.

"Nothing there about his being the initiator of the Atlantic slave trade in 1562 – and he wasn't just following orders, he wrote the book on the slave trade; and I don't mean that metaphorically, he literally wrote a handbook for slave traders; how to set one lot of African people fighting with another, then taking the losers as slaves, sowing rotten legacies. One of the ships on his second slave voyage was called 'Jesus'! Hawkins died in his own shit, like Drake after him, eaten up from inside by what was called the 'bloody flux'. Like so many of those pirates, he couldn't live with himself on land."

He leaned over the wall and patted the chains he had left.

"Maybe that will make them think," and he wishes me well and leaves.

Hawkins was not just a slave trader; he was a designer. Another in the devil's footprints of designers.

I think I get the 'Behemoth' point; the sea and the land are here at war.

A space ripples, the dancer has reappeared; from the pocket of her furry jacket she takes a copy of Lepecki's thin book *Exhausting Dance*, holding it curled up like a scroll in her hand, dismissing the guide and lecturing me in ideas from Heidegger and Fanon and the crawling of William Pope L., straight from the book. For her, the ground is rippling, disturbed, she explains. She cannot stand for long. She sees the wound in every quarry mark; not just in the old buildings, but displaced into the new. A society filmed from the neck down. She keeps moving, trips often, occasionally squirms on her belly. "It's the same surface for everyone, but it only trips up the being of some. Yet it is objectively rippling, for both you and me? How does that work?"

She is adamant that I should say this is not about appropriating an identity; that when she crawls she makes very sure that she cannot be observed. In woods, behind walls, in empty buildings or busy buildings after hours, with and without permission. "I now know some good corrupt janitors", she laughs. That also is not her phrase.

"I can't imitate William Pope L. in Brooklyn. On the Royal Parade, for god's sake? I can only walk *in relation to* that oscillating space."

She spits out the word "relation" as if its spine were baited with chilli sauce.

"How can we walk, when for some the street denies them being?"

She stumbles as we attempt to amble over the windblown square between a suspended screen, an outsized sundial and two blocks of retail; nothing is giant, everything is moderately obese. I fear for her. She has an arm in plaster; "fractured, possibly more".

I have not realised at this time that I am in the thrall of a Tree of Life.

"It's not about my identity", she insists as I help her up by the good arm.

"But you're a.... woman of colour? A black woman, aren't you?"

There is no point in not saying it.

"I'm a mystery. My parents were white, I had assumed they were, designated 'white', it wasn't an issue until I was born. But there must be something in our history. That's all that I'm fucking interested in. History. Not the names or 'on whose side' or anything. I'm not interested in identities and memes. It's the ground..."

"...the fundamental...?"

"No! Yes! The fundamental... You're right. You're right! That's how it presents itself – as Plymouth limestone, as pavements, from far, far, far back in the day, old buildings made from fossils... billions and billions of dead molluscs piled up at the feet of an architect. How do we dig up and replace shit that old? How do you get rid... of the *geology* of racism... wipe away its strata? That is what we *have to* do. Otherwise there's no hope for us... we have to become a geological force..."

This time, picking her up, I could see that there was an equally thin book curled up inside the Lepecki.

"Isn't there a danger of re-writing the past?... like Orwell says..."

"No. No, there isn't any danger from that."

"Don't you think..."

She put her good hand on my arm.

"If you're swimming in poison, don't sing."

And she walks away.

She turns a corner ahead of me. I see people running, but I don't follow them. I know it is not meant for me to see. I have become the malevolent gazer in all this; suspicious that stumbling and crawling are just two more ways to appropriate the pavement from those without a Claude Glass to frame it. Like the tripper, I can see no way out of the cycle, but I am not doing anything about it.

I have another appointment.

The statues on the side of the Guildhall are troubling. One, a stone sculptor, sculpts his own stone head. Another, a god of cornucopia, surrounded by fruit, is succumbing to moss. An astronomer observes the stars through a nest a bird has built in his eye.

On a square between the courts, what Salmon describes as the headquarters of ConSec, administering the Ripe programme for the distribution of ephemerol, two students are standing, shivering and walking on the spot.

"Cold?"

"No, we're imitating the herring gulls," says the girl, "but instead of worms other things come up."

I want to stay and question them more, but I am already late at the market.

Outside the theatre, one of the patrons' metal stars has been removed from the pavement; I wonder if this is the ghost of some other now-disgraced celebrity; there are so many. Does anyone see a pattern? Inside the theatre, in the star dressing room, Salmon claims, a mural painted by the imprisoned entertainer Rolf Harris has been concealed, but not destroyed.

I lose my way and end up asking directions to the Pannier Market; a modernist curio, all concrete waves, a great swell rolling out across its huge ceiling above stalls of bulk fabrics, cheap clothes, second-hand books and dvds, cheeses, organic foods, drug equipment and guns, a comics shop – "Captain America's joined the Nazis!", the super hero emerges on the front cover of 'The Titans' (£2) with a group of men in coal scuttle helmets hurling grenades: I buy it, just for the cover, Trump is just getting up steam in the US Primaries – the owner, who has to be fetched from somewhere by a security guard, is carrying a copy of Richard Littler's *Discovering Scarfolk*. I remark that I did not like it; that I thought it would be like the lovely *I Know Where I'm Going* or Chris Lambert's *Tales from the Black Meadow*, but it is horrible, like being stuck in one of those terrifying public information films from the 70s, 'danger deep water' or whatever. That it is brilliant in that way. I hope he will smile in recognition, but there is no flicker. Instead, as he takes my fiver and first long-changes and then, when corrected, short-changes me, puts the comic in an unnecessary brown paper bag despite my protest, he harangues me as he writes out a receipt (I know, £2, but I'm registered self-employed!):

"All this 'Scarfolk' and the rest... the nanny state!"

He reads from a leaflet by the till.

"Sustainable development will not be brought about by policies only: it must be taken up by society at large as a principle guiding the many choices each citizen makes every day."

"No wonder, eh? And now the whole thing's shaved so thin, like movie cowboy towns there's just a front with almost nothing holding it up, you turn up at A&E and there are ambulances in a queue to get in, try to get in touch with who's in charge and they put you through to a call centre in Timbuctoo! Armies that no longer fight, all drones, 'Scarfolk' is here... all we have left of all that welfare or whatever, libraries, can't afford to use the buses... you speak to the people who come in here and they're paranoid about their kids being given LSD skin patches, it's stupidity..."

And he waves his copy of *Discovering Scarfolk* at me.

"They get it off the Internet. This is their 'self-expression', but they don't have nothing to say, just this mush – we let all those painting clubs go, 'Scarfolk' takes the piss out of us, the "superfluous", "undesirables"...

He lowers his voice.

"...food that isn't food – "fibreglass candyfloss"! "Shingles Cakes"! Then it has a pop at political correctness and multi-culturalism and foreigners just as you were thinking that was the kind of attitude it was getting at! – that's its genus..."

I think he means 'genius'.

But where is the stallholder coming from? Would a mixed-race stallholder have a "pop" at multi-culturism or, rather, at a book that had a "pop"? We are being dragged into the mire of the book. And the book is the mire it is having a "pop" at.

"...and the endless roll call of accidents to kids... it gets inside that mentality, *the* attitude, there is no escape from it, baby! Everything is a stupid gag; it's not funny for us. This *is* Scarfolk!"

He gestures up to the huge concrete waves of market roof.

"You ever see old photos? Who *were* those people? In this book you can live in pessimism forever, it's bloody black magic this book! The piss-poor jokes... it's like being trapped in a room forever with Bernard Manning. It's real!"

He is a character. As plotted as a bit part in 'Mister Robot'. What kind of stallholder quotes from European Union documents? All these characters, with their liquidising monologues; even when someone is trying to be on your side, they drag you under with them.

Upstairs is a shelf of greasy spoons serving close-to-identical menus, and then, dotted about beneath, unusual and highly edible Jamaican and Thai food.

I meet the pair for Thai Pad; perched on stools, elbows on formica, the food sizzles in pans a metre away. We hear the food before we see it.

They announce themselves as an odd couple in a complex set of introductions; I feel I am being tested on some level. As if they are taking a cultural capital reading from me. She is from the States, Japanese American, third generation immigrant, here on a year's research leave; he is from "a small coastal town in North Wales" which he does not name. There is no Welsh in his voice. He seems to have drained a lack of belonging into his body; all the time nervously looking about as if for a cap and scarf and an exit. It takes me a while to like him. She is quite different; she has a calmness that is almost oppressive, almost entitled. She is a Professor; he a writer of small pamphlets. Her thing is cities, he is only for the old ones. He plots the ancestors and she reads Dupuy, Graham, Weizman, Massey, Anderson and Castells; she talks about Doug Farr and smart growth, balancing her Coke on the most recent edition of *Critical Cities*.

He says that if it has anything to do with ethnicity, that is because everything does.

"Even the Large Magellanic Cloud?"

"Particularly the Large Magellanic Cloud."

They laugh, and he takes out a black and white print; it looks like it might have been an illustration from a book of fairy tales. She passes him her A-Z; he opens it at the page we are on, and he lays the line drawing over the map. The paper is almost as thin as tracing paper; I can see the lines of the map running beneath and entangling with the trunks and boughs of the forest.

"'Cosmopolitan canopies'? Zones of civility, usually in the centres of large cities, places where a truce has been declared around race and culture, normally in the interests of commerce, retail, and so on? The idea of Elijah Anderson, the sociologist...

"Rubbing along..."

"Getting by, getting along... jokey, negotiated, easy going..."

That's why they've brought me here. To listen to the lippy Janners lovin' and darlin' the sharply beautiful Thai woman boss; who takes their conservative orders with a politeness that does not give a single hundredth of a femtometre to subservience. Snapping them on to the women in the bouffant caps. The menu-fumbling of uncertain locals who are beginning to doubt their adventure; it is this awkward space, between uncomfortable and relaxed, where no one gets angry or upset, inhibitions are brusquely dissed.

"Maybe there's something older and more frightening going on? Elijah Anderson is no one's fool; all the qualifications and contexts are in place, he's fully aware of the reactionary spaces between and within the canopies, and the spasms and breaks that threaten to tear the canopies apart. But the driving narrative is..."

"Is resilience..."

"Yes, the canopy is resilient. That's the narrative, but..."

"We could hear another."

"Could you get me another Coke, babe?"

"For sure", and he bobs around on his stool trying to catch the eye of one of the cooks.

"There's so much salt and chilli in this... it's good though..." She shakes her head at his twitchiness. "Putting an urbanist and a mythologist together is less remarkable than you think, Cecile. In Finland the planners consult folklorists, to avoid trouble with trolls. *Feng shui*, of course. That's why we brought you here, especially..."

There is no booth selling chow mein.

"Not for the canopy?"

She looks up and laughs.

The concrete above our heads continues to break in rollers and white horses.

"Though I do adore it. No. Not for the canopy. Partly, maybe. It is such a wonderful exception here. Nothing in the whole central rebuilding is anything like it. It does not fit with the Portland stone of everything else. This is where the locals put up their resistance, right here, built their barricade against everything that Abercrombie imposed on them... Abercrombie..."

She pronounces "crom" like "crumb". I imagine an architect with remnants of his breakfast stuck to his shirt.

"...studied *feng shui* in the 1920s; his designs were influenced by abstract and ideal forms; he was some kind of neo-Platonist, possibly... His first model for the rebuilding of the city centre is as close to a Kabbalah 'tree of life' as you could smuggle in without a whistle being blown..."

272

"I've seen one of those..."

"...in fact it was quietly scrubbed away, a polite, behind the scenes kind of viciousness, his vision watered down so much it was drowned! It was Vico who had me question "canopy". I had imagined it as something like this; airy, tall, a space to breathe, to expand, to liberate yourself, but with something of the labyrinth, pushing strangers together in a shared tension. But for Vico the literal canopy is something else; it's that roof of twigs and boughs and nests that blots out all of the sunlight, the roof canopy of the Grimm forest, the never-existing fairy tale forest... or, at least, which *was* never existing until modern forestry came along! The canopy is the primal memory of the trauma we never had. The great shadow, the night in the day. Until the lightning comes..."

He rips the ring pull and hands the fizzing syrup to her.

"It's the screen of barbarism pierced by lightning at the very birth of civilisation; according to Vico..."

"The Italian philosopher?"

"*Neapolitan* philosopher! Probably never stepped inside a forest in his life!"

He folds his arms.

"Is there any worse narrative than civilisation? Isn't it for civilisation that we bomb and bomb and bomb and bomb?"

"You're saying that the cosmopolitan canopy is a new kind of..."

"European nightmare forest."

She drinks a sip from the can and looks hard at the prawns in her bowl.

No.

Wrong.

Has to be.

They guide me back through the centre; through each genus of space – square, monument, temporary booth, flower bed, fountain. For each they have a dark, old myth; I think they must be caught up in a nostalgic *folie-a-deux*, but it becomes clear that their *folie* is *nouvelle*, they are making them up, awakening structures that never stood before, never worked, never flexed. They are enacting a fundamentalism that they have detected in progressive urbanism. They call this performance 'satirical urbanism'; they plan to take it on the conference circuit. Hunting urbanists.

In the grinder
Only the tiny gesture will survive
The blades.

I lie about a midday train. I follow them out of the station, keeping a discreet distance. When they turn off, I keep straight on.

Queen Street, Hele Road, St David's Hill, Exeter St David's Station, train to Plymouth, Glen Park, steps from Glen Park to Winston Avenue, North Road East, James Street, Portland Square, Glanville Street, Drake Circus, Drake

Circus Shopping Centre, Eastlake Street, Old Town Street, St Andrews Cross, St Andrews Place, Royal Parade, Armada Way, Royal Parade, Derry's Cross, Royal Parade, Courtenay Street, New George Street, Pannier Market (City Market), Cornwall Street, Armada Way, North Cross, North Road, Plymouth Train Station.

I turn inland in search of water. The thought of a sea full up of behemoth submarines, designed to deliver nuclear payloads, has filled me with a dark kind of enchantment, and I am excited and determined to find a deeper level to the supercilious sex and magic I keep finding just under the surface of the manifestos and *flâneries* with which I am being repeatedly and oppressively presented. I would like to find something of my own again.

Looking back to check that I have not been spotted and followed by the deadly duo; above the station lobby there is a clear rectangular box crossed with a metal structure and more polyester sails, as if the sea must constantly be asserted. I am doing the right thing, walking away from this.

I spend the afternoon, the night and most of the next day doing two right things rather than one. Three if I count the drinking. Mostly local beers, in halves, never more than one in any particular place. But I visit many places. I am becoming a little exhausted and delusional; but very, very careful. I know that there is some writing about this city and how deceptively the various gazes work here; quiet places suddenly filling up with eyes, great patches of invisibility and generosity in the big market where I had Thai Pad, and then thin attention on the esplanades. When I eventually get to see the Hoe later, in rain and low light, its slightly bowed blurriness suggests there is something unclear here, an unhelpful veneer cloaking the giant figure of Gogmagog, Madoc the Great, defeated by a hero of Brutus's (Britain's) army, becoming two figures simultaneously, at once on and under the Hoe, Gogmagog and Corin a double monster, Gog and Magog, enemies of the Old Ones' utopia, one an idealist and the other a slayer, Fasolt and Fafner, each a hero but in different revolutions. I realise later, looking out across the Sound and imaging the prehistoric river course in the submerged bed of the contemporary estuary, that it will be very difficult to tell fiend from friend.

My second activity is a slow reading of a thin book – *Flâneur* by Frederico Castigliano – slow because it is hard to stop all the words from sliding together into a single slough of melancholic male entitlement. I hate this book, but I learn much from it, more than many of those I loved during my preparatory reading.

I had already guessed that *flânerie* is individualistic, egotistical and male. It comes as only a mild surprise when Castigliano reveals that for him it is the 'Game' of the street pick-up that is the apotheosis of *flânerie*. More surprising when he deigns to mention the possibility that *flâneuses* exists, not that he mentions anything they do. (I had read Lauren Elkin's fabulous book *Flâneuse*; I know I have not invented this sense of grievance.)

More interesting is what Castigliano's book reveals about *flânerie's* "reading" of the urban text; how the atmosphere of a space one day will have disappeared by the next. But what if the opposite is true! What if ambience is how we experience the resilient affect of a revelatory totality?

I think it's remarkable how often I share the same perception of a place's atmospheres with someone else. About which way to go we can have opinions, but about atmosphere we have feelings that accommodate like clouds. Perhaps ambience, the softest thing of all, is what we should be anchoring our walks to?

How we make that happen could be more like Deleuze's idea of thinking in 'n minus 1' dimensions; the "1" (that's taken away) is, then, not anyone's particular intuition, but rather is the dominant way that "mood" structures our intuitions about the world; minus that and we are on our way to a precious and fragile sensitivity even more vulnerable than 'minus'.

Maybe artist walkers should be more aggressive in their vulnerability; insisting that in order to subtract the oppressive "1", every meeting, every interview, every date, every work of art, every work assessment should be organised as a journey, guided by the mutual interpretation of atmospheres; that every gathering, jury decision or assignation, boardroom meeting or wage negotiation be subject to the changing ambiences of an enigmatic route?

Pow! What a city this is! Released on my own, this is my most intense walking so far. There is just thing after thing! Why did people tell me this is a dull city? This is not a nice city, nor a picturesque city; plenty of artifice and design, but so violently jumbled, bombed, amalgamated, redeveloped and rebuilt that it bursts with meaning, destroying sense as it makes sense; it brutalises in a totally different way from a Northern industrial city. Despite the differences, it heaves with excesses that I recognise. And friendliness; I would expect the villages and lanes to be where people are most friendly, but nowhere do people speak to me more than in this city.

No sooner am I across the bridge from the station than the details impinge: the bloody (not real) handprint on a window, a black guy in a back-yard peeling off his top and sipping tea, he nods, a consultation of posties I do not interrupt, a cat posing on a "fairy girl" dressing table. The concrete has fallen away from the wall at the end of the road to reveal a slate structure filled up with orange, bluish and burgundy rocks. A torn sticker over the municipal coat of arms reads:

NO ONE HAS (EVER?)
LOVED ANY(ONE?)
THE WAY E(??????)
WANTS TO B(E LOVED?)

I am not convinced that this is a correct translation of TURRIS FORTISSIMA EST NOMEN JEHOVA.

A colder, darker thing kicks in: the pubs and shops and chapels are dead here. The Patna, The Archer, JETS the Unisex Barber's and Hairdresser's, St Peter's. They come very quick; a number of what are clearly now unloved flats still sport windows or doors that betray their retail past. I cross a park with six arrangements of a tree and four short stakes, each in blue, green, red and yellow, sinister in meaninglessness; unnecessary topmast and rigging. The sign for The Archer Inn has survived; wearing on his chest a cross of St George, an archer stands and fires a stringless bow from within a stockade of sharpened pencils. Beneath, more 'bloody' handprints. This will become a theme with more handprints in blue and green and then, again, 'blood'.

Penrose Street frames the Guildhall's Italianate tower, far off. From the top of Harwell Street, a huge block of flats stands guard over the distance. The edifice of All Saints House faces a road that ends in two towers, one needle sharp, one stumpy. I am sweetly horrified by the way windows are blocked up in different ways, by fluffy toys, by super-hero eyes, by union flags, by chipboard, a lion cloth, curtains that are never opened, I see the unpromising sign for Ocean City Place, but the road swings round into what the developers called 'The Arena', with two basic housing types 'The Winchester' and 'The Alexandra'. The development is the work of the Guinness Partnership who create and manage homes that are mostly let at "social"/ "affordable" rents; if this is indicative of their work, then just hand the whole housing sector over to them. The way that the architects have used the shaping of the ground, the way that there is privacy and public space and liminal space, it feels epic and like a 'real place' at the same time as being domestic. I am just going on the most superficial of feelings, but unlike other new builds I've walked past where people have had to put some meaning on their space – a pixie or a Green Man or an eccentric house name – here the space seems to welcome different identities.

Such spaces need a dirty secret; an excess that can hold the everyday on the creative edge of excess. I find it very easily. Beside the top of the sweeping access road there are twin sets of steps, both gated and fenced. I am surprised that the thick black gate is without a padlock; beyond it, parallel with the steps to the abutting and conventional contemporary estate of incoherent, un-dramatic, off-the-shelf flattened properties, is a mural of geometrical shapes: a split circle, floating triangles, a giant pencil tip, two orbs bursting with spores; as the ground rises and the wall is shortened the design seems to become more fiercely symmetrical. Oddly, this is all concealed from the actual residents on whose behalf, presumably, it has been painted; an act of generosity to the few users of the adjacent estate path, and those like me, very few if any, willing to scramble up the narrow grass bank where the steps run out.

Caught at, partly made by, the crossing of vectors, something like a fish.

In the parking spaces a huge blue football blown about.

A thick black fence has cut off access to and from the next-door estate. When I was growing up on a new estate with Ma and Dad and my little bro, a few years of acid rain rusted away the wire fences that divided our back garden from our friends' gardens and we kids made tracks that connected them up. The children here will long be dead before these fences rust. In morose irony, the fence is hung with glistening webs.

Back on the road, the bright sun has picked out the white-on-white lettering UNISEX. Next to the former shop, its window steel-meshed, is an in-between space, probably left by a bomb, obscurely shaped by raised flower beds and seats so that although it is very small the whole of it is never visible from any one point within it; a place of anxiety rather than relief. Exploring it for a moment, although I know I want to be off and checking out those 'towers', there is an odd rumbling dialogue within the place. It takes a while of discreet edging in and out before I find the source: two men, one very, very drunk and the other drunker. The second man is doing the Freddie Frinton walk (from 'Dinner for One'), raising one leg to step forward while falling backwards, while the very, very drunk man repeatedly catches him; the two converse in a submarine tongue of swallows and gulps.

Opposite the derelict St Peter's chapel, to which someone has stencilled a speech bubble: NO HOPE, a group of potential buyers gather for a pre-auction visit to an empty property. A man, with family in tow, says to me:

"15,000 in cash and it's yours. In cash and you can have it now."

"The chapel or the house?"

"The chapel."

"I can let you have fifteen."

They all laugh. We chat about how long the chapel might have been closed. The work around the top of the door suggests a subtle Egyptifying of the neo-classical columns, as if it might have been a club since its closure as a chapel. A ten-foot band of white paint around the building has obliterated the JESUS NEVER WENT OUT OF BUSINESS graffiti and the two giant hairy testicles added at the bottom of the tall thin Romanesque window.

The front of the chapel is piled with rubbish; a record deck inert. Behind the chapel, in a fenced off jumble, is an oarless rowing boat adrift on a sea of moss. Running alongside the chapel is a straight and narrow cobbled lane, just like the one that runs through the university campus. I wonder if these are the urban equivalents of hollow lanes? On the cobbles is the paper outline of a submarine, packaging from a toy.

I chat with two old guys outside the startlingly-green tiled and pillared pub, matching the moss that is beginning to climb the chapel opposite. They seem joyful in a modestly bloated way, bulging their tight jumpers, crinkling their faces puffed with the years of booze. They are very enthusiastic for the landlord who owns his building and "is here to the end". They hold their rollies studiedly in the backs of their fingers. The sun warms them through the briefest miasma of smoke. I feel I am catching them at the end of something; two rogues gently playing sentinels to a redoubt.

A black rubbish bag has split and spills food and packaging. The blue of the statue of the BVM in a niche on the side of the Catholic Cathedral of Saint Mary and Saint Boniface (the axeman to the sacred oak) has greened. I peep inside the cathedral and a crucified Christ hovers. In the connected building, residential flats have been built inside the bombed shell of a convent, the building is troubling; according to all the official online stuff the building was constructed from scratch in 1865 in a neo-Gothic style; yet some parts of the building look much older than that. Is that because in 1865 they faked age to get the mediaeval Gothic effect, to rub out the years since the Reformation? It is a queasy place. I peep through an open doorway where an electrician, I think, is making a repair.

"Just being nosey."

"Come in, if you want."

I do want, but not massively.

"Is that the Bishop's Palace?"

"Bishop's House."

"Ah, big isn't it?"

"I often don't know where I am."

A space in the car park:

RESERVED

BISHOP

Personally, I prefer them eccentric and outgoing.

In a niche high on the old convent, the saint has been replaced by buddleia.

Two galleons navigate a window sill, Christian crosses on their sails. Flats have gobbled up half a chapel. Across the square, a house is chopped in half to make way for modern flats. Blitz architecture. I suspect that a large piece of stone in the middle of a lawn might have been thrown there by a bomb blast.

In the church in the middle of the square, Christ does not hover, but arches over in a swan tail droop from the crossbeam. Where Christ had transcended suffering into nobility, here he drops into it, his hair flopping over his face, his divinity lost in animal defeat. One church is Catholic, the other Anglo-Catholic. I suppose it is by such contradictions that religion does whatever it does; something different for everybody. And why it is evil to impose it on those who do not wish to be imposed upon; to be forced to imitate a contradiction is to be ripped to shreds.

I am surprised. I expected Plymouth to be all about Protestantism: the Plymouth Brethren and that.

The base of a bed, folded in two, blocks one of the pavements, on the other side of the road another bed leans against a garden's metal fence. A huge grey wall stretches as far as the eye can see in both directions. At a corner there is another malevolent tower with a flag of St George. In the shadow of the tower I stop to admire the jumble of a junk shop and am shocked bitterly by what I see among the old milk jugs and quaint ceramic ornaments: a display of Catholic icons – Pope John Paul II, Virgin Mary and Baby Jesus, Saint Anthony and the Baby Jesus – dominated by anti-semitic portraits of Jews, most in a *kippah*, some with *payot* curls, all counting money or entering figures in a ledger. I discover from the shopkeeper that these are made by a Polish woman.

This is my 'Theroux moment'.

When I got the 'job' of documenting the Paignton conference, I sent out a call to friends to point me to preparatory reading and one of the suggestions was a book by Paul Theroux called *The Kingdom by The Sea*, which I read until I could read no further, brought to a halt by Theroux's description of a covert porn shop in Llanelli, which he unknowingly blunders into, then realises that the publications on sale feature underage girls. He records this, but there is nothing about alerting care groups, the police, women's groups, anyone.

That night in my B&B I cobble together a short note with an image I take of the obscene 'icons' and email it all to a friend up in Yorkshire who prints them off and posts them to four local agencies. (A month later I emailed the tweedy guide who said he'd looked in and couldn't see them there.)

There is a huge, apparently amputated, chimney in the lane; twenty metres high, used to disperse sewer smells into the 'upper atmosphere'. I am attracted by the concrete infilling, into which has been carved:

DAWSON
Steeplejacks
1992

But what really draws me in is the doorway opposite, blocked with collapsing boards and slats and broken slates, an implosion in a barrier, leaving a crack to peep through to a dank space of naked umbrella-style clothes dryers and chairs placed against the back wall. A cul-de-sac of miserable lives that have lost their way, or a lovely sunned sinking into the pleasure of regular company.

Going back to the main road, the wall runs out at the edge of a park; at the far end I can see a subversion of towers: atop abandoned railway bridge piers is a squeezed topology of red steel. Easy to mistake for a piece of genuine industrial archaeology. This end of the park is the meeting point of the three towns that were amalgamated to create the single city, driven by convenience for war-making. Jealously guarded local identities evaporated in the heat of the colonial imperative; distant property retained by a tribute of blood on European fields.

Cakes and Cuticles, Shine Nails & Beauty, Koko Hair.

I find my way to another of these narrow, cobbled lanes with walls that have turned into Rauschenbergs. It brings me out on a main road, on the other side of which a huge broken tree trunk lies across a thick stone wall, like a slain pachyderm. Two women observe my surprise.

"Exploring Plymouth for the day?"

"Yes! Looking at that big tree..."

"It covered the whole road when it fell."

I expect them to elaborate, but they sail on slowly and happily.

The park from which the tree has fallen is not a park. The first thing that catches my eye is a small construct on pillars at the far end. I make my way along a slippery path through the grass. It takes a moment to realise that I am walking on glistening, levelled headstones. A handful stand against a wall; the sun picks out the letters and carved images. One is particularly striking; a catafalque loomed over by a giant plant, its fronds enveloping the stone casket. Another to a soldier shot dead while on guard aboard a convict ship in the Sound.

The pillared thing is enigmatic. As ambiguous as the concrete cone dogshit bins. An altar for Nothing. A young couple wander by; a balance of desperation and organisation. Her made up meticulously; him in ruins.

A man hovering; I decide to take a chance that he is benign. Turns out he is waiting for his child outside the nursery beside an old, locked, church. What are they trying to protect? The two Christs of Wyndham Street cannot be stolen; one is transcendent, the other has already lost everything. These locked buildings are indictments of secular society's failure to create equivalent spaces. Later I come to a raised viewing platform on what looks like a large gun emplacement: it has something of the layers of resonance and the possibilities of sanctuary.

In the graveyard, a sign celebrates the planting of trees by the local Play Group, but is surrounded only by piles of ashes.

I cross a bridge that was once part of a railway station with a convoluted line to London; all that remains are elaborate railings. Then I semi-circumambulate "our field", which the residents of the Georgian villas, one the birthplace of Guy Burgess, spy for the Russians, with fine views of the nuclear subs in the Sound, are seeking to prevent being turned into housing. There is a hole in the hedge and I take a diagonal route across the grass, past the former Devonport Municipal Art, Science & Technical Schools building, now flats; carved compasses wreathed in laurels remind me of the predatory stone shrub. At the junction with Devonport Road is the mouth of an old railway tunnel, fenced.

I should be exhausted by this onslaught of meaning and meaninglessness, of grand designs and global histories rendered ordinary and ripped and ignored; perhaps it is being out on my own, choosing my encounters, that keeps me so geared up. If anything, I am avoiding finding any walkers, taking parks and alleys where I can. The walk so far is preparing the ground for a corner of Devonport Park, where the jumble of wretchedness reaches heights of tangled ecstasy it could never own up to. The lodge there is occupied after renovation and this gives a fizz to the place, the washing on the line crackling with the *lehrstücke* of the whole operation: its arts and craftiness inlaid with tendril initials, with bifurcated gods and a looping obligation:

THE CARE OF THIS PARK
MADE FOR THE USE OF ALL
WITH PRIVATE AID AND
PUBLIC FUNDS IS
CONFIDED TO THE PEOPLE

This is flanked by a twin-tailed and muscular Dumna or Melusine, a female knucker, admiring herself in a hand mirror, moonish, reflective, her hand pulling back or combing her hair – comb and mirror the symbols of female wealth and social power – her face reminiscent of Queen Victoria's, the great mother looking down on the world and finding her reflection in the ocean. These primaeval myths are made imperial on land reclaimed from the Navy; part of the defences, the Devonport Lines, still evident in the park. While the tips of Dumna's two tails are remarkably floral, perhaps most interesting is the liminal region that is both tail and thigh, plant-like, but also like the bruising of giant veins; the integration of the ocean city; sea and floral ornament. Dumna is gridded by the tiles, in some variation on the Master's Square, while her flanking image is a twin-tailed Poseidon who turns his back on her and us, averting his gaze and scolding us for not doing likewise, testing the sharpness of the trident against his fingertip; turning from the reflective to the warmongering. As well as the twin fishy tails, he has the beginnings of a mammal tail at the bottom of his spine. This is a shattering machine, moving around the rare, open renouncing of public duty by authority.

And this is only at the gate! What I now see, and I only have energy to see two things in any detail in this corner of the park, I fancy almost no one else notices, though there is no disguise of what is there, simply that what is there does not fit with what one might expect to see. The first is a headless (this is a detail, nothing significant in this) beast carved in stone clearly taken from some exploded church or abbey; but when I circle it I begin to grasp its odd and meaningful inconsistency; on one side the animal has feet like hooves, like a pig, and on the other it has claws, like a lion. Divided by the backbone visible through the skin, one side of the back is smooth, the other ribbed. A chimaera. What it was once symbolic of, or meaningful about, I have no way of knowing; it pre-dates the bio-tech sciences. Beyond the jumbled memorial to Nelson, Wellington, Churchill and others, its plaque inscribed…

> Elle & Ryan
> Forever in
> Love (heart)

…and various Veitch imports, is another stone piece that takes the hybridisation that little bit further; something like a tree stump, shrouded in the leaves of an ivy-like plant. Expectations are disturbed by a curled tentacle and then overthrown by two bird's feet poking from the trunk. The serpent-fish-god hybrids at the gate are intense, but this fragment is off the scale! I would never have noticed these things before walking, before reading the tactics, before at least in theory recognising the arts of noticing, but this is almost insane; before I might have noted some stone remnants of a chapel or an old garden ornament, some generic understanding would have been enough. Yet the moment I begin to look, there is a language here of the most perverse and transgressive world on the surface of the most conventional and tedious things. I begin to doubt whether there is anything straightforward to how things are governed, to how things are settled, to how things are organised. That I live in a country quite foreign to the one I think I live in.

It does not calm down.

A startling white egret rests on the Napier Fountain; a monument raised by the rank and file when the Naval authorities were ill-disposed to recognise their champion, now fanfared by twin-tailed satyrs.

Giant female heads lean back in the grass.

I take an 'ordinary' road; even the triangular Catholic Church on the slope and the tower blocks, towers and pillars on the horizon do not diminish my relief. The spectre of a green paint spill, a skull-like face and the trace of limbs, I take in my stride. I reach an immense monumental arch, amputated from whatever it once opened into. Cut off by a wooden fence and an estate of flats, it is both sealed up, windows long closed with breeze blocks, and open. Inside the main arch, under the stare of a psychotic heraldic stone lion there are more arches. The graffiti...

M
O
O
N
HEAD

...reminds me of a Mooner encountering aliens in his park, in his head and in his bed in Newton Abbot. But now I am having my own encounter.

The limestone blocks that make up the giant arch have been depredated by acids in the rain and the breakdown of organic materials gathered in the roof, long streaks of white lime have coursed down the face of one of the arches in humanoid form, looking as much like an archetypal spectre as an archetypal spectre can look. The ghosts in groups march out of the stone.

As I leave the arch that leads nowhere, a couple, their faces drawn by the same insistent vortex of substance abuse, turn in; they might be twins, almost.

By the huge sports facility, I turn right and transition into another zone. Through an incoherent mini-park on the site of a long-gone theatre and past a Co-op wedged inside an old chapel and a side street dedicated to a former leader of Her Majesty's Loyal Opposition, I walk in the middle of the road, running a gauntlet of smart cars, between two streams of modern terraced properties. Their parallel lines meet at a neo-classical Temple of Diana, naughty Diana, wicked Coade-stone Britannia, the world for her armrest. Massive columns, forbidding steps, a spaceship from another culture, flanked even more incongruously by an Egyptian House (formerly the Devonport Classical and Mathematical School) designed in trapezoids. ODD above one of its columns. The information board at the bottom of the street promised a missing Zion chapel in "the *hindoo* style" (how much appropriation in that!), but beside now empty space a column rises some 40 metres and ends in more empty space. A huge school name in stone is all that remains of what I presume was bombed here. Behind the temple is the house of the masons who built the dockyard, a smartly painted empty pub.

OK, I know I am channelling the details in the park back there, that it takes a certain 'eye', that I have peeled so many layers from my senses in the last few days, but this assemblage of buildings is an unmistakable, unignorable epic tableau! So where are the coach parties? If this were in Italy it would have its own resort; the former centre of a displaced mini-city now rendered ornamental for a place on the elbow of gentrification. It is good to see that the Egyptian House is a social club. I eat immaculate baked goods – salmon and cucumber slices and an incredibly light and tasty sausage roll – in a café in the basement of the former Guildhall. Getting lost on my way to the loo, passing a busy office where I imagine regeneration is planned, I end up in some prison cells converted to exhibition space; I particularly like the drawing of a lady who is wearing an octopus on her head. Or maybe the octopus is wearing her as a dress. In the City of Destruction.

Following things downhill I crab along the giant wall of the dockyard where a clumsy graffiti artist has splashed the cartoon shape of a submarine and a trail of foam behind. It ends at a cove, long ago made into a small harbour. Along the side of the wall, of what in revolutionary times would have been an incendiary barrier with sedition discussed both outside and inside, are small numbered stone bollards, and cut into them along with the anchor of the Navy is the broad arrow of state, the latter taken from the family coat of arms of Sir Philip Sidney, straightening the sides of a pheon, and given to the Office of Ordnance (of which Sir Philip was Master in the mid-1580s). Today, this symbol (I got all this from Salmon) is still used in a distorted form by the Ordnance Survey, is visible on a huge but decreasing number of buildings, carved above the benchmarks used by the OS mapmakers prior to satellites and GPS. Sir Philip came to Plymouth to make himself an "exploit" person of the predatory leisure class by joining Sir Francis Drake on a voyage to the West Indies. He was recalled by the Queen before he could set out, firstly in order to renew his administrative post and then to be sent as Lord Governor to Flushing. So Sidney is remembered not as a slaver and pirate (though he seems to have aspired that way) but as the epitome of the Castiglione courtier: calm, studious, heroic, of good posture and speaking with art. He appears in the novels of S.J. Parris as a companion of Giordano Bruno, cosmologist and theorist of the 'art of memory'; his love poems – in which he embraces symbology and cosmic imagery – are examples of an artist whose reach is across the planes of myth. According to his *Defence of Poesy*, the function of poesy is to be an inspiration and tutor to heroic action. And for a single act of that Sidney is remembered, when, wounded and dying, he offered his canteen to another wounded soldier; "your need is greater than mine". Water is again and again the way that, the medium through which, meanings here are made.

In the old covered dock, I am shocked at the cartoonish King Billy figurehead gesturing across the Hamoaze with some stick of office, a herring gull on his head. The sun is low and a thing ploughs through the green and gold water; a cross between a troop carrier and a farm vehicle. It bowls along at military medium. The men at Mutton Cove eye me suspiciously as if I take too much notice of the line of their iron huts.

I cut off the pier and up steps to a grassy knoll, passing the yard of Knights Surplus, selling ROPES, FURNITURE, RACKING, AND MUCH, MUCH MORE, and above the abject breeze-block playground, shaped like a battleship. In the wall of the Knights Surplus (an excess of knighthood, like Sir Philip's, perhaps) is a broad arrow and another, slightly distended, on the company sign. I climb the hill towards a huge viewing tower with a radio mast on top, built over a network of tunnels and a nuclear bunker. In the grass an information board, recording the habitat of butterflies, has perished in the sun, the text cracking open in the shapes of spores and blooms and unlikely insects.

The Sound opens out and to my left, where I can see a string of giant yachts of the gin palace variety, and beyond them the tall chimneys and grey expanse of the Royal William Yard, once eyed by Nazis for conversion to something very sinister, according to the Crab Man's speculations. In a city where over 20,000 houses were hit and almost every civic building was destroyed, it *is* surprising that this giant military supply complex went unharmed during years of raids.

Around the base of the viewing tower on Mount Wise are the traces of various gun emplacements and stores; ground plan outlines and metal signs.

TIE FOR BARRAGE BALLOON, WORLD WAR II

The tie is still there. I imagine the rest.

I climb the stairs and under a giant metal octagonal shade, the thick wood panels beneath my feet almost burnt through in places, I contemplate the notional outline of the Royal Laboratory; an 18th-century armaments factory. On what is now housing and Knights Surplus. This should be the city I am escaping from; but it feels like the nearest to a Heavenly City I am going to find. I see a man enter the complex; he does not strike me as being the heritage sort, but looking for some quiet spot for a call that should not be overheard. I skip away across the grass and into a grove of exotic trees, elegant and twisted, where I stand for a moment, letting the desperation of others slip away. I need these meetings with the trees.

I scramble down the grass to the road.

TO SEEK
AND NOT TO YIELD

In cold brass a tent piled with snow, a cross wedged in the top.

I head back towards the centre of the city. The Towngate is another arch to nowhere. Passing the Princess Yachts yard, makers of those gin palaces, barely surviving the ravages of the 2014 storms, still arguing with their insurers, then the road where Conan Doyle failed as a doctor. At the Genesis building, I howl uncontrollably with laughter at the public art; people turn their heads, but they do not look surprised. Along the sides of the building, a sculptor, with great skill and fine working of the stone, has represented, to my aroused eye, a man carrying a plank through his head, two men sawing themselves, and a craftsman beating his erect penis with a mallet. It is a worthy lobby for the faded excesses of Union Street: its 'gentlemen's club', its giant theatre decorated with before and after scenes of the Spanish Armada, its chimærical architecture, a scribbled obituary on a utilities unit, decaying art, and the vast 1930s' Gaumont Palace cinema – which opened with 'The Ghost Train' starring Jack Hulbert, a film remade ten years later with scenes filmed along the rail track I have been taking back and forward between Dawlish and Teignmouth – now taken over by God TV, but as yet undeveloped into its promised Christian revival prayer centre. God TV is currently seeking a revival of its own, after the resignation of its founder following his "moral failure" with "the divorcee daughter of a farmer in South Africa". According to his wife, the "devil got in very, very easily".

He is always "in" in Devon.

Next door is The Two Trees, a pub; at its far corner is the faint shadow, screw holes and raw plugs, where a plaque has been removed or stolen or fallen off; it had named William Friese-Greene, who had a photographic studio on the site, the man the British film industry fraudulently attempted in 'The Magic Box' to claim as sole inventor of cinema technology, the movie camera and projector. The reality is that cinema was invented simultaneously and far from independently by a number of individuals and organisations in a number of different countries.

Looking for a B&B for the night, I have a feeling that the city is presenting itself to me as some kind of exemplary space: a theatre of memory in which each element of the scenery stood for something else, and that if I can stand up all those secondary meanings they will spell out a new alphabet.

Passing the Athenaeum, under which The Beatles once escaped their screaming fans by running down a tunnel that is still there, I think about trajectories; that we are only the journeys we take. Something is communicating to me through a web of lines, casting a nest of arrows around me, bending backwards over a brutalist department store all the uneven streets with their faint trace of mediaeval twists, untangling the junctions of a chequerboard city, making a gridded playground. Yet everything I have learned since this morning is that I am arriving late at an event that is no longer happening, that I am to look for the fluid, the curving, the leaking and the negligible. That while there may be sciences swinging around me, offering patterns and quick routes to answers, they are of no use to me unless I can wrap them around a funhouse field of intuition, unless I can morph out soft new organs looping back into the sensorium at the 'back of my mind', forgetful, distracted and seeing from the corners of my eyes the shining symptoms of the molten core. Which leaves unanswered the question: what is this thing that is presenting itself? ...that stands behind the veil, clothing itself as a city, seeking to convince me that its Tron-like city-body, its arteries all lit up across the volcanic rocks in its old walls, is the thing made of such a thick authenticity that it is becoming part of me?

Once checked in, I go out again, to drink. We can do these things, we abandoned women.

During this walk of doubleness – re-walking Exeter in my skin's memory and mind's imagination, while walking Plymouth in my feet and bones – I also am a Player in the Game. I see no reason to write about it. But there is a place for screwing, fucking, banging oneself into and onto a place, hanging over a wall, or balancing with one hand on a concrete post, feeling the squeeze of the moss, hearing the bark of distant dogs over the panting of a temporary partner, feeling the tremor of a passing train spring the beat of your own heart, seeing your sweat turn to mist and rise up into the sodium flare of the playing field lights. Feeling the feel of the place as you experience the blood surge under the skin of your surprised and surprising encounter; what s/he felt I felt, but didn't ask, I didn't either. Both drunk, we told quick lies to each other and parted. Keeping hold of the moment; which is now stitched with this space and her/him. And I have a fancy for a friend to make a whole geography of such consecrated sites. The concrete seemed to melt and there was nothing brutal about it at all.

On the back cover of Castigliano's book, his author's note says that he believes himself to be "one of the very last of the *flâneurs*". I do not mean him any ill, but I hope he is right.

Reading *Flâneur*, I realise that what sets the worst *dérivistes* apart from the best *flâneurs* is their willingness to savour the vulgar, the populist, the rough, the lay, the sentimental.

When one of the walkers I had met saw that I was in Plymouth, she posted on her Timeline an image from the first plan for the redevelopment of the city's centre after it was levelled by Nazi bombing. Just as the couple in the market said, it is very like a Kabbalah 'tree of life', very like the shape in the Ringmore parking space. Yet, the great plan never did get built, like Wren's for London, or Constant's for New Babylon; if they had been they would probably have been nightmarish, fascist. The city is too vibrant for any single plane, always dropping down through or pushing up against, and the contradiction between the perfect and the vulgar, like the shifting of faults in the surface of a planet, is what generates ambience. Even in a new town like Cranbrook? We can measure it across our whole body; because there's a mathematically accessible quotient of aspiration and realisation, and beyond the equals sign is an atmosphere.

I lay my head on a cotton pillow and do not care about the furnishings.

Footbridge over Saltash Road, Bayswater Road, Patna Place, across play park, Archer Terrace, Wyndham Street, Ocean City Place, Wyndham Street, Wyndham Place, Stoke Road, Wyndham Lane, Stoke Road, Victoria Park, Hotham Place, Edgcumbe Avenue, Fellowes Place Lane South, Fellowes Place (footpath), Paradise Road, Stoke Damerel (former) churchyard, footpath to Stoke Damerel Church, through churchyard to Kings Court, Paradise Road, Devonport Park, Fore Street, Raglan Road, Madden Road, Raglan Gardens, Mills Road, Chapel Street, Theatre Ope, Ker Street, Bennett Street, Mount

Street, St Michael's Street, Mutton Cove Pier, Richmond Walk, Mount Wise Park, George Street, Clowance Close, up the steps at the end of the close, follow path straight ahead and left along Mount Wise Crescent, right down Devonport Hill, Stonehouse Bridge, Edgcumbe Street, Union Street, Derrys Cross, Princess Way, Notte Street, Lockyer Street, Alfred Street. Next morning: Alfred Street, Lockyer Street, Notte Street, left across the square between the redundant Civic Centre and the law courts, Armada Way, North Cross underpass, Saltash Road, Plymouth Train Station.

On my walk to the station, an early morning start, I try to close my eyes without tripping over living things. I need to get to Exeter by the evening and there are places in between I want to go to. But I cannot help noticing the plaque in the square between the redundant civic centre and the law courts; a gift of four Imperial Locust (!!) trees from the people of Plymouth, Michigan. Yet there are clearly only three left.

WE WOULD HOPE THE QUIET INFLUENCE OF THESE TREES WOULD CAUSE YOUR PEOPLE TO EXPECT OUR PEOPLE TO REPLACE THEM AT THE END OF A LONG LIFE AND THAT OUR PEOPLE WOULD CONSIDER IT AN HONOR AND OBLIGATION TO DO SO.

Later I will email the city authorities in Michigan.

I walk through the rough Tree of Life to the train station.

Half an hour later our arrival at Totnes is signalled by the artificial symmetry of the Saxon castle mound.

I want to walk around the mound to the old timber yards on the quay, to intuit like one of the timber merchants there who could see a rudder or a roof beam in an uncut tree. I want to walk to Sharpham House, to see how the land is painted in grass and trees and sheep. I want to get a sense of how real was the vision of Maurice Ash, who lived there; his 'new monasticism'. The more he tries to explain in his *New Renaissance* that there would be no enforcement of common beliefs, the less you believe him; is his the establishment's Trojan Horse in the alternative movement? Is there anything to be said for a secret monasticism of walking, with no requirement to seal oneself away but opening the body to the somatic, to a general, gentle eroticisation of space. This is what is happening anyhow, it doesn't need anyone or any institution to organise it, does it?

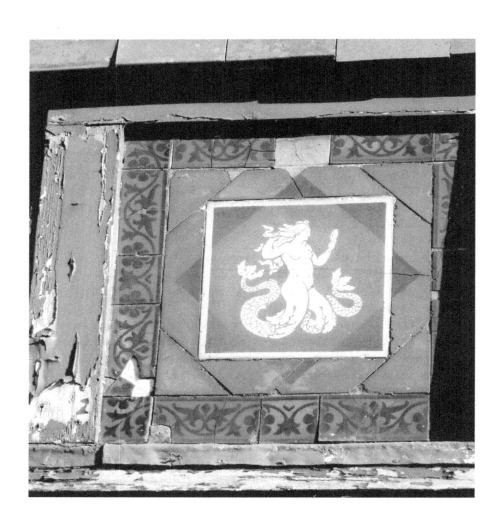

Chapter Sixteen: Dartington Estate and Venus

On other levels, the monastic disciplines are still evident – their ordering of the day into prayers and services and work is still there in our bus timetables, bin collections, opening times and libraries, structures around which to build things anyway. But always, at their heart, there is a solitary practice within the collective practice, anchorites that slip anchor to escape the relentless visual chatter of the Spectacle and the mountains of published theory; each walker is on a personal quest, the singular self is only ever denied in order to multiply and complexify it; walking artists and psychogeographers are a hidden disorder of undercover hermits of selves-indulgence. So is there any point in planning such practices strategically; because the non-planning of their tactical proliferation and the undirected dispersal of ideas and practices are already a strategy?

I have arranged to meet a former theatre lecturer from the now defunct College of Arts. I meet him for coffees in the White Hart pub at Dartington Hall, the pub where the 1945 Labour Party manifesto, the blueprint for the most radical transformation of British society, was drawn up. Then we walk through the gardens and the Tiltyard, on its green table-top Jooss dancers had once exercised with actors under the tutorship of Michael Chekhov, the psychiatrist in 'Spellbound' – drink up your milk! Among the performers was the daughter of Dorothy Elmhirst (along with husband Leonard, then owners of the estate), Beatrice Straight, who would go on to win an Academy Award.

Above the Tiltyard is a reclining female sculpted by Sir Henry Moore. It seems to be this particular piece that Sir Reginald Blomfield singles out in his *Modernismus* as exemplifying the trait of modernism which gives him most concern: thing-power and the privileging of materials. Blomfield worries apocalyptically at Herbert Read's suggestion in *The Meaning of Art* that a sculptor intuits a surface "situated in the centre of gravity of the block before him. Under the guidance of this intuition, the stone is slowly educated into an ideal state of existence", which Blomfield interprets to mean "that if the stone could carve itself it would present a 'reclining woman' exactly as it is presented by Mr. Moore... We seem to be slipping into the abyss".

At the opposite extreme to Blomfield is Dame Sylvia Crowe, key thinker in the sculpting of the nuclear landscape, something recently re-prioritised by then Tory Energy Secretary Amber Rudd: "we're hoping to build new nuclear plants and I think it is a reasonable ambition to make sure that these big projects have aesthetic appeal" (*The Independent*, 6.6.15). Dame Sylvia was very enthusiastic about Moore's "extension of the organic world"; she saw his work as a rejigging of the human senses to meet a cosmos in which "experience has penetrated into regions which were inaudible and invisible... The cavities and solids of Henry Moore's figures are less an idealization of the human mean than... [a] groping for his position in the universal framework, while his mind and experience has attained a new mobility which enables his consciousness to travel over the whole gamut of creation."

Is that what the College was? Just as a new farming was pioneered here, so also here was the cultivation of new kinds of feeling, sensing and experiencing? Not so much an engineering or planting of new ideas, but the nurturing in anarchic experiments of new, un-designable 'structures of feeling' for a hypermodern economy.

Not that (other than at very broad policy levels) there was any manipulation of the college, for that would be to destroy its experimental productivity, but there was observation and harvesting. Initially hostile to the Elmhirsts' experimental mix of foreigners, hard-left rank and file politics, mysticism, radical arts, community involvement, experimental ruralism – the Soil Association which was, at least in its early days, in danger of becoming a Blood and Soil Association, was influential here – and big foreign money (to MI5 at the time this must have looked something like the Strasserite wing of English fascism), the deep-politicians had come round to seeing the usefulness of these innovators as an extended experiment in a new art of living.

Only when the system itself had fully adopted these innovations – and begun to organise on the bases of shock, precarity, chaos and rupture – was the experiment deemed expendable.

Though my companion confirmed the gist of Salmon's account of the security services' interest in the place – "London", he said "has always had a direct connection to the college" – he had little time for my speculation.

Beyond a giant yew is a tower left behind when the church was rebuilt outside the estate grounds in the late 19th century. The discarded tower, one of those malevolent sentinels I keep finding, was used for US military communications in the 1940s. It is the opening, the crack that Dennis Wheatley prises to site the ritual actions of his trash novel *The Haunting of Toby Jugg*; he would have found the site when he was sent here as an intelligence agent for MI5 to spy on the alternative school at Dartington: "the school authorities had converted the crypt of the Abbey into a Masonic Temple... a Lodge of the Grand Orient... Fellowship of it gave one lots of pull in the political and financial worlds... pupils who had proved satisfactory were given a special course during their last term to prepare them for initiation."

Wheatley had no personal belief in magick or witchcraft, though he was happy to affirm the popular misapprehension that he did; when people began to copy the occult practices he pretended to reveal, he opportunistically authenticated them in a feedback loop powering his paperback sales and skewing neo-paganism. In *The Haunting of Toby Jugg* he mixes a narrative of demonic possession with a spy thriller about Stalinist subversion. The whole is coloured by anti-Semitism: a German Jewish agent seeks to infiltrate and influence the Labour Party (an interesting coincidence given the White Hart's role in the 1945 manifesto): "the coast resorts in south-western England... were packed with Jews... how is it that there is always such a high proportion of Jews in the 'safe' places where there is good food and soft living to be had?"

It turns out that the 'Grand Orient' and infiltration stories are a cover for the work of a Satanic Brotherhood: "It is Socialism, but on the highest plane... through the agency of Communism, my master, the Ancient of Days, the Archangel Lucifer, the Prince of This World, will at last enter into his own again". When one of his characters expresses surprise at an apparent contradiction – "It was so obviously absurd to think of the masters at Weylands dabbling in spiritualism. They were all dyed-in-the-wool materialists" – Wheatley is pointing to a tension that becomes pronounced at Dartington. (The novel ends with a Giant Spider being vaporised.) I knew all this because Wheatley's biographer is Phil Baker, who writes so well on psychogeography.

I noticed at the conference that Dartington was often associated with artiness and marginality – at Babbacombe Model Village it appears as Artington – but it feels more important than that to me. A place where lightweights like me would get gobbled up. I wish I had an ally here, the birdman maybe. Someone who would recognise the signs of a social experiment still in progress. The former lecturer does his best to disprove my theory with descriptions of his students' radical experiments, but these only add grist to my mill.

We pass studios once used by the now defunct College of Arts which was sent to Falmouth and quietly strangled there, vaporised in an unsympathetic institution. Then we visit a patch of ground that was the location of Michael Chekhov's rehearsal studio, subsequently converted for the pioneer battery farming of chickens, before demolition.

I want to know more about the closing of the College. People at the conference muttered darkly about it, but then changed the subject, perhaps because they were embarrassed at knowing nothing. My companion does not want to tell me much, but he does talk about what was lost for walking when the college went. He has written a paper and promises to send it to me, yet never does.

We double back so we can walk through the gardens. Then we turn out onto the road down towards the Schumacher College, named after the "small is beautiful" man. Almost immediately we're out of the gardens, on our left is a gate and the most remarkable straight path, double tracked for vehicles, across a huge field. It is stunningly formal in the rigour of the line it traces down and up the basin of the valley, inured to its contours. My host notes my reaction; many students, he says, created performances of walking, crawling, running, carrying on this path. I wonder what it does to land to suddenly take away such years of attention. He nods slightly but ignores my question.

At a fork in the road, we turn away from the Foxhole buildings, where students stayed during the College years. In the 1980s, according to Salmon, when the institution was struggling with its finances, a call came in from London, sounding out feelings at the College about the buildings being used to train pilots on fighter plane simulators for the Saudi air force (or maybe it was Ceaușescu's?) We take the right fork down to the entrance to Schumacher College.

My companion is a disciple of Latvian-American scholar Edmunds Valdemārs Bunkše. I like his idea that "stories can fill in for the missing rituals". The big Stonehenge-era landscapes were major adaptations of natural terrain for journey or procession rituals, the evidence from seeds and other vegetable waste points to people travelling from all over the island for them. But when the religious system those rituals sustained fell apart, probably due to famine, landscape-spirituality became less invasive, more orientated to small natural features – springs, streams, trees, groves, woods – and in a way the landscape (at least the parts regarded as religious) became more unnerving, less manipulated and more disordered. When Christianity arrives, it has no connection whatsoever to the landscape at all: it's a story from the Middle East, so the alienation from scary places continues in the centuries up to the Romantic break. Prior to that, for the vast majority of Christians the non-urban and non-farmed is a 'waste', a chaos to be avoided at best and survived when necessary. So maybe fairy tales, urban legends and ghost stories are filling in the gap between people and the grand and authoritarian ritual landscape, between people and the local intimate but frightening micro-magic?

With the fading of organised religion in the UK over the last century or so, the idea of the church building as holy sanctuary, as a place to seek haven from a disturbing landscape, has receded for most people. Is this (obviously technology plays a part) why there is so much drama? Ancient Athens had a couple of drama festivals a year, today some people watch four or five full length dramas a day. Is part of that appetite to immerse in performance a desire to find a story that will put the viewer back in touch with their, now largely imaginary, spiritual terrain? Similarly, the explosion of non-necessary travel? Both of which, sadly, avoid the very encounter that might make such a new relationship possible; and so, the absence of resolution generates a renewed appetite for yet another 'story' – and then another.

I had thought the teacher had a specific walk to take me on, but he suggests we just 'follow our noses', so we turn down the driveway of Schumacher College and find we can walk directly through its linhay at the back of the house, cluttered with gardening and other materials. Out through their garden and into the North Wood; an unfeasible boat hangs in the tree tops; it reminds me of the ark the birdman spotted. We cut up a narrow concrete path, absurdly straight, before we turn through the trees; the teacher compares it to a written or typed slash – he is very keen on "reading" the space and "writing" our journey – separating or joining the binaries here: nature/artifice, anachronism/ modernism, co-operation/institution.

The trees are massive, Coast Redwoods some of them, the canopy so dense the temperature drops a few degrees. It feels melancholic here.

"The students would fall in love at first sight with these woods; the immediate impact they make, the students assumed that everything they did would be enhanced by its spectacle. Boy, were they wrong! I saw almost nothing that was successful here. A forest like this drives out life, fabulous trees planted like this pretty much kill off everything else, they kill off the forest floor, they shade everything out, it can be pretty quiet in here. The best performance I saw here was about trying to survive."

There are small wooden structures, somewhere between sculptures and dwellings, in various states of collapse. As the ground falls away we follow a path down through the trees, and the teacher recognises a signed path to one side, he is surprised when it comes to a halt after no more than a few metres; a gate in the hedge is now locked solid with brambles and nettles. On the other side of the tangle is a wide field. The teacher explains that there has been a field walking project here for a few years; repeated walking, collecting artefacts from a large flint scatter on the surface and logging the finds; flint that probably came from the Haldon Hills, flint on which I had stumbled on my way down to Lidwell Chapel.

Flint starts out as sponges and plankton; even here, on the experimental estate, is the ruin of the ocean.

Apparently we are looking, on our tippy-toes, at the 10,000-year-old abattoir of an early Mesolithic people who poised themselves up here high above the river and harvested the large herbivores moving along the valley north to south, migrating from their higher summer pastures to their lower-lying winter shelters. These mass mobilisations provided an opportunity for a 'collective kill' and it seems that this is the site of one of those; it is odd to feel the shaping of the land that provided this place of repeated ancient slaughter.

This is much, much longer ago that when the Dumnonii were here; these people would have been as strange to the Dumnonii as the Dumnonii would be to us; or as familiar. Such prehistoric industrial-scale slaughter is perhaps appropriate for an estate where new elements of industrial-agriculture were trialled.

We drop down where the earth is boxed into steps. The teacher swings under the wooden rail and we climb down a snaky path on rock and under a bough to the dry edge of the river bed. The teacher leaves me at the ford, where a bunch of lads are kicking up the water. I see how far I can get by following the exposed river bed, ascetic and momentarily bleak in its thick scatter of smooth pebbles. I slip.

A place where terrible things happen. A poet says it takes one person every year, this river. In some way or other. Cutty Dyer. Cutty Dyer come down on the Ashburn in the form of a male swan. A bad river from a bad movie: 'The River's Edge' or 'KM31'. The route of the river, changed by the roads; the drowned turn up on verges. We have messed too much and all we have are stupid monolith-myths to go by; we might as well be paddling with dumbbells, requiring a myth to solve any mystery: a body, naked, found in a 'pool' of the river, a mark on her neck consistent with the attack of a male swan. The victim, who had been sunbathing, just seventeen years old, had been taking an impromptu Kung Fu lesson with demonstration of pressure points and throws onto a blanket, from an expert, a local school caretaker she had coincidentally met there. The reading at her funeral was from the Book of Revelation:

a "world in which all things can be made new, which [she] discovered for herself in so costly a way"... what on earth does that mean? That there was some transformation of the world in whatever violence it was she suffered? At sixteen, she had taken part in Maori occupations, at four she had been identified as a future Prime Minister, she was an heiress, she had partially deconstructed herself both racially and hierarchically, "she had gone fishing with a great bone hook baited with her own blood and pulled up a whole new continent".

The flood channels soon run out and I am back on the path, parallel with the river, which is much deeper and darker now. Salmon:

The school building has been long closed, but is opened now for various New Age practices that will not worry anyone. This was once one of those quiet places where massive things happened. The security forces always took an interest in what happened here. Today those trees that were planted around the open-air swimming pool, to shield the estate workers from the naked bodies of the children, have been cleared, connecting the Hall again with the (dead) school and the (dead) college. Now they are both defunct they can again be seen by all. Here is a gap, an affordance, a space into which things could move, criminal, sexual, para-political, this rich mix from which the future makes itself: Jewish dancers on a Green Table, an alcoholic actor-trainer integrating "atmospheres" into character production, the massive money of Dorothy Straight. These were serious players. Dorothy did not mess about with fey-liberal causes, she went straight to the rough Wobbly heart of bad-white America, those Trump supporters and kingfishers when they wanted to raise a red flag over the White House and burn the Kremlin and the Lubyanka too. She was on fire with the people inside, but outside she never threw off her subservience and ended up planting flowers in the garden, some revenant of which remains, to exorcise the disappointment of not leaving Leonard for Hollywood. Her daughter Beatrice wins an Oscar for her part in 'Network', the Trump-predictor: "I'm mad as hell and I'm not going to take it anymore!" It is de rigueur that these populist things are partly worked out on the jousting grounds of failed stately homes. We could call that irony a "farage"; a mirage that has a real, material and misleading effect. The idealism here was always bifurcated: the headmaster Bill Curry declared that "the system" must be radically changed, a new elite would be required! Wobbling between radicalism and fascism. The old elite did not take kindly. An MI5 file was drawn up, entitled 'The Case Against Dartington Hall': accusations that an Elmhirst house in London was used by Aleister Crowley (who had his first mutual sexual experience in Torquay, nothing exceptional in that) as a Satanic initiation temple, shipping its novices to Dartington. The sources for these accusations were super-reliable, including Captain Arthur Rogers (military intelligence) of the Nordic League, Chairman of the 18B Detainees (British) Aid Fund (supporting jailed British fascists), a member of the League of Empire Loyalists, an organisation set up by Arthur K. Chesterton, the Editor of the Torquay Times and one of the founders of the National Front. Their accusations linked Curry to communism, Crowley and, most interesting perhaps for now, European federalism.

Why do these men want world government? What is the matter with self-autonomy?

Dorothy's son Michael spied for the KGB. One of the Apostles. Privilege, like Blunt's, protected him.

Satanism, then, was Communism and Communism was anti-Christianity; a flip would happen later and anti-Christianity would become a Far Right thing, the ideology not of empire loyalists but pirate-rebels with authoritarian desires. When Rogers and his allies broke cover, dragging in accusations against a proto-EU Federal Union of intellectuals, like William Beveridge, formed in 1938 in anger at the Munich appeasement of the Nazis, the Elmhirsts took Rogers to court and he backed down. The other defendant in the case was Lady Alexandrina Domville, wife to an Admiral and jailed fascist, founder of 'The Linl' promoting closer relations between Conservative Britain and Nazi Germany. This could all have ended very differently.

Rumours were harder to contain than minority extremists. Much harder to censor; the Right was learning the lessons of the Spectacle – that was what was really being experimented on here. By who and for whom were those experiments conducted? Lies and fictions, if strategically placed, can curl round on themselves and become unanswerable. That the cognitive mapping of the dispossessed has been repossessed as digital populism; UFO's, pyramids, lodges, Masonic squares and the 'Protocols of Zion' have been re-appropriated from the hippy Left of the 1960s, de-hippyfied, entrepreneurialised, and, then with added alcohol served in shitkickers' bars and on campaign stalls? Whatever it started out as, was this place a looking glass for what Mark Pilkington calls the 'Mirage Men'?"

I want to take a look for myself at the school and college buildings. A steam locomotive sounds its whistle nearby and I hear the harrumph of its engine.

I arrive at a tiny wooden bridge; the wooded land banks steeply up ahead of me and the path splits. I fancy I should turn away from the river if I want to find the buildings, but something starts crashing in the trees, as if someone, wrapped in silver foil, the Dawlish mummy-shopworker maybe, had suddenly fallen and rolled. In the sound box created by the hill and the meeting of paths the sound roars like thunder. I am staring into the gaze of a roebuck. Neither of us moves, scared of scaring the other. The beam between our eyes is as solid as a wooden plank. It dissolves when a roe fawn skitters to my feet from the path to my left. I start, the fawn starts, the parent starts and as I step backwards across the bridge the two deer zig zag haphazardly up through the wood's undergrowth. The adult had seemed big, felt angry. I am wondering about taking the right-hand path along the high wall, when a terrifying and unearthly barking breaks out from the hill. I can see nothing, I can imagine Nothing; a chasm of imaginary giant animal. What kind of dog makes a noise like that? Images of huge Wisht Hounds chase me down in my head and I run away back down the path, and scamper up some steps until I find a path back to where I want to be going.

I come out of the trees and find the corner of the wall – so high because it seals in what was a 'deer park'. I had forgotten the aristocrats who lived here for hundreds of years: they've been squeezed out by the industrial Mesolithic slaughter and the drama warm ups on the Tiltyard grass. Following the path running along the wall, I come to a metalled road dotted with modernist experiments in house-building and then the school and the college buildings. There are some (Bauhaus-inspired) two storey offices; a doorway with the year 1933 as its sign; not a doorway I want to be going through right now.

Behind the school is a dry swimming pool; this must be where the children and youths swam and sunbathed naked. It is smaller than I expected. Most of the blue paint is still in place; in one corner of the pool, leaves have been joined by cans. I know from the teacher that long after the school had gone and the pool drained, there were many performances here; the intention and function of holding absent water as seductive as the dark woods for performance makers.

Opposite a hexagonal studio space is my favourite thing on the estate: a rough concrete trough with obscure symbols on each side; a functional thing had to be made meaningful. On one side is a fist, one finger pointing to the things above.

Trying to find my way out of the estate, I take a footpath around the back of the old college studios, a fallen branch with the head of a dragon, and end up in a 'cul-de-sac' of barbed wire where someone has carved deeply and unevenly into a fallen tree trunk the lines of a rectangular box; the almost-symmetrical perspective and the green mould on the tree generate the illusion that the box floats free from the trunk, as if it realises its ideal form. I retreat and take a path over a big field towards the Hall and then back down the road to the station.

A forest of border posts is built in the suburbs, while
All the garden fences are torn down to make way for a labyrinth,
Whispered plans are signed off and prisoners become sincere,
Defensive jokes lose their value on the exchanges
And tangled levers flail; then, the machine stops,
The temperature falls and the city enters, left, a glacier.

I have not a clue what these poems are about.

I had overheard some talk among one of the walking groups about asking people to pull down their garden fences, so that the Right to Roam could be radically extended across back gardens, interweaving public footpaths into ornamental paving. That will be popular.

I think Keble Martin's mother was a Champernowne; one of the last of the aristocrats here.

What closed the college and brought the whole project – radicalism and intelligence – to a close was simple practicalities, the teacher told me. Chinese students were streaming in to study at Exeter University, bringing with them their security advisors and, in turn, attracting monitoring by the domestic intelligence agency. In term time, the Chinese students constituted the second largest ethnic group in Exeter; I remember the ludicrous fear of the old man in Stoke Canon. Dartington's plan for survival in the 'noughties' was to focus on revenue from foreign students, specifically from China. Could the security services afford doubling up, spreading personnel thinly? When the College had first been threatened, a mystery donor from the deep establishment, never revealed (some say Paul McCartney), had saved it, but the second time around no one came forward; the deep political structure had shifted. Logic did not apply; arguments about how easy it would be to build new accommodation were ignored. Protests were counter-productive; everyone was swept up into the spiral.

It was at Dartington that James Anthony and William Froude endured their "loveless, cheerless boyhood". While William made death in miniature form and wrote the formula for scaling up model battleships, toot toot, and a law for a scalability that "requires that project elements be oblivious to the indeterminacies of encounter" (Tsing), his brother James Anthony wrote a scandalous novel, *The Nemesis of Faith*, published in 1849, in which the pressures upon the literal truth of the Bible created by the findings emerging from Kent's Cavern and the Windmill Hill Cavern on Berry Head play out in a young clergyman's life. What provoked less scandal was Froude's writings on the British colonies, celebrating Drake and Hawkins as "freebooters of the ocean in one aspect of them; in another, the sea warriors of the Reformation" while decrying a lack of similar contemporary British heroes as comparable to the absence of Ulysses: "I do not believe in the degeneracy of our race... but we are just now in a moulting state, and are sick... the suitors of Penelope Britannia consume her substance, [but]... They cannot string the bow". According to Froude, the British Ulysses had deserted his Penelope and left her to suitors who had lost their "unbridled thirst for space".

Where the Dumnonii, according to historians, had 'failed to Belgicise' and adopt a centralised agriculture, James Anthony Froude was keen for Devonians to adopt, in the manner of his brother William, a formula for colonial scaling that *is* recognisable as Belgian: "exterminate local people and plants; prepare now-empty, unclaimed land; and bring in exotic and isolated labor and crops for production. This landscape model of scalability became an inspiration for later industrialization and modernization" (Tsing).

The black islanders subjected to this scaling up and down were not beings with agency – no, according to Froude they "would infinitely prefer a wise English ruler to any constitution which could be offered them" – these beings were subject to the economic equivalent of William Froude's 'Law of Steamship Comparison': their local ecologies treated no different to the materials of battleships, their behaviour predicted by the square root of their linear dimensions.

Froude's narrative of race and degeneracy is not metaphorical. For him the indigenous people of the colonies and the descendants of slaves "had little more sense than a monkey, perhaps less... curiously suggestive of the original from whom we are told now that all of us came... Morals in the technical sense they have none... there is sin, but it is the sin of animals... They have no aspirations to make them restless... If left entirely to themselves, they would in a generation or two relapse into savages."

There it was.

Quite explicit.

Pure white supremacist ideology.

For all of which, the Trinidadian linguist John Jacob Thomas, a son of liberated slaves, would call Froude a "negrophobic political hobgoblin" in his *Froudacity: West Indian Fables* of 1889 (one of those great books that transcend their provocation).

Like a seaborne pincer movement from either side of Torbay, the nascent positivism of the excavations in the dark, deep in the limestone, were combining through a pseudo-classification of the human being, with the needs of capital for a scalability of human and plant. "The blacks" were at best one of the lower animals; the evolutionary trail was quickly turning into a hierarchical scaling; and Trevena, Mallock, Heaviside and Froude were political hobgoblins haunting every lane of thought. From now on I would be vaulting fields like Widger.

I was feeling very peculiar indeed. I had drunk so much of the world alive that I had begun to dilute myself in jelly. I found it increasingly hard to tell inside from outside; I was no longer an academic with an interest in the journey narrative in northern European 19th-century Symbolist Theatre. I was no longer a mother in the conventional sense. I was no longer a woman. I was no longer a citizen. I was with the jellies, at home in acidic seas if so they would be; I was pulsing while appearing only to float.

A train is pulling into the station and I climb aboard, sitting on the side I know will face the sea. Then I get off again. I have seen the steam from a locomotive at the alternative station. There was another line like this at Paignton and I ignored it, missed it. My last chance now. I hear the doors of the train slammed along the platform as I find my way over the bridge and to the river, then walk along the bank to the bridge over to the steam station 'Totnes Littlehempston'.

Totnes train station, cross car park beyond Signal Box Cafe and follow alley there, take the footpath that hugs the west bank of the River Dart, turn right along Dartington Lane, Dartington Hall, via White Hart to Tiltyard and gardens, left down the metalled hill, take the next right fork, Schumacher College will be on your right, North Woods, Staverton Ford, Deer Park Wall, Warren Lane, Park Road, footpath, bluebells, Park Road, Dartington Lane,

retrace your steps via the footpath to Totnes train station, cross the bridge over the tracks, leave the platform and turn left through the car park, follow the footpath straight ahead, turn left at the river and turn right over the bridge to Littlehempston Station.

The train follows the Dart much of the way and I recognise some of my journey in the woods and at the ford. The nostalgia of the service exhausts something in me. An energy I had when leaving the mainline service is draining away.

Getting off the train, I wander listlessly out of the station; the dumpy shunting units, model shop and wheel-less carriage do little to amuse me. I wind under the elevated road and up into the town. Moonstone House does not intrigue me. Is there a kind of imperative and overbearing menace inside this hyper-sensitised walking?

I am mooching aimlessly in the town; vaguely aware that somewhere there is a giant cavern that is rarely open, a church burned down by Satanists in 1992 (after an unsuccessful attempt in 1849) and a tomb around which you can walk thirteen times, insert your finger and get a nip from a wicked squire. And an abbey of monks who pull in £8 million a year selling a caffeine-heightened fortified wine that fuels domestic violence in parts of Scotland. None of which interests me much.

I had expected a rather dour moor town, but there are small signs here and there – like the poster for Jellyfish Productions – that suggest the place has a bohemian strand. I order poached eggs at a brightly lit café and sit wondering how to get back to Exeter; tomorrow I am supposed to meet with the Crab Man, and I should be writing up some of my experiences. I have my notebook and my images; but how do I remember all these feelings? How do I stop them in memory morphing into something like the dull feelings I had before?

I write feverishly in my notebooks, trying to record the qualities of emotion I have felt in different spaces; the fear of vulnerability to my own fear, an unexpected calmness when another person's crisis overlapped with my own, some deep connectedness when after meeting the four airmen in folding chairs I saw the rising mound of Denbury Hill, the repeated rush of tiny discovery, rising horror at repeatedly tripping on the spills of canonical and doctrinal race theory, the sense when walking alone, down long lanes, of being surrounded in a protective cloud of butterfly feelings.

A figure, neither male nor female, watches me from a corner table; sharing a gaze between the street outside and my rabid scribbling. When I check something in Salmon's guide, running my finger along one of the hand-drawn maps, the androgynous figure resolves itself and draws a chair over to my table.

A pilgrimage slowly unfolds. While before I have walked with others who have an agenda or a premise for exploration, this is the first time I am walking to 'holy' spots. We have a 'holy book'; "but not wholly reliable" my companion quips. "Are any of them?" I retort, and there is some knowing shaking of heads and sinuous gestures.

The shrine we are seeking is the field up on the moor where – if we discount the fictional Cedric Allingham's encounter (fabricated by Moore and friend) and George King's neo-theosophist Aetherians – the very first nuts and bolts alien-human encounter on UK soil took place between a local handyman working at a Newton Abbot care home and three aliens from Venus, including one calling himself Yamski.

My accompanying enigma hands me the source: *The Scoriton Mystery* by Eileen Buckle. A woman author. I am pleased to read inside that the contactee, Arthur Bryant, was interviewed by two young astronomers, Gerald Aspin of Exeter and Hedley Robinson of Teignmouth; the latter later donating the telescope belonging to his father (of the same name) for the observatory within the kitchen garden I had been invited into at Teignmouth. The one opened by Sir Patrick Moore. I am pleased by the mesh being woven, it might hold me up for these last couple of days.

As we walk out of the town towards Scorriton (it can be spelled either way) and the moor above it, I hear the different narrative strands of the book and see its pictures too. Photographs of Bryant, with Eileen Buckle with her back to the camera, in the field above Bryant's house where the spaceship came to visit him a second time; the mechanical fragments that he found in this field and in the lane beside it, with a glass "phial" filled with silver sand and a fragment of paper on which, written in classical Greek, were the words "Adelphos Adelpho" or "brother to brother". There were also sketches, like police photo-fit images, of the aliens; these were based on Bryant's descriptions and adapted under his instructions. At first the aliens had appeared in "diving gear" spacesuits; the sorts of early aquatic envelopes developed by John Lethbridge in his orchard on the edge of Newton Abbot.

The entity wants to take me on to a mine in King's Wood on the edge of Buckfastleigh, once we have paid our respects at the two landing sites. I am relieved when, later, the light begins to fail and, to avoid walking in the dark on narrow lanes, we return to the town without visiting this adit; dug in search of copper, it had turned up highly radioactive pitchblende, rich in uranium. I wasn't sure I really wanted to brave the uranium rich dust of its spill.

As we walk and pass the book to and fro, I notice, thanks to the heavy underscoring of one paragraph, that this whole story only really kicks off when Bryant feels obliged to respond to "a certain lady living in Buckfastleigh, a gatecrasher at local council meetings, 'ban-the-bomb' type" who had written to the local press to suggest that "a flying saucer... had come down in the area of Scoriton, the ground was highly contaminated with radioactivity". This provokes the locals: "they came in their dozens, cars came from all directions". Did the anti-nuclear 'busybody' know that there was already a radiation source nearby?

There are a lot of hypnotic objects to be dealt with in Buckfastleigh before we can get out. The brutalist church with a chain running out of a gutter and down the back of the building and through the grille of a large drain. We decide it isn't mechanical, but there simply to guide the stream of water into the drain. A thin drizzle is starting to fall, we watch how the water flows from link to link. On a wall:

> this wall
> has been left
> intentionally
> alone

And then an old chapel filled with the parts of organs, large and small, and other clutter. In the hall next door, the organs are being made. The craftspeople there are remarkably tolerant of our interruption; we ask them if the glass phial in the photo in our book could be a musical instrument, a pipe?

No.

I am surprised that so many of their organs are made for private homes, rather than churches.

"Cambridge colleges. Oxford colleges. Choirs. And private homes."

"To the Glory of God."

It just pops up, like that.

"And... do you source your wood locally?"

"Yes. Jewsons in Exeter."

We all laugh and laugh, all of us.

To the Glory of God.

A dustbin, by a chapel, labelled:

> METH
> CHURCH

Preaching Bad.

A vast expanse of industrial yard; sheepskins. Turning animals into rugs. In the centre of the giant yard is a piece of classical 60s' modernism, an office so functional it has transcended its ugliness; the precariousness of its overhang come back into fashion as things all go wrong.

The chapel is a visual illusion; it looks concave, it is convex. Bryant struggles similarly with the shape of the alien saucer's tele-screen.

Above the Catholic Church's front door, half the crossbeam of Christ's cross is missing. My enigmatic companion somehow deduces the Steiner identity of the 'The Christian Community' by the font of its list of services:

Enquiries to last door on the left.

Which explains why one of the services is called 'The Consecration of Man'.

Above a house in Jordan Street a carved wooden plaque depicts an oak tree, its trunk ringed by a crown, sigils at three points, the one beneath its tentacle-like roots broken like the Catholic cross. A ceramic house plaque includes a representation of two fields with a blemish that might be a spacecraft. A window installation of pens and a golden hand. A decaying wooden arch that looks like it could be a rotting whale jaw.

The mural painted on the street corner might have been specially prepared for us: owlmen, foul bats, a pig-cow hybrid standing on a ruined part of the wall, a snake made of railway track, and a robin pursued by hybrid sky creatures, part flying saucer and part spider.

Taps in walls. Conduits.

A giant tree house; flat metal gates deterring peepers.

Coming out of the town, geese gather on a hill, and we head into the woods across Holy Brook. I imagine there were baptisms here; that children bathed here in the summer. There is ludicrously elegant metalwork for a serviceable bridge; this was somewhere special once.

Around a tree, by the water's edge, a sash is wrapped; we unfurl it and it reads GOOD BOY. The void laughs long. I hadn't expected to laugh so much, hunting aliens.

The hollow ways are overgrown around here.

After a couple of miles we find the best spaceship ever, right on the lane. Probably a water tank, but it has become an interplanetary prop for some unspeakably unfunny 1960s' film starring Lionel Jeffries made by British hacks incapable of taking futurism seriously; a cylinder with a cone stuck on the top, caressed by ivy. It is the most beautiful thing I have ever seen, keeling slightly; a drunken moonshot. I want to hug it, but I fear toppling it.

Ants' nest built into the embankment. Orbs on the gateposts to Hawson Court. We are getting close. Piles of black, hospital green and fairy pink silage bales.

Then...

Stumpy Oak. How dare they? (I'm not very tall.) I stand inside its hollow and I feel Oak, I feel tree. I stand and fuse with its entity and nonentity. The space oddity has turned into a stone cross; tree and cross keep company on a tiny traffic triangle. The diminutive Oak is a gesture, an ignition of splintering boughs and twigs, while the trunk is as hollow as a hill; this is as rhizomic as a tree could get.

The cross is much less evocative than the black ivy-strangled missile. It is somewhat abject here, if it had arms they would be clasped behind its back, in frustration, no more symbolic than a blank signpost, a crucifix crucified; there is nothing of the floating Christ, nothing of the flopped Christ.

Suddenly we are there. The gate of Hawson Farm Cottage, home of Arthur Bryant: "I wheeled my motor cycle up the little drive from my cottage to the lane and was about to start the bike up when I noticed on the ground a piece of metal of rather an odd shape... It seemed to me that the metal was glowing. I picked it up and put it in my haversack together with some other pieces of metal which were lying close by, and off I went to Newton Abbot".

I look about in the hope that there might be some scrap of metal, glowing or not. Nothing. Meanwhile, the nothing has wormed up through a gap in the hedge opposite the gate, hanging onto thick, springy boughs and prising off the crazed stones lodged in the bank. I follow, fearful of slipping. In the field the sheep panic, then stand in a group, a hundred strong, and bear down on us with two hundred ridiculing eyes.

Now what do we do? What do you do at the site of a hallucination? How do you respond appropriately inside the symptom of a tumour?

I think I had expected somewhere like the infected zone in the Strugatskys' *Roadside Picnic*, source of Tarkovsky's 'Stalker', where a brief visit by aliens has left behind the trash of magic; a labyrinth at the heart of which is a sphere that grants your deepest wish. But Tarkovsky's pilgrims do not know their deepest wishes, and the deepest wishes of the Strugatskys' characters have been decided for them by the sphere.

We are not even sure we are really here.

We hold the photo of the field, Bryant and the back of Eileen Buckle, up to the vista, comparing the field boundaries in the distance with those in the photo. It cannot be right. Instead of the "tiny" cottage, there is a substantial property. Where is the big clump of conifers? The field shapes only approximately match. It is the water tank alone that convinces us, just as we are about to leave the field. Bryant's cottage is just identifiable inside all the annexes and additions. We have to climb a little higher up the field to get the boundaries in synch.

Being certain is no more magical.

Later, on reading the book more thoroughly, I realise that we failed to explore the second field, through an ungated gap at the top of the first, where Bryant and the young astronomer from Exeter, who took away the mechanical parts, found burnt patches in the grass; and in my head now this is the 'second field', the vastness of anything that is always unexplored.

The anonymity produces a small purple silky pouch from which is drawn a small black coke-like lozenge; this is the residue of a meteor strike, tektite, it's not part of the meteor itself, but the hardened black glassy sludge that coalesces when planet and meteor meet. I hold it in my hand. I am transported.

A dog barks nearby.

When we clamber back down into the lane a fuzzy German Shepherd is heralding the approach of his owner, the present resident of Hawson Farm Cottage, a tall man with 'flu who asks us if he can help? We explain and show him the book; he is not phased. He explains that he gets many visitors; even a party from Japan once.

"What do you think of the theory?" he asks.

We qualify, we are sceptical. The narratives are unreliable, the investigators less than systematic.

"Have you ever had any experiences here?"

"Not here", he explains, "but in Plymouth one night I heard a humming sound, like a spinning top; when I came outside the sound was still there, but there was nothing to be seen."

This is Arthur Bryant, here at Hawson Farm Cottage: "I was on the point of going to bed when suddenly I became aware of a low humming noise which gradually increased in volume until it became quite loud... I ran out of the house to see what it could be. In the sky I observed a blue light coming from the south-west in my direction. It came right over the top of my house and then became stationary. Suddenly there came from this object a noise which I can only describe as like the slamming of the door of a castle with a long corridor behind".

This last turn of phrase is just that little bit too much like the famous description of James Cameron's (the journalist, not the film director) of a Bikini Atoll nuclear test: "like a great door slammed in the deepest hollows of the sea".

Always back to the sea, even in the plasma of fire.

We show the cottage owner the photograph from the field and he dates the various extensions to the cottage since the Bryants' departure. The owner was responsible for the removal of the conifers, which had confused us more than anything else; then, he describes how a previous owner had closed off a path, a hollow way, running along the side of the Bryants' cottage, and that – and this is breathtaking – the cross by Stumpy Oak had once been here, right at the gate where Arthur Bryant had found the metallic residue of his visitation.

The landscape lights up, with its meshwork of drivel, rubbish, tumour, green lanes, stone markers, lights and humming.

"What do you make of all this?" The void waves the book.

"It's a big universe", says the man behind the cottage gate. The dog chews on a blue bone.

We walk on, fraying.

An alpaca observes our turn towards the village from the end of its long neck.

In a back garden a trampoline is upended into a radio telescope.

After lunch in The Tradesmans Arms, where many of the meetings between Bryant, Buckle and her companion Norman Oliver took place – I have a shepherd's pie while the void picks at a sandwich – we set off up a wide and solid track towards Scoriton Down, the edge of the moor. We both inhale sharply at the sign for:

SCORRITON
DOWN ORGAN
FARM B&B

Brambles have grown across the IC of ORGANIC.

At the end of the lane are two wooden gates. The landing field, where the saucer came down and Bryant was invited aboard, is to the left between these two gates. At first, we think it is too large, but then detect the trace of an older fence that has been removed. The nonentity paces out the seventy feet with delicate steps. We are satisfied that we have arrived at the first meeting place of Venusian aliens and Newton Abbot handymen.

While the ambiguity sets up a tape recorder, I stare at the mists and sheets of rain drifting down the valley. We are high up; this is where Bryant came to reflect on his life, able to look back down the valley to his home. Somehow tufts of mist defy the general tide and swirl around in their own space, hovering above the dark treetops on the opposite side of the valley before snagging on their leaves. The field, full of sheep at the time of landing, is now planted out with small saplings. The bracken between the white plastic stem-protectors is brown.

We leave the scene, to let the tape machine do its work.

A tape recorder plays a major role in the mystery. It is operated by Eileen Buckle's colleague Norman Oliver (who would later publish a sceptical pamphlet on the encounters); after one recording, Norman announces to Eileen that "I've got an insertion". A 'voice' has been superimposed over part of a previous recording instructing the pair where they should go to next to search for ufos. The "weird voice, slow and deep, speaking in a virtual monotone" communicates in rhyming doggerel, as aliens (and Joanna Southcott) do, sending various messages that instruct Eileen to accompany Norman on wild goose chases across the hills of Sussex and Wiltshire. Had Norman Oliver assumed that a bond was developing between himself and Eileen and was trying to give it a nudge? Eventually, Norman would 'betray' Eileen's faith in Bryant; after she received an assurance about the truth of the encounter from Arthur on his deathbed, Oliver visited Bryant's widow who told him she had first heard the story from her husband as the plot for a sci-fi novel; the metal pieces left by the saucer had been purchased from a Navy Surplus store. Perhaps Knights Surplus at Mutton Cove?

Bryant died as a result of a brain tumour; the effects of which he may have been suffering at the time of his encounters: "you see, because at the time I was beginning to get a bit red about the eyes, accompanied by severe headaches... it covered most of the front, more than an ordinary headache. I would hear a sort of drumming noise."

We open a small metal gate in a larger structure that lets us onto the moor. The metal bulges outwards, as if some great force has been hammering itself against the bars, attempting to escape the moor. We wander up the tracks, letting the spools revolve. On the far side of the valley, the mists that have been sliding sideways, gather themselves up. A deer hide towers up, wreathed in murk; we decide not to risk its rotting ladder. Cloud now tumbles down the valley and across the bottom, rising up towards us. Like in a bad dream, like in a movie; one of those 'mixies' with glowing light inside; except there is no light, only the dull white wall of mist marching relentlessly towards us and, just as it is about to engulf us, thins to almost nothing. We retrieve the tape and I look one last time across the saucer field.

My wet jeans stick to my legs, my jacket drips; I work at dis-illusion.

I suddenly see through Bryant's tumour: on the hill across the valley, the thick mass of dark treeline rises only so far up the hillside. What it leaves at the top is a strip of bright green grassland under the sky: saucer-shaped. Checking the times in the book, Bryant would have been looking at this with the sun low in the sky to his left and shining up the valley; the grass would have been a startling green against the sky; with the fiction already in his head, and the location becoming a flying saucer, what more invitation would 'space brothers' need?

Is Bryant not the beginning of something? Is he not the Internet before there was one? H.G. Wells's 'World Brain' as jellified production? He invents a commercial fantasy with the naivety of the mildly talented autodidact, in the belief that the literary industry works according to his own idea of imagination, but before he can be disappointed he pre-empts his disgruntlement and turns it into 'reality fiction', going to his deathbed believing in it enough to lie about it. He is driven by media, both popular and official, by TV and local journalism, but also by the web of letter writers to the press, by young enthusiasts and by the sublimated romance of those who write as if they should know better, who by their pseudo-literary-science are most prescient in their wonder-becoming-paranoia. It is all here; fifty years ago here was right now everywhere, we are right here on the door between moor and conspiracy culture.

Bryant describes his aliens as wearing "suits of a silvery colour, which made a sound like tinfoil". The lead alien told Bryant that his name was "Yamski" and that, like Bryant, he was "of Romany origin" and that they had a message for "Des Les" and would send "proof of Mantell" (all half-correct names that would trigger recognition among ufo buffs). "Yamski went on to say that he and these people were going to bring proof of a wonderful existence and life beyond our understanding", but there was a darker side: "the dangers of forces from another planet which were taking people from this world for what he described as procreation purposes... they were already here in the guise of what we termed poltergeists" and tells Bryant of a disappearance (already the subject of a TV report) of a family from Yeovil.

Pretty much mapped out is the next half-century of paranoid ufology, abduction therapy and conspiracy theory. The *bricolage* of a handyman from Newton Abbot, amplified by the 'mirage men' who repeatedly emerge through poor Eileen's narrative: a fake 'atomic physicist', two Desmond Leslies (Des *and* Les), Devon youngsters, hard-boiled journalists. No wonder then, that the last online trace of Eileen Buckle is a post from a fellow investigator into the activities of the shadowy Aerial Phenomena Enquiry Network (APEN), a kind of 'Men in Black' set-up manipulating ufology groups: "over the last two weeks, two people waited in the car park of the flats where she lived and tried to hedge her in closer and closer each time she returned home at night... She then disappeared from the UFO scene... I've tried to trace her over the years, but to no avail". Space had run out for Eileen. Outside the gate to the saucer field we find two pieces of tinfoil.

Walking back down the track, repeating is reflecting; how Yamski's message embodies a magical mixture of idealism and hypersensitisation that borders on paranoia. To pass over the border, as the shadowy and not so shadowy APENs in multiple fields would invite us to do, is to end up hemmed in at the side of a car park unable to get home.

The void asks me about my work as we clump around a derelict caravan; a tear in its metal side is the same shape as the 'frog' above the door of the Heavitree pub. I am very happy to float away from the tumours and space vehicles; perhaps the void notices. I talk about Oscar Wilde's Symbolist drama of Salome and John the Baptist; how the crucial dialogue is between Salome and the decapitated head of the prophet. Horrified, the tyrant Herod cries out:

"I will not look at things. I will not suffer things to look at me. Put out the torches! Hide the moon! Hide the stars!"

Where the track runs back into the village, we confront such a dialogue, as Salome's with a dead head. On a cottage gate in the village is a head. Carved in stone. It is *identical* to the forensic drawing of Yamski approved by Bryant! We hold the 'photo-fit' drawing alongside the head, they dialogue in a silent manner; human head and representation of an imagined alien. The same.

To avoid retracing our steps we turn off before the Stumpy Oak and take a path through woods. The ground is saturated. If this goes on, the cliffs will crumble and the railways will fall into the sea. Dumna is returning to retake her realm. Until the whole thing burns up in the charred arms of Percy Seymour's ugly sun.

On one side of us, the big holy brook races, on the other, moss-covered remains of quarries and mills. We pass a 'nothing'. The nonentity is obsessing on hollow hills; wants to take me to the giant chamber of a slate mine just a little south of Ashburton. The world is Swiss cheese. Sinkholes are coming. Assad, Trump, Putin, Duterte, May, Erdoğan, the ground will open and swallow you up.

Back in the town, we meet a friend of the void's. He is rushing from feeding his solitary duck, the sole survivor of a fox raid, now forced by government order into solitary confinement in a shed. Bird 'flu has landed on a farm in Lincolnshire. Somewhere, someone will be taking out the list of morgues and checking for availability.

The void walks me to the bus stop, bids me farewell with a hug. Unsure who I have met, I doze for a few minutes in the steamy bus to Totnes.

On the train back to Exeter. I wonder whether Bryant's visions were caused by his tumour, or if it was the other way round. What if the tumour had been a new kind of sense organ, the body-adopting-the-spectacle, attuned to flying ships, but no one had recognised it in time, and eventually his body had rejected it?

Over the sea a battleship sky shimmers with inner light. As if someone is holding a torch behind a thin curtain. One of those perception experiments by Kardos Lajos in 1930s' Budapest; shining lights on white paper makes it look black.

Things hover in this light, coming in and out of existence, dreamy, Tanguy-like, dolphin grey. I come awake with a jolt. Four hundred metres offshore a white vector is making its way through the grey, leaving a foaming wake. The white thing glows. I stare from the rushing train, but the whiteness will not resolve itself into a boat; there is no right angle for the cabin. If anything, it has the shape of an upturned hull, yet it seems to be making steady progress through the wrinkled grey steel of the sea. I stare hard. I fix it against the horizon and the shore. It is big. Ghostly. Perhaps an Aspidochelone, a serpent-turtle.

It seems to be thinking.

Is this one of those "watery creatures, barely distinguishable from their surroundings" which the ecocultural theorist Stacy Alaimo suggests are proposing to us "the need for a more aquatic environmentalism... from some scarcely possible engagement with the heretofore unknown and still barely known if not potentially unknowable forms of life that inhabit the depths?"

A dim light bulb in the ruins of a dead city, an old woman left solitary in a bombed and abandoned waste land.

The train passes behind Langstone Rock and the white is gone. Blotted out by the Point-in-View.

Buckfastleigh Station, Dart Bridge Road, Station Road, Fore Street, Plymouth Road to St Luke's Church, double back to Fore Street, left into Chapel Street, Jordan Street, Merrifield Road, about 400 metres out of the town and, opposite a junction with two turnings on the left, go through the metal gate on your right (like a kissing gate) and follow the path immediately to another gate, through that and through the woods, keep taking any right/upwards path in the woods and you come out on, and turn left along, Oaklands Road, left at next junction, straight on along Hockmoor Hill, past the Stumpy Oak and stone cross, at next immediate junction ignore the sign to Scoriton and take the middle (straight on) road, Hawson Farm Cottage will appear on the right hand side of the road, the rough clamber up to the field on the left brings you into the field of the second encounter, continuing back on the road, at the signpost showing Holne one way and Buckfastleigh the other take the left unsigned road, at T-junction in Scoriton village turn right to The Tradesman's Arms, then double back and take the next right, this metalled road becomes a dirt track, after three quarters of a mile take right hand turning, follow to the first gate you reach, through gate and on your left hand side is the first encounter field while on your right hand side is a large metal barrier with inset gate onto the moor, follow the moor path to the deer hide tower, then turn back, back through metal barrier and follow the track back to Scoriton village, turn right at T-junction, and immediately left at the war memorial, then right at the next T-junction (you are retracing your steps this far), past Hawson Farm Cottage, take the next left hand turn, after about half a mile there is a sharp left hand turn in the road and a brook directly in front of you, take the bridge over the brook and follow the path through the trees, at the junction of paths take the left hand path, through gate and walk to metalled road and turn left along Hockmoor Hill, straight on at crossroads, at next junction take the right hand turning along Oaklands Road, Silver Street, at the Sun Inn junction turn right, Bridge Street, Market Street, left into Chapel Street, bear left into Fore Street, immediately right in Plymouth Road, catch bus back to Totnes from the Victoria Woodholme Mardleway Car Park. Bus to Totnes Railway Station, train to Exeter St David's.)

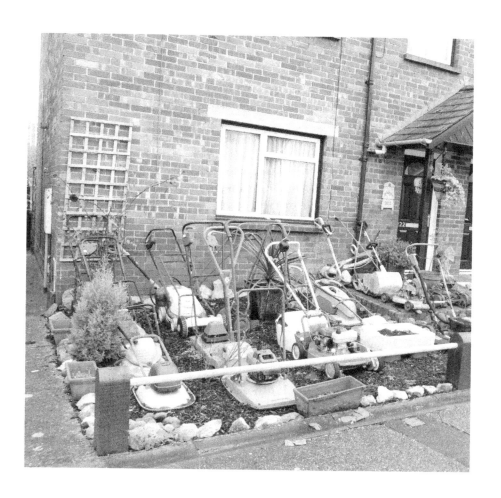

Chapter Seventeen: Whimple, Cranbrook, Crab Man and home

First thing the next morning, I catch a train to Whimple. I nearly get off too soon. There is a new station which is not on my map: Cranbrook. It is not in Salmon's guide, either.

On the platform at Whimple two freemasons are swinging thin black cases by their sides.

I am looking for the storyteller; we are to walk with one John Palfrey in mind. The author in 1892, under the pseudonym of James Bathurst, of *Atomic Consciousness*. Recently hailed in the *Fortean Times* as a possible 'Founder of Modernism', Palfrey proposed that everything is dual; if you think something then somewhere else in the cosmos, and probably in a bit of it not too far away, something else would think the same. It was a little bit like serendipity: there was the same need for sagacity, someone has to spot the coincidence. And the vehicle of transference for this duality is all at the atomic level; not the one with nuclei and so on, but the atom as imagined prior to sub-atomic physics: as fundamental and irreducible fragments of matter.

These atoms are the stuff of fields; not points of view on arcing trajectories, but factors with equivalencies in other spaces responding and reacting without the time of reaction, because the spaces of a particle and its equivalence (the duality of everything) is already entangled. When one particle responds, the field is already reacting, no time separates them. In Palfrey's case, his was an act of largely unfounded speculation, he was going on what his hyper-sensitised and only-just-contained-paranoid senses were telling him; which was that the coincidences all around him were not without some mechanism, but rather the effects of a displaced cause, an ablative relationship, the particle and its equivalence as always and already the thing itself and its effect.

There is no one on the platform that I recognise as storytellerish...

Then I see him, in hi-viz jacket, crossing the car park. We are already in enfolded characters!

The storyteller has come by car from visiting a string of hospitals in the South-West where he has been taking sick children into the patterns, narratives and skeuomorphs of a never-existing but nevertheless real folklore with multiple folks and lores anchored to space; then ripping up that anchor from its bed of dreams and setting fresh sails.

We dither around a huge former coaching inn speculating idly on the average speed of travel over various centuries. The coach from Exeter to London, passing this way, was once attacked by a lion; a Palfrey-prefiguring of our later discovery of Tash in the Cranbrook pavement. We talk about jellies as we walk through what was once council housing, and I stop to photograph two dropped shoelaces that have turned into a tendril-thing; we get trapped under a tatty union flag where a void has been opened by something, probably forensic. We backtrack out of the dead end.

The storyteller has an address for the author's home: The Green.

We walk under the railway bridge and past the school to the church; in the graveyard there is a gravestone for a John Palfrey but this one dies in 1902 rather than 1921; possibly his father?

The derisive critical welcome to Palfrey's first edition of *Atomic Consciousness* drove him to write his own reviews: "There, at last, the victory was won" wrote the imaginary Professor Scripture in *The New Psychology*.

Inside the church there are panels which are illuminated by a motion sensitive cell; one of Apollonia carrying the instrument of her torture and another of Sidwella with the scythe she used in the fields, taken and wielded to behead her. Not only does Sidwella have a head on her shoulders, but she carries another, detached, in her arms. She could play both John and Salome. Bathurstian dualities, released from chronological and hierarchical linearity by right of the suffering that would come to define Christianity as a religion of persecution; a release that John Palfrey, who believed that the cosmos conspired to "generate from any sensitive organism the greatest amount of suffering possible", did not ever receive.

Comfort and peace, to which the Christian religion might seem to aspire, have always been fatal to it.

English church spaces are remarkable things, now; I think when I started out on my walk a few days ago, and opened the first church door, I did that as if I were visiting some mixture of museum and forbidden space. But I know now there is no mixture; these spaces float in a magical (in the best sense of happening and open) way between different meanings. They are spaces to come to, to be away from 'meaning', spaces where symbols are released into the imagination again; where we do not believe in the elves anymore, but the elves still have their effects. That is the Bathurstian duality; releasing a single other to a field of multiple others.

Just as Sidwella's and Apollonia's martyrdoms cannot quite hide that they are gushing water and blood, that they are openings up of the dark wells and cavities and darkness that are at the heart of the sense of everything, and, subsidiary to that, are necessary for both the simple survival and the sophisticated individuation of any soul.

It would be harsh to say this to the face of anyone who maintains these buildings, but it is their *lack* of faith (in the sense of them not trying to enforce it, with the

311

exception of the Jollyween evangelicals) that generalises their thin faith generously. Evangelism collapses the wave. Enjoy it while it stands.

We ignore the shop and carry on up the road in the expectation of finding The Green. We are taken aback at the scale of the Heritage Centre! Expecting something like a small hut, the converted and restored linhay has a large modern annexe, each section of which is separately dedicated. We peer through windows. It is unequivocally closed. Two rooms are piled with second-hand books, while a third room has some diminutive cider-making equipment in it and numerous bottles. Behind the heritage centre is a small tree, hedge-side of a large, but ill-attended, orchard.

> WHIMPLE WONDER
> This cider apple tree is a graft
> From the only Whimple Wonder tree
> Remaining in the village.

We loop around the village. Later I forget to ask at the shop where the sole Whimple Wonder is.

Why is the church open, yet the heritage centre closed?

The power of these churches comes from them being places of performance where the show is over; they have the quiet spirit of theatres when the actors and audiences have left and the technicians are discreetly attending to things. That thing a Benedictine monk once famously said, when asked how his order sought spirituality: "we ring the bells, we say the prayers, we sing the psalms". Spirituality is a technically realised process; to the side of doctrine, zealotry, ambition, emotion and captivity to a milieu or a style. If it doesn't creep up on a person, it's something else; simulation and self-deception. That's how these spaces have achieved something, in this moment, unusual. The ambience of lost performance has replaced clunky creeds, psychology and ideas, and something different is dominant. If museums and other secular temples could stop performing at us; drop their doctrines of progress, liberalism and supremacism confusing around each other; open them up and let people wander in them alone, without invigilators or curators, take down the information boards, and they might reveal how they work to create structures of feeling and ambience at odds with their statements of inclusivity and, instead, release something numinous and democratic.

The road, after forbidding topiary, is leading us out of the village. We turn left and look for a next left to take us back to its centre, but the road takes us further out into the fields.

The storyteller explains that, increasingly, his stories are formed and reshaped by journeys. He is planning a special journey, walking with a companion made of faked human relics, a palæontoillogical version of Shelley's people-monster Demogorgan which translates its quest, as it goes, into local myths and legends. This will take the storyteller from Piltdown to Brittany.

He talks of how, although he never reads from a book, never learns a script and spontaneously changes stories as he goes along, his audiences persist in thanking him for "reciting" or "reading". This is one of the last revenants of authoritative text, which is fading as creed is fading in the best churches. We discuss whether the mush of the web will bring back a pre-Gutenberg storytelling of unreliable sagas and quest-dramas of cosmic indifference. And whether storytellers will emerge from the bleeding, dancing, revealing and transforming of everyday performance to exorcise the Trumps and Farages. The post-truthers have exploited the confusions of the moment of crossover between text and saga, but a story can double back and undermine a hero as quickly as promote them, showing them up for a mere doorkeeper.

We pass a hollow way. 'Plum Tree Lane' says the signpost. Under wooden gates, a huge head of a dog observes us. An ornamental milk churn embossed with DRIED MILK PRODUCTS. A sign promises a farm shop, but we never find it.

We see a line of houses across the fields and take a left-hand turn, passing a long and tall cottage. Alongside it a channel is overflowing with frosty water. A car approaches and we stand back to let it pass, but the driver winds down his window to chat. By accent he is a local. He peremptorily dismisses any idea that the long building was once a mill and that the stream is the remains of its race. He puts it down to run-off from the fields; "sometimes the goyle blocks, runs down yer and floods 'The Jays'". Neither of us had heard that word before: a "goyle"; a ravine in Devonshire.

The driver re-directs us to The Green, suggesting we take a turn off, once we find it, "to the Square"; and though we misinterpret his direction it takes us to our best moments of the walk.

Around a turn, from the opposite direction a tiny mechanical digger, piloted by a large man, is making absurdly slow progress. Before it can reach us, we turn into an odd bit of cemetery, the village's overspill. The sloth-like machine pursues us into the burial ground. We stand back among the stones to let it pass.

"Come to dig a grave?"

No. A recent burial has sunk and he has come to add extra earth. He guns the machine up a precipitous pile of earth and leaves.

The storyteller tells me a foaftale that happens to be true; his friend had been responsible for digging up the body of Benny Hill – "he was in a bad way" – and reburying it under a half ton of concrete. Apparently, there is a widespread belief that the comedian – the son and grandson of clowns – had been buried with treasure. Unlucky graverobbers had dug right down into his rotted coffin and disturbed his putrid bones. Hill had been one of those comedians whose work referenced then authoritative texts, performing an absolute certainty about the fixity of race and gender and sexuality, a text which is performed more slipperily now.

A young woman passes and the storyteller wonders what life is like for her in a small village.

We cross back under the railway bridge and end up retracing our steps past the coaching inn, ignoring the enclave of former council houses, in which we had earlier become trapped, and turn down The Green. We speculate on which of the more modest cottages might have been the Palfreys' home. The lesson from Hawson Farm Cottage, however, is that now is no guarantee of then.

Unsure whether the "goyle" man said right or left to The Square, we take the right and the path winds around a property, across flood-washed pebbles, over two stiles into an orchard. There are enigmatic grey buildings at the top. We climb towards them; they could be anything. Sheds for farm equipment, government laboratories. The closer we get the more abstract and unreal they seem.

The orchard is apparently neglected. The trees surrounded by their falls. Just one tree still bears watery-yellow apples and another some brilliant red ones. The storyteller collects yellow ones to make an experimental sauce. He bites into a red one and reacts, beckoning for me to try. They are exquisitely sweet and we discuss the effect of a fruit like this on someone unfamiliar with chocolate or refined sugar.

I remember reading in the bible, when I was a child, about wine. In psalms and exotic tales, wine was always made out to be thick and syrupy and rich; when I came to have my first glass it was disappointingly thin and sour.

They are water tanks. We assume. Three rectangular blocks, inviting more fantasies of hollow hills. The storyteller describes the many variations on the story he tells of waiting warriors dozing beneath the ground. The concrete tanks fulfil the role of stone slabs, laid across the entrances to the in-between spaces of the storyteller's hollow hills. But these are water portals, pylons to the lair of a sleeping jelly-warrior. Here on Eden, we take in a fort's view across the whole valley until it rises up in one long escarpment to the east.

Retracing our steps from the orchard and its oblongs, we take the left path, through a bleak playground with television-headed graffiti figures, arriving at The Square, which we had passed through earlier; we have coffees at the general store there and chat with the owners who know nothing about John Palfrey. But they can tell us that this was once the home of "Muffin the Mule's Mum"; not the woman who sat at the piano and chatted to Muffin, but Muffin's maker and manipulator, Ann Hogarth, who retired to Whimple with her fellow puppeteer and husband Jan in the 1970s. They established a small puppet museum at their home in the White Barn, displaying the puppets from their neo-Cubist production of Macbeth and their "genial minstrel puppet Wally the Gog" – bloody hell!!!!! On children's TV!

We also get to hear about the big abattoir and the cidermaker's that once kept the village prosperous, which explains the empty space in front of the station for bringing goods for loading.

"The post office has been in six different buildings!" We had passed signs for 'The New Inn' (now superseded), 'The Old Fire Station' and so on, but how could we be sure how many times such borders of identity were crossed, or in which direction?

Heading back to the storyteller's car we cross the stream for the third time; this time we notice the collection of different coloured footballs round the culvert, escapees from the primary school playground. The footballs are like a conceptual illustration of atoms from a science magazine; perhaps a revenant of the day when an accident at the cidermaker's flooded the playground with scrumpy.

The storyteller drives us to Cranbrook, a new town parachuted in to the nearby fields.

The duality continues.

From a 7th-century Saxon village to a town without an authoritative text. A 21st-century new town. Inside its single civic building is a long stretch of paper on which young people have drawn their demands: KFC, SKATEBOARD PARK, SEALIFE CENTRE. Even here there is a sea inland. An adult impatiently demands a pub before the first McDonalds.

There is a good-looking café and the school, which at first seems over-familiar and sinister, comes alive as children pour out and mothers shout one to another, arrangements for meeting up later. People look relaxed, the children are not cowed by us; a child warns us to be careful on the frost, others want to wave goodbye.

Yet there is a moment that worries me; as we are crossing what passes for Cranbrook's 'The Square' a young man emerges from the Co-operative chewing on a sandwich and begins to rehearse obsessive angular movements in the parking spaces, proceeding by a series of a crabbing movements. He seems shackled to these turns. Beside him, a woman steps from her car, oblivious to the human geometry, and comprehensively sprays her coat with something. In among the rush of children and young mums it feels hopeful, but what is there here for you if you fall through the usual nets, where is your anonymity?

Just as John Palfrey fell through the texts of village, church and schooling, or James Lyon Widger dropped into hollow hills, will Cranbrook produce its own minority of unhappy eccentrics?

Not much has been retained from the fields, with the exception of a fabulous muddy, woody recreational area on the edge of the school.

In Whimple the storyteller had described his tale of a knucker, a water dragon, and its bottomless watery knuckerhole. Why its proximity to the office of Nigel Farage was germane, I didn't grasp. The storyteller often threw in these 'easter eggs'. Now we find a broken dragon, in pieces in the small gravel portion that passes for a front garden; what happens in Whimple has its duality in Cranbrook. The two are entangled across the same fields.

Is this the beginning of the 'quantum walking' I heard mentioned but never explained?

Have the snowflakes and the "MERR CH I" letters been up, and slowly falling, since last year?

There is something not right. Oddities about the architecture: each house is an amalgam of existing styles, fishing village clapperboard wed with Scandinavian stone cabin, bungalows with supermarket roofs, the larger gateway properties have Georgian porches and Johnsonian postmodern rooftop twiddles. Throughout there is a sense of variety and difference from house to house; it lacks the pseudo-egalitarianism of some estates and the callous zoning of others. There is nothing flash about the inequalities, but nothing dishonest either.

On a number of the houses we pass there are fantastic figures around the doorways; an elf, a Green Man. This feels like a town that has been given a chance; it will be partly up to those shouting mothers sustaining their early enthusiasm. We come across a threat to that, a local BBC Spotlight team: grizzled cameraman joshing his young female colleague for forgetting her mic.

"Are you making a documentary?"

She explains, with surprising care and detail, how the provision of nursery care is being reduced for the Education Campus here; that there are young mothers who are threatened with losing their jobs, even those who can afford to pay for the childcare are struggling to find local child carers who are already over-subscribed. The kind of mismatch of resources that Cranbrook was intended to overcome; affordable housing for those in junior management and semi-skilled office work, reasonably close to their workplaces. All about to be planned out of the meshwork.

The reporter encourages us to watch at 6.30pm, as if she were a member of a tiny touring theatre company rather than a national broadcasting organisation.

On a wall, children have painted, perhaps by accident, a vibrant and shining pop group in handfuls of mud.

On a pavement, some frost has first melted and then partly dried again to make a silhouette of Tash, the Satan of C.S. Lewis's *Chronicles of Narnia*. O, he draws you in at ten years old with his lion, his witch and his wardrobe, but then seven adventures later he hammers you with his tale of end times. In *The Last Battle*, Tash, the devil-god of the Calormen comes racing through the forest. That engraving filled me with such fear for years. What is so terrifying about Tash is not his multiple arms and many talons or his bony but powerful legs, but the miasma that shrouds his limbs and follows along behind them, containing every unspeakable and unthinkable fear. Written and published in the same years as the Suez Crisis, it is not so difficult to guess who the Calormen of *The Last Battle* might be: "dark-skinned, with the men mostly bearded, flowing robes, turbans, and wooden shoes with an upturned point at the toe... the preferred weapon is the scimitar".

At first I think our water-Tash is without a beak; then I see that just above his head is floating a beaked mask; the devil is a performance.

Theories of performance and mimesis destroyed John Palfrey of Whimple, the self-proclaimed "human wreck", retrospectively re-proclaimed as the "founder of the New Psychology, New Age, New Mysticism and Modernism". A working-class man, the equivalent of more than half of Cranbrook's population, he was plagued by coincidences. He turned this haunting into a pseudo-science, rearranging time and space through atomic consciousness, bringing his thoughts into narrative and action.

A skilled contemplative like him could reproduce these stories to himself unendingly; but he was trapped by the same thoughts; they all had polarity, and a negative charge can loop back on a thinker and destroy her intentions and then herself.

Repeatedly a terrified Palfrey tried to destroy himself, sometimes in parts and sometimes in total. Like John Ruskin (Mallock's 'Mister Herbert'), hoping to blow up the railways and Wolverhampton, Palfrey sat above an industrial town and considered "as to whether a few thousands of particularly developed minds, with strong will, may not cause some plague or fire to devastate 'civilised' countries". Palfrey's misunderstandings, more akin to Southcott's than Robert Graves's, about the relationship of an imaginary totality to a material world, as a duality rather than as an entanglement, leads him to the dispersal and fragmentation of himself rather than the 'magical-causal' effect upon the world that he desires; it was something like the magic of those four men in folding chairs on the moor above Teignmouth talking down a "mixie" that he never understood.

For the storyteller and me, Cranbrook is the co-incidence of Whimple.

At the station that had surprised me earlier, a huge concrete semi-circular wall has been built around a large oak tree; the bark looks tired and mossy, it is hard to tell how healthy it is. Have they trapped too much fluid around its roots, is their protection rotting it from the bottom up? And when the tree has gone and all that remains is the semi-circle of concrete, will anyone guess the point of such a skeuomorph? Will Cranbrook one day become similarly a skeuomorph?

"What does it matter what remains to those who have gone..."

Mid-sentence the train is pulling in and I break off and run for the train. The guard smiles and then, sweetly, she compliments me on my sprinting.

The Withey, Talaton Road, Broadclyst Road, Orchard Avenue, Orchard Close, Broadclyst Road, School Hill, Broadway, The Square, Church Road, Woodhayes Lane, Grove Road, Broadway, School Hill, Broadclyst Road, The Green, right up footpath, follow signed footpath through orchard to top of hill, back down footpath and take footpath on the other side of The Green, past playground and under railway bridge, left into Webbers Close, The Square, Broadway, School Hill, turn right up footpath alongside stream to Station, catch train to Cranbrook (one an hour), Burroughs Fields, Younghayes Road, St Michael's Way, footpath to boundary of St Martin's C of E Primary School, Younghayes Road, Hayes Square, Younghayes Road, space by Younghayes Community centre, to London Road roundabout and back along Younghayes Road, Burrough Fields, Cranbrook Train Station, train back to Exeter Central Station.

I hurry out of Exeter Central Station, go to collect my rucksack from the hotel, check out and then head on down to Exeter St David's Station where I am to meet with the Crab Man.

The corner of the Cathedral Close is still smoking.

It is as though Mary P. Willcocks's "white figure of the old divine with a wise book on his knee" takes leave of his plinth and rises into the grey clouds; then it turns a darker colour and I see her critical thoughts, more striking than her novels, first form a column and then drift into obscurity; the hypocrisy of the English unable to grasp a great theme, Dickens satirising "red-nosed preachers" but incapable of seeing or saying what is "big scale production" in his world, or "the sentimentalist... a creature who plays the vampire just as zestfully as ever the egoist did, but each time he drains another life-blood he draws round himself a cloak of holy purpose", and on Symbolism: "a perpetual interchange of the physical plane with the mental... usually we only see the material unrolling as it is woven, but now and again we catch a glimpse of the loom itself... the lie sexual merges in the lie economic and that again in the lie political". In the miasma of depression she sees from where change will come: "it would be woman, not man, who would first awake and find her own soul... if an honest world is ever to be built, we must begin with the springs of life". All this in 1926, *Between the Old World and The New*.

He is much older than I had expected. I tell him so and he coughs up laughs.

He is much bigger in girth than I had expected.

"I am twenty years older than I expected! When I was 15, I didn't expect to get to 40, not without a nuclear war. Only on having reached the limits of my expectations, did I finally turn away from art – while practising it secretly, of course – and got into this. Hypocrisy is necessary to genuinely do new things. But for the purposes of public consumption I have turned towards everyday life..."

"Are you serious?"

"Am I laughing?"

He is.

He tells me the place we are walking in is blighted. The unsolved murder of a teenage girl twenty years before cast every man in the district under suspicion. The police had DNA'd the lot and found nothing. No one has ever been charged. Most likely it was an attack by a stranger who had never been to the area before, came once, killed, never returned. Like a misfortune or an inexplicable mutation. The police lab subsequently contaminated the evidence, the chance of a conviction now is nil. What hangs about the place is a sense of a threat that is both real and absent.

"If you assume that meaning is made by reference to environmental conditions, social relations and so on, there is no sense to it. It has nothing to do with here. But it put a hole in here for everyone to throw their fears into. There is nothing magical about these moments – I hate the Rippercrap of some London psychogeographers – the effects are social and visceral; women are terrified and men suddenly, and without anything in the least liberating about it, feel the gaze turned on themselves."

He seems to be avoiding the new suburban part, joking, as we pass, about a pub called, generically, 'The Village Inn', which he says could be something from the movie 'Xistenz'.

I have not seen it.

"Pity it doesn't sell 'David Kronenberg'."

I don't get it.

We have entered the area via a level crossing, stepping over the naked tracks of the lines to London and Bristol; I had crossed them just a little further north at Stoke Canon. The cool shaping of the flood defence system, a church made of volcanic rocks.

Icons in a virtual space.

By the bridge over the river, on a concrete post, there is a small ceramic Rapunzel-like figure with long blonde hair and in a white dress, framed in a triangular leaded window.

We have to find a hidden gate, obscured by the apparently private space of two driveways: one to a modest cottage, the other to a mansion. This is the entrance to an old hollow way. Crab Man probably thinks he is showing me a novelty here, but I know this network well now. Certain 'secrets' are very quickly open to anyone willing to give more than a cursory glance to things. Crab Man explains that this was a packhorse route and a coffin way for a village with no church; the exposed slate in the wall of the lane is 'Crackington Formation', it goes underground here and comes up again somewhere in Germany. We sink below the row of modern suburban houses. In the cold and shadowy dip, although we climb steeply, the eyeline never changes.

We find an installation that gives the lie to the assertion that children no longer make dens. This one has its own gibbet. A chair on its side, beneath a washing line noose hung over a branch. Whether this is a piece of informal play equipment or a warning to the psychogeographically curious, who can say? Crab Man pulls down the noose and throws it out of the lane.

"You write a lot about paranoia..."

"Limited paranoia..."

"Yes, but what if it's really pronoia?" I worry. "Paranoia puts you in the same camp as the pessimists, 'life is short and quickly snuffed out', but what if it's worse than pessimism? What if its brainless complacency, this idea that the landscape is conspiring to give you pleasure?"

"Why would that be bad?"

"Depends on the landscape?"

"You think the landscape is against us?"

"Might be... You never come out and say that things are actually conspiring on our behalf!"

"I remember seeing Stella Rimington, MI5, talking about James Bond movies and the interviewer asks her to comment on the similarity to an actual operation. Her response: secret services don't comment on past operations."

"You do that a lot – use mainstream ideas and turn them to your own uses. Like 'counter-tourism', you say it is more like the diversionary interventions of security forces than the subversions of revolutionaries. What if you just *are* reactionary?"

"Thank you very much! Let me put the question back to you – what if my hypocrisy and complicity are signs of my good faith?"

I laugh, he smiles.

"Are you OK now?"

"I've been ill for a few months. Not a bad thing, maybe. I've had to drop out of things, I want to be more anonymous again. Facebook forced me to reveal my real name; and publishing was the same. That meant that I got to know some of the walkers who were coming forward at that time. I don't know why people want to come to walk with me, but if they do I bring them up here. The place is so apparently unpromising, it guarantees a miracle."

"People like *me* come?"

"They are usually going to do something; change their lives, go on an epic journey, never just for a walk. I hear some fascinating things, I give them some irritating advice – take blister plasters, take Vaseline, study noticing, certain kinds of mental things. I'm irritating *myself* just telling you! Anyway, we look at things together, discuss stuff we find. I'm not sure they always get that the route is meaningfully woven around what we are talking about."

"Point taken."

"Perhaps my mistake is that I never properly spell anything out. I never fully generalise what *my* project is; what *the* project is."

"Then why don't you? Now? Why don't you try giving *me* the big picture; then we'll see?"

That makes him laugh a lot. I am being "Cheeky".

We hear some indecipherable cry from the estate. The streets here will turn out to be emptier than anywhere else on my walk.

"Good! The present system, this variant of capitalism we are experiencing and reproducing right now, the predomination of lifeless property over the living, the interests and rights to profit for a minority – this really is very old stuff, for heaven's sake – this is driven by an exploitation not just of labour, but of the whole of life itself. It's in your meditation time, in your holidays, in your sport, in each and every pleasure, leisure, recreation, relaxation – those are its grounds for exploitation. Partly, this is what digitisation has brought to us, but the mental mechanics have been in place ever since the first mass media and the founding of the modern mass societies in the 1920s. Digitisation and globalisation are the technical realisations of the integrated Spectacle, they are not fundamental transformations, they were already present in ways of thinking before they came into operation in practice. Today the system is easiest seen at work in social media; not only are we charged rent for our use of its imaginary space, but we are also its unpaid workers and its raw materials. The social media system puts us in a relation of exploitation with ourselves! Meanwhile the electronic field constantly and algorithmically searches out our preferences, looping our desires with its marketing department, hollowing out our inner lives for information fuel. The resistance starts, the progressive resistance starts – because pessimistic reactionaries have been aware of this for a lot longer – with the International Lettristes and their first *dérives*, seeking out spaces in Paris that were uncongenial to the system's youthful tentacles, making spaces of disconnected pleasure. Never work! Play! Those 'Naked City' maps that were produced by Asger Jorn and Debord, they were visual reports of unalienated walks; they were the remaining contrary spaces, stitched together; maps for an internal defence of the city, from which they intended to advance outwards increasing the hold of aimless pleasure on the city. Why did they not? Have you read Andrea Gibbons's paper?"

"I think I know the one you mean: how the *dérive* came to an end for the situationists...."

"She paints that moment as a betrayal of their Algerian comrade-drifter; and she may be right, I wasn't there! At very best it was an immoral preservation of the group. They had learned – their Algerian comrade the harder way – that to drift at that time was to directly confront the racialised meaning of presence on the streets of Paris; to defend an Algerian was to become Algerian. And they couldn't hack it; they were out of their depth. Jorn's and Debord's naked map did not apply to Abdelhafid Khattib, for him the map was completely blank. He had nowhere. Their conspiracy... woosh..."

He blows through his fingers.

"...disappears! That's how quickly! When Gibbons and others say "psychogeography is just a safe space for middle-aged white males", it doesn't matter whether the accusation is strictly true or not, it is the responsibility of the *dérivistes* to do something about it: 'safety to drift for all means all'. The secondary threat is that now, given the prevalence of hand-held devices, on one particular level, it's the same for everybody as it was for Abdelhafid Khattib; there are no spaces left. But the consequences are *completely different*; being threatened with adverts is not the same as being clubbed to death and your body thrown in the Seine. And so, likewise, the project has changed; in some ways it is much easier now. It is no longer about defending localities, mini-communities, regions or blocks of space and building out from there, with all the pitfalls of nostalgia and territory; on the other hand, it is much harder, much less promising, it is about very thin layers and about individuals and about subjectivities and about collectively standing up for them and about things no bigger than your hand. That is the battleground: subjectivity, the agency of imagination, the inside of ourselves that should remain unknowable to others. Just as the bastards have forced it down to the basics of a racialised body on the street under threat, so they have digitally got it down to the basics of a threatened soul online. In response, in consequence, walking has been forced to regroup romantically; the question is: around what kind of 'spirit'? Do we mean some kind of universal humanism or something newly made from the surplus pleasures we can win back in tiny engagements from the machines, stealing items here and there from the myths in everyday space? That's what driving all this Chthulucene and re-enchantment and vibrant matter stuff going on right now. Almost none of that is possible without quests, nomadic meanders, repossessing the imaginary 'old ways'. By which I don't mean hollow ways, pilgrim's ways. I mean the old way of walking, because walking is always old..."

"Isn't that in danger of turning walking into another kind of universalism?"

"It is another kind of universalism! It means taking 'universe' at its word – this is not about normativity or common traits or shared origins – bullshit to that! This is about a theory of everything slowed right down to walking and crawling and limping and wheeling pace, out of step with the system. It doesn't have an ideal revolutionary agent standing above it, no Hegelian Spirit or Marxist proletariat – in the 1920s you could join the Clarion Walking Club or whatever was organised to destroy the Nazi walking groups... *Edelweisspiraten* or whatever... now you have to learn to relate to something more disparate, more fluid..."

The hollow way ends abruptly at a fence, but a trace of the old path is still visible as a 'shadow' in the surface of the field, then runs out to nothing, ploughed under.

"Jelly-like? Tentacular?"

"If you want. But in order to connect to the other fluidities we have, at least for a while, to do it ourselves, as the Irish nationalists have it, "*sinn féin*", we have only ourselves to be revolutionary with. We cannot drift on behalf of anyone else. *That*, at least, the situationists were honest about..."

There is something moving in the field, beyond the flock of sheep; it is within sight, but at a distance that makes it fuzzy; fox-like, but it looks bigger.

"With mass radical politics gone, the Arab Spring over, Occupy evaporated, we have to be honest with ourselves, there is no special political space any more; Occupy and the Arab Spring came out of the everyday and took over iconic spaces; but power re-grouped and re-took our icons. We mustn't become like those cartoon characters who run over a cliff and for a while their legs whirl and they hang there – those spaces are closed to us. Now, we have the everyday alone as our terrain, and also the possibility of interior spaces; the virtual offers us very little. The test is to make layers and micro-spaces within the everyday and within ourselves that are *like* those areas in the Naked City maps, but that don't apply to actual geographical boundaries; what is contrary to the Spectacle is what post-truth discourse inadvertently offers us, the chance to make imaginary space that is not subject to the authority of a fundamental text – no Marx, no Heidegger, no Deleuze, no Debord – that is our terrain now, and somehow we have to win that battle inside as prelude to taking it onto real streets and into real fields and have it readable, visual, impactful. We haven't even begun to work out how..."

"'We'?"

"That imaginary and hopeful 'we'... I don't know who I am talking about. I don't know any such people, do you? It's *ludibrium*-speak; saying it in the hope of it becoming real. The ones born in Internet times, that's who I mean. Anyone can walk in places beyond or hidden within the malignant gaze, making it readable for others without producing a new personalised Spectacle for each of us... that's something else."

The fox-dog-calf thing is still not resolving itself. We try to define it for a while.

"But let's distinguish this identity-making from the nationalist inflection; paranoia and pronoia reflect the nature of the things on the ground right now, how some things conspire with us and some against us. We need to know how to tell which is which, what are our allies in Thingworld, in Meatworld, in Cyberspace, in the meshes of them all. We need allies for this conflict with the invasive economy, we need to develop hyper-senses, any body can do it – in any body and with any other body – through training in the field, something like a sociable urban guerrilla training, specialised knowledge passing from one cadre to another without charge, through chatting, woolly stories, exemplary adventuring together.

"I've felt the way that particular sites – whether they are seaside resorts or Georgian stately homes or model villages or hill forts or factories or UFO landing sites – they help you out, act with you, make a space between becoming and being where things help you, a space that lends this transformative frisson, which, if knowingly and sensitively harnessed, gives you a way to understand things and a strength to change them. This is the basis on which we could move forward... or rather, move sideways: by surplus energy recognisable by pleasure. For what we do now in small numbers, if we can restrain and retrain ourselves, we can do sideways and then, it will be everyone's..."

"Everyone?"

"Which is the point! Isn't this the lesson of the situationists' failure? It can be a mass thing, but only if there are no exclusions, starting with the most marginalised. Only then can it become like rambling used to be – massive! Imagine if we could map the places with *chora* – and then map them with the interiors of individuals, entangling serious and unrespectable knowing and feeling with abject and scared spaces..."

I wonder if he has been speaking to some of the people I have been walking with. This sounds like the Crab Man's exegesis of our walk around Denbury, our conversations about conspiracy, the meaning of the hill fort and the amoral force inside the hollow hill.

"Each person would make their own map. You could never make such a map for anyone else. But they could be readable by others... Imagine if people had these in the same way as now they take it for granted that they have a passport, or the collection of photos on their phone... all they need to do is walk it, use it... the *chora* will do the rest..."

"Ring the bells, say the prayers, sing the hymns..."

"Yes. You've got it! I think that some kind of inward-looking of the body is necessary in a time of Spectacle. Without any external revolutionary force, the generator has to be re-found within, until new myths can be formed and the process ritualised..."

The fox-dog-thing exits the field; the lens on my camera is not strong enough to capture a sharp image.

"Rather as William Beckford did with the memory of the young Earl of Devon, turning the boy into a tower, is that what you mean?"

He laughs.

"You characterise it with the worst possible analogy!"

"But even so," I press, "is that what you mean?"

"Of course it is. Disgracefully. That's why *Mythogeography* and the other books back away. The generator is so easily made mystical, made ideal, made reactionary."

"What is it then? The generator?"

He laughs again, derisively now, and fingers a group of nails hammered into the drooping bough of an old oak. For one horrible moment I think the gesture is intended for me; that all he is prepared to say about the machine is inside the machineless. But he is gathering his thoughts.

"Against my better judgement, this."

We set off away from the ghost of the hollow way.

"The generator is that dark nothingness... unknowable... or, rather, the darkness or nothingness best unknown – the part of ourselves that is best activated within the loops of the road's narrative; where we can hide in plain sight..."

"S – I – G – H – T?"

"And S – I – T – E."

Dew on the blades of long grass is soaking into my trouser legs.

"Activate the private nothingness that every self has. I'm not talking about some kind of madness, or religious ecstasy, or 'id'... and certainly not a 'collective unconscious'. I mean a genuine nothingness inside; that space that is beyond the event horizon of ourselves, from which, incredibly but genuinely, faint traces of information escape, that are genuinely mysterious... no system of interpretation will make any sense of them without collapsing the information wave and destroying it..."

"This is within oneself?"

"NO! If it were just interiority it would be immediately invaded. It survives by connection to distant things – roads, nebulae, oceans, everything. We're talking about planning on a really simple level, organising what we do on the map by our intuitions of that mystery that is escaping so faintly."

"And this is what the Spectacle is after?"

"Of course. It's where our preferences come from. But we can protect it, shore it up. Then we can *really* work our darkness. Make own maps of our own naked cities, inside and out."

"How would that work? Technically?"

"Protecting stuff and letting it do its own work – connecting up to it and then ignoring it – it will throw off all sorts... do you know Matthew Barney's three stages of creative production?"

"No."

"I've forgotten the names he gives them..."

Situation, Condition, Production.

We drop down a recent path between the houses and follow a road of brutal design, voided, tank-like parking spaces, collective pagodas that no one uses, big arched entrances that feel out of scale. The road drops steeply again. There is a laminated handwritten sign on a lamp post, a warning about the repeated scattering of screws to puncture the tyres of cars and the local school bus:

> An old woman and an old man have been seen walking their large dog
> in this area on many occasions and acting suspiciously... If you spot
> these individuals please do inform us. THANK YOU.

At times the streets seem crowded, at times deserted, but there is never anyone else walking them.

"One is your original idea, your inspiration; two, you shape it into something in the physical world; three, that hardens into a publicly shared commodity. One, two, three. Pretty banal, the usual model of a commercial production. But what Barney is doing is to say "stop at number two and go back to number one", again and again and again until that creates a loop between one and two, whirling and spiralling until they throw off a wholly unexpected number three. That is creativity – the making of an obtuse object, an oblique angel."

"Angel?"

"Something to stand up on the point of a pin and be counted. That's how we make the dark space work for us. By refusing it production, denying it access to the market and the market access to it. If we can do that in our own walking minds, we can do the same to everyday space. Creating private dark space in public places – and I don't mean private in the sense of property, but private in the sense of being driven subjectively, disruptedly, not by memes and algorithms – fucking algorithms! Does it not strike you as sinister that there were all these neo-situationists in the 1990s who were drifting around using simple algorithms to determine their *dérives*? That what they did back then might have served what is happening to us now?"

Like Dartington? I wondered.

"If the Israeli Defence Force can train its officers in the ideas of Debord and Guattari..."

"Let's do the opposite of that! Shutting down the connections to commerce and exchange, dimming the brightness of the Spectacle and advertising, reprogramming the behaviours of the users to obsession with texture and standing still, to the 'small dance', to the dance of falling dust and humming electrics, draining the system of its power. To difficult initiations that are easiest for the marginalised."

"Does it *require* initiation?"

"I suppose it does... but then, when you initiate people, many say 'o, I think I am already doing that!'"

"Do they all say that?"

"No, but it's heartening that so many do. Any successful revolution will be largely based on something that is not new, something that is almost already happening, already nearly dominant, but not quite noticed, that needs to be given a stage. Revolution is too rarely described in terms of how a change in the landscape gives space for a longstanding, mostly ignored and low-status activity to become revolutionary."

In the narrow grassy interregnum between pavement and building are handwritten notes on ripped cardboard; someone has been researching the business affairs of a famous restaurateur with an establishment in this city and those of a prominent funder of the national Conservative Party:

£1.4 billion... Dubai based... private equity firm...

"If a duality that keeps collapsing into messy classical systems can effect a molecular change, a lever between incredibly weak but still meaningful forces, like the earth's magnetic field and the thumping great molecules in a bird's eye, then the same weak forces can speak to us as they do the bird: there's the road and there's the arrow of direction!"

"It's only robins, actually, not other birds..."

"OK, robins then. But the process is totally clear and simple for the robin! That's how the darkness can work for us, its instability and weakness is what makes it powerful, because it's supersensitive to certain forces that have no status in the Spectacle; forces of suffering and defacing, forces that are antique and pedestrian... engage them, in numbers, across populations, personal maps that are ubiquitous, everyone on their own pilgrimage... then dark nothingness is the lever that sustains the superposition, that establishes entangled equality before the collapse, and you have an action. When the Spectacle arrives on the doorstep of the subjective darkness it's like a giant version of itself arriving, a stupid cousin with dictatorial limbs. It's like having a fascist round for tea! You kick them out – your indifference collapses and you take action, the universe turns blue and you have the arrow of direction. Then intuition, a sense of the ambiance ahead, takes you one way rather than another, without you even needing to choose, that is the entangling of darkness with the landscape, collapsing your giant cousin, indecision, asymmetrically."

"It all sounds rather solipsistic. I can't hear anything very popular or general."

"Ah, but what if we had social relations like that; indifferent to social distinctions? What if we take our lever from trash culture and from old stories, things with resonance that the Right think that they have first claim to? What happens if we now attach this asymmetrical lever to both popular culture *and* the landscape?"

He stops. I think he is going to touch me.

"What if *you* annihilate your one within to become part of many tangled ones? What if you serve as a knight...?"

I had mentioned 'Sir Constant' earlier, he quotes it back at me.

"...a questor, ringing the bells and singing the hymns, but this time the bells and prayers are of darkness, of privacy and hyper-sensitivity?"

We get entangled in a mini-edgeland, a giant verge of trees and the dry bed of a water channel, running up against a back-garden fence and twisted clothes.

"We proceed with a hope..."

By the Community Association building a sign warns about air rifle shootings of pets; a newspaper cutting from the local paper quotes a local "cat lady" and "trained mental health professional, who has asked not be named for fear of reprisal" who warns that "if the individual behind these crimes is not caught quickly, we may well end up with a fully-fledged psychopath in our community".

"...but more with real people. The colonised, the angry, the disgruntled..."

"Are they your knights?"

"They are everyone's knights. There is nothing special, nor totalitarian about those kinds of heroes. They represent points of destabilisation – by marginalisation, age, class, disability, vulnerability..."

We are losing height and must be almost back to where we started, then we turn sharply right and up a steep climb between houses that are as generic to suburbia as 'The Village Inn' is to village inns. It feels like we are entering a meta-narrative.

More laminated signs; an elderly man protests the refusal of the authorities to allow him the right to visit his invalid wife; he protests his innocence of their claims of abuse.

"Everyone will be on a quest?"

"Yes. That's the harder part, perhaps, for the people involved. It involves a certain breaking away. Even Christ said that anyone who came to him, but had not first rejected their mother and father, they could not be a disciple of his. A gospel of peace is stuck with stasis to begin with. In order to meander we break with certain networks of destination, function, intention; there's an element of violence there, not to people, but to behaviours. Particles emerging from a quantum vacuum, which must borrow energy from elsewhere to pop into being before paying it back and returning to the void of potential: there is a certain theft in that borrowing..."

He is talking about the thievery in shipwreck modernity.

"...and there is a certain responsibility as a result to pay it back in reparative, depressive action."

He races on as we climb a steep hill. I forget to question him about depressive action; but elsewhere he has drawn on Eve Kosofsky Sedgwick's *Touching Feeling*, so presumably that is included in all this.

"The point of leverage is a hill of pessimism which we cannot climb, which we have to tunnel through, without a tunnel, of course, only the potential of a tunnel. When Kierkegaard said... but you know...."

"What?"

"His leap is not a leap *of* faith..."

"...but *into* faith."

A large derelict site behind tall metal fencing, service roads built, foundations for a children's centre, long ago abandoned due to government funding cuts.

"No one leaps to their destination; they break from the network and into the meshwork. Those who don't come back – the Ivan Chtcheglovs – they are under medical supervision. That is why, after the initial leap, it is necessary not to keep leaping but to settle into your pace, follow the timetable that the field gives you, sing the hymns, ring the bells. The tactics – the hymns and bells – are already out there; there's no excuse any more for using the wrong map and throwing in a little occult spice; anyone who has been at this game for more than a couple of years and cannot write down more than thirty tactics, more than fifty tactics... well, fuck 'em! Because they are frauds. Pardon my French."

We had reached a point where there was a view to the two towers of the cathedral.

"It's very simple really. I am proposing that there is an emotional and philosophical discipline..."

"That in previous times you might have called a religion..."

He howls with laughter.

"Yes! Yes! Brilliant... this is nothing to do with the dark against light, the good against the evil, or any other such binaries, this is only about darkness, remember? Facing the cosmic amoral power of things..."

Now I am thinking that Oak's Law might be a real one.

"Face that inside yourself, see its absolute unflinching scale and indifference. And then you have a choice: on the one hand, you can take it as a horror movie, a heralding of the setting of one against another, of survival of the fittest, of the two sides of slaughter, the rising of 'the children of the sun', as the only meaning in a meaningless cosmos. Or – and this is what such a dark-mindful walking in the world is really all about – you can face the darkness as unflinchingly dark as it is and be inspired by its nothingness, as a kind of humility before the world, an attitude through which to entangle with others with only a shared meaningless in the face of the cosmos. All this is done with the modesty of a one-mile-an-hour stroll, and the mass mobilisation to provide the safe and transfiguring space for everyone to take that stroll."

He sighs with exhaustion. We stand in silence looking at the vista. The twin towers of the cathedral stand out startlingly above the roofs of the city below.

"It's a dog's dinner of a building... I heard the tourists' oohing and aaahing, but it's a mess," I say, "half Romanesque, half Gothic."

"Do you see the street names?"

I look around. Canterbury Road, Gloucester Road at the junction, Truro Drive, Winchester Avenue behind us.

"Cathedral cities. Look behind you." I turn round. "Looks like the drive up to a private place? That in fact goes to a locked gate and then it directly connects to Exwick Lane, which is the main route out of the old village and away from the city;

now look in front of you. The road stops at Gloucester Road just in front of us, but the route..."

"Is that a path there?"

We cross the road and we walk straight into an alley running behind the back gardens. A "ginnel" I would have called it as a kid. By the tangle of collapsed fences and weeds underfoot it is rarely walked.

The branches of overhanging trees part and the cathedral appears again, less than an hour's walk away.

We choose not to double back to the old village or take the road down to 'The Hermitage', but follow the alley around a concrete bend, tracing its line to what must have been the ford, near where the railway station is now, and where the river must once have spread out, slowed and gone shallow. Crab Man points across the river, divided now in two for flood defence.

"...and that takes you up Clement's Lane, along Howell Road, for a mile and a half, over the valley that is now the other railway, into the city centre, heading straight for the cathedral. But here's the thing: what were these pilgrimages? What were these through ways and thoroughfares? In the end, they are all linked to Jerusalem, a city that was never 'ours' and was repeatedly held under siege and occupation, the tyranny of a centre, of a destination. The model of pilgrimage was always poisoned by an early form of religious colonialism. The only way to put it right is to dissolve the shrines, but the whole Grail thing did that, so that doesn't work! Much better would be to make holy the way itself and the way of going on it. The things of the road are what is holy and the road is the shrine; there is nothing final to find, setting up new paths along which to practise hospitality towards strangers, with no occupied capital at the end of it."

"What about strategy? You are very keen on conjuring up these imaginative tactics, but the overall picture..."

"O, I thought I *had* been talking strategy."

"O, OK..."

"Maybe it's better this way; sharing experiences, sharing practices, swapping tactics, it's sometimes been thin, but it's thickening. Anything strategic now would necessarily be prescriptive and dictatorial."

I look across the rooftops and wonder under which one are the fragments of spacecraft collected by Arthur Bryant in the Scorriton field and taken away by the young ufologist. The broken pieces of hope.

I explain how I have been frustrated when I read the posts on the Walking Artists Network. I expected to find an intellectual to and fro, a dialogue, but the whole thing is so intensely practical. A walk here, an exhibition there, technical advice with audio, news of talks and presentations and radio shows and films; invitations to walks, but there are no real disputes or debates. Dialogues are short-lived.

The whole thing is accumulative, he says.

We walk all the way back down, almost to river level, passing the volcanic rock church where the Crab Man promises remarkable ceiling paintings, unappreciated by its evangelical congregation. Then we walk up through the centre of the old village again, once more passing 'The Village Inn'. As he puffs up the steep rise of the old lane by 'The Hermitage', laughing at a sign for 'The Square' next to a pointedly wedge-shaped stone, Crab Man struggles for a strategic approach.

"We are in a war, not of our own choosing. The Spectacle declared war on our subjectivity, and we fight back as individuals, against the representations and against the machines that make the images. I've said this already..."

"Guerrilla bands?"

"No, I was hopelessly wrong when I wrote about that. I was so wrong. We need to get serious about subjectivity. It's both the game board and the piece; that gives it enormous power. What seems like self-indulgence is exemplary altruism. To walk through a space and remake it by force of imagination; that destroys Spectacle. Offer that free, on tap, in pubs! In the schools!"

We cross Knowle Drive and I recognise the road from before by its sharply stepped grey brick wall; we are looping inside the loop of our second walk, tripling things up inside the suburb, we are tying it up like a knot. This must be our state of Condition now, but then we flip back to Situation...

We pass the barely recognisable remnants of a portion of cut-and-laid hedge, grown out but hanging on in a children's playground; its abjection is a sign of how little of the sense of this as a place of agriculture has survived.

...and all the repetitions and all this going back to basics in the conversation is planned by Crab Man to create the moment for a spontaneous Production.

Opposite a topiary knucker, we climb down through a hole in a steel fence and mooch about on what were the floors of a demolished school, treading down broken glass and running around on the playground together in what only feels like spontaneity. We dance together, competing to make the loudest crunches.

We go back to Situation; attention to the place. Just a little further up the hill is the new school, heavily fortified. We follow a footpath around the school to a pair of heavy gates; peering through the gaps we can see how the road inside the gate once linked up with the view to the cathedral one way and the other way to the old lane leaving the city.

Our way blocked, we skirt around; a curling dimension, parallel with the pilgrims' path, and, in turn, curling around that, spiralling into the middle of the darkness at the heart of this Production. The route is meaningfully woven.

I feint to turn up the hill again, and the Crab Man overtakes me, but I turn again and he neatly steps, with the feet of a dancer, behind me and goes in front; he is not leading me, but following me from in front. This is my spiral.

The thirty-eight stab wounds that could not kill 'Fat Dan'.

Dropping down off the suburb's hill, on the boundary road of former council houses, one of the diminutive front gardens is a museum of small lawnmowers, green ones on one side and orange on the other. While we have been getting nowhere, these lawnmowers have got somewhere, without a hint of meaningfulness.

"I think I've been too quick to seek the comfort of a few faint echoes on Facebook. I should have been more daring, more self-destructive. Don't be like me. Do as I say, and not as I do."

"A hypocrite?"

He giggles.

"I'm a mystery, Cecile. Officially! The consultants don't know what is wrong with me. 'Listen to your body', my anti-medical friends say...."

But I stop listening. I stop looking. He has already told me that he is shaping the walk to make the sense he wants, but I am bailing out of his flight of fancy. I am inside my own head now. I hover above the river footpath, I ignore the hollow way in the side of the playground, I float over the steel bridge while inside my head there are three knuckers spiralling around each other. His mouth opens and shuts, but I hear nothing; for some reason it reminds me of the 'Wallace and Gromit' thing, ripped off from Buster Keaton, when they are building the track in front of the train engine as it goes along. We have been walking in parallel with ourselves.

The Rapunzel icon has been smashed while we've been walking.

"I hope you get better soon."

I try to get away politely.

"...what in the end gets to eat us is the mystery we have been seeking all our lives..."

I lie about having to catch a train and we part with a bungled handshake.

I understand it all now. The bastards.

They want me to be their wader through the Slough, their intellectual machete, happy conqueror of Giant Political Despair, one of the Shining Ones to clothe their melancholy.

Stuff 'em!

Exeter St David's Station, footpath and car park to Station Road, right along Exwick Road, ignoring the left turn to Kinnerton Way a left hand turn into Hamlyns Lane hollow way (entrance obscured by a driveway), at the top where the lane once went on into a field slip to the left behind the houses then sharp left between the houses onto Farm Hill (off the path and through the trees as the road drops down), Kinnerton Way, Moorland Way, Knowle Drive, Gloucester Road, up Cleve Lane for view to cathedral and back down again, down footpath opposite entrance to Cleve Lane and parallel with Truro Drive, Cypress Drive, Rowan Way, Exwick Road, Exwick Hill, Higher Exwick Hill, Gloucester Road, Exwick Lane, Peterborough Road, Winchester Avenue, Exwick Road, New Valley Road, footpath to Station Road, Red Cow Village, Exeter St David's Station.

I give it ten minutes, then double back on myself, only narrowly avoiding him. He is stood at the bottom of an abject footpath in animated conversation with a smartly dressed Asian man. By email I later discover that they have met by chance; the man is lost, and the Crab joins him rather than directing him up to the centre. According to Crab, the man had represented the Bradford mosques during the Rushdie fatwa and book burning. He and the Crab amicably discuss blasphemy, the anti-Catholic outrages in Cathedral Close on bonfire nights. They stand outside St David's church and contemplate its splitting into two parts; built partly over an older church, the ground beneath is moving at different rates now and is dragging it asunder.

> *To touch a coat strokes the boiler inside,*
> *To roll a bowl prods a heart to beat,*
> *A worm turns into a stick*
> *And a planner-god makes armour for a soft armadillo.*
> *To turn your back invites a flower to open.*

These were not poems as such. They were notes. I'd re-read each one of them a number of times. Attention to rhythm had yet to come, but it was not any worth in them that I was supposed to think about. Rather I was to consider what the point of *any* product might be that did not make "a world that gives one the desire to get lost in it" (Jappe).

I was fed up with principles and instructions. I felt an old-fashioned itch for an Eliotine 'objective correlative' coming on, not for metaphorical sticks and worms, but for a real worm in the real grass, skewered with a real stick by a real child.

To feel that in at least one of the crockery fragments that we had cracked underfoot in the hollow lane a spider pattern of distress had so darkened that it would scare the next child who scrambled there to build a gibbet.

The gibbet was the poem.

Trash installations and what Wrights & Sites call "ambulant architectures", transitional and transient. Scary not because the kids mean that much by it, but because the structures are barely there at all; the creations of digital children.

I am easing myself into the cold water of a planet of thinking jellies.

I am going to go to Plymouth one more time and then that will be it. I can easily find a B&B in Plymouth and add one last day to my walk and let that be the completion rather than let the Crab Man define it. Why should he determine my walk?

I want to get out into parts of Plymouth that the walkers have told me about, away from where the remains of the Navy's grip are still visible, to the place where a tributary has made a tangled Tanguy-landscape of wheels and prams and bollards in uniform dark sludge. I want to see the thick doughnut of big houses.

It is one of the slow trains. A glorified bus really. The man opposite me is reading a lurid horror movie magazine, *The Dark Side*. He is very keen to tell me about movies I am not interested in.

"I'm not very interested in horror movies."

"You are. You just haven't seen the right ones."

"I'm afraid I haven't seen any of those... I did see 'The Exorcist' on dvd – I thought it was disgusting."

"I'm not interested in the Devil. Real evil is mechanical, not supernatural. The point of movies is the screen – have you read anything by Stephen Barber?"

"No."

I lie.

"You should."

Later, once I'm finally home, I get Stephen Barber's *Projected Cities* from the university library to remind myself of the passage where he juxtaposes a visit to see "an anonymous American thriller" in the Sõprus cinema in Tallinn built in Soviet-style, late 1940s, with "obsolete hammer-and-sickle emblems at roof level surmount[ing] a huge carved-granite screen... its grandiose surfaces intricately impacting historical memory with the void interval of the contemporary" and a subterranean Hamburg gay porn cinema just before dawn where "pornographic films flickered on the screen while bouts of anal sex were unsteadily executed among the collapsed rows of seating". The seating at the Sõprus is waterlogged from its leaking roof, in Hamburg the seats are semen-sodden: "cries of orgasm from both the screen and the spectators' space split the dank air... the cinema's clientele... would never understand that Europe's cities had ostensibly become 'digital' zones, that their culture had evanesced and vanished".

I love that strange resistance.

"The screen defies the digital swamping of the world..."

...the movie man bangs on the window of the carriage as the black wrecks in the Exe hove into view.

"Have you seen 'The Mist'? The survivors in the supermarket make a break through the haze to get to some medicines in a pharmacy..."

Please, not half the movie...

"...they go in single file one by one disappearing into the white mist. Then they are all gone, and just for a moment there is only the mist on screen – except mist is white, so there is nothing. White light simply illuminates the screen, it does not hide or disguise or cover it. The movie disappears. And in that moment, in a moviehouse, you realise where you are and what movies do. You see the screen itself. That's why secrets and hidden drivers are right there in plain sight in trash movies. 9/11 was 'Godzilla' and 'Independence Day', the US invaded Iraq because of a Michael Bay movie, 'Possession' and 'Spring' prefigure everything that's happening with trans-sexuality, do you know how many kids no longer identify either male or female? The last scenes of 'Super 8' are a premonition of the coming American Civil War..."

He gets off at Starcross. Turning and backing down the aisle between the seats, bowing slightly.

"Stay restrained. Don't show, don't perform. Treasure the little things. 'One Hour Photo'." Then, he winks, and is gone.

When the Chilcot Report came out it was noted that part of the information on 'weapons of mass destruction' supplied by shadowy sources had been taken from 'The Rock'; a thriller directed by a man that Donald Trump has playfully mooted as a possible member of his Cabinet, Secretary for Visual Effects.

Only by thinking of the granite screen in Sõprus do I feel better. Then I feel worse.

And why was the horror fan so unnerved by the Devil? As if such an entity, even in celluloid form, would have any remaining power? We were soon due to be coming up to the Parson and the Clerk after Dawlish, the frozen forms of the gullible. None of the films the fan had referenced – and later I would, for my sins, watch them all on Netflix or dvd – had any connection to the terrain we were in. Yet together they do constitute a strange and queasily organic landscape, an amoebic terrain where apocalypse is at work in the fibres of bodies and in the relations between them.

Approaching Langstone Rock from the Exeter direction, I notice how flat the Exe is this morning; a pool of mercury, the 'South Coaster' wreck half-submerged, no mast to mark it now. It feels like the past is disappearing, eaten by Langoliers. That this is a place where history comes in order to be forgotten.

I remember the strange white shape in the bay last night. I had meant to mention it, tell someone, ask their opinion, post it on Facebook for comments. To register my own anomaly, a little nervous that others would see it as an enthusiastic delusion. But once back at the hotel I had entirely forgotten that it had happened.

I see the tail first. Then the whole thing stretched out on the thin strip of sand left by the high tide. A huge bleached and beached whale, with flashes of red and blue. I shout out! And burst into tears.

I tell my story to the passengers in the nearby seats. A young guy in the seat in front: "so sad". He saw it too. The young woman across the aisle searches on her phone and finds a BBC Devon report. The journalists are saying it is a sperm whale; I do not think so. Its jaw was big, open and distraught, not that small hinged thing. Ringed around it were people. Stood about like carol singers without a Christmas.

I get off at Newton Abbot. At Dawlish I had dithered. Along the Teign I finally decided to abandon re-walking Plymouth; that can wait for another life. I catch a train back to Dawlish and begin to walk at pace along the front in the direction of the cadaver. Why do I walk so fast? For fear that other eyes will suck up all there is to see? A thin crowd drifts along the sea wall. I can see the maw, dark against the red sand. The bodies ringing it.

The 'Wrekin Tristar' access covers on the reconstituted sea wall under my feet are like the masks that a sea serpent might wear to hide its tendrils. Something very bad is coming. The waves thud relentlessly; reflecting directly out to sea again until they are overwhelmed by incoming waves. Rebuilt, after the storms of 2014 ripped out the ground here and left the track and sleepers strung across an abyss, the white concrete sea wall is warming slowly in the sun. Salmon's 'ghost house', shots of its empty iron window frames parcelling up the sea, is shining white now, an 'as if' Mediterranean brightness, glowing red beach towels hanging from its balconies. More uncanny than when it was unoccupied.

Some of the sandstone cliffs are smooth from peak to base, single dunes that must have stood in this same shape in the deserts where they formed 300 million years ago. Time stretches itself out along the prom towards the cadaver.

As I get closer, I can see that a square of beach is roped off around the whale. The BBC is wrong. Witnesses stand at the tape. Young officers in Council and Wildlife jackets sit, taciturn and superior, under the sea wall. It is immediately clear that if what I had seen last night was alive, then this is not it. A huge bone protrudes from a slush of decayed jaw. Its filters are exposed. Its back is like worn linoleum, its eye is wax.

I brave the stench down wind, gagging a little, to speak with the experts. It is a fin whale. They think that what I might have seen the night before was a slick of oily decay left by the whale's body giving the impression of a moving animal. They are polite, but I feel as though I am reporting a ufo sighting.

Despite the huge realness of the dead whale, last night is returning to its original ghostliness. I am surprised how moved I feel.

When I broach the significance of this, one of the wildlife officers, a young woman, qualifying her remarks as speculation, describes this anomalous beaching as part of a more general pattern of shifting relations that we can barely grasp: "we don't see much of the reality, very little of the oceans is surface. But far down something far bigger than this baleen whale is changing; over-fishing, rising world temperatures, the effects of excessive nutrients like nitrogen and phosphates running off the land, they have to be having an effect, a complex gathering effect..." (I thought of the sign where Dawlish Water enters the sea, not to bathe close by, the Devil got in very, very easily) "...all kinds of other pollutions..." (Salmon mentions three children dying of e coli poisoning picked up on Dawlish Warren) "...the rise of plague species and the obvious disappearance of others, anything with teeth basically, and, soon, with the acidification of the waters, anything with a shell. Unless we do something, very very soon..." Pause. "...we have probably run out of 'very very soon', actually; so we better get ready for the 'rise of slime'."

I ask her what she means and she recommends a book called Stung!

And I read this: "so, then, what is left? After the big fish and the marine mammals have vanished, after the clams and the worms have suffocated in the bottom hypoxia and the snails and the corals and the calcified plankton have disintegrated, after the birds and the mussels and the sea cucumbers have choked on plastic bullets, and the macroalgae have succumbed to the shading of the dinoflagellates, what is left? ...lots of jellyfish. It might seem outlandish and farcical to think that jellyfish could rule the seas. But they've done it before, and now we have opened the door for them to do it again. Jellyfish are weeds. They are opportunists. When they have the opportunity, taking over is probably, to some extent, just what jellyfish do" (Lisa-Ann Gershwin).

We have to get back in the sea. We have to get rid of the defences. We have to make allies with the beautiful, sophisticated and dangerous slime; like buddleia we cannot fight them and win.

I get myself upwind of the whale again and back to the witnesses, exchanging little parcels of lay expertise and online information; lacking a Bishop or a procession

335

of the priestesses of Dumna to lead us in prayer. Engineering myself into conversation with a local middle-aged couple, they tell me that the French authorities have been monitoring the corpse off their coast for a while. A bronzed and rosy-cheeked local butts in to tell us, uninvited, that the French are glad to see the back of it as they have enough on their plate "with all their other arrivals".

I am unreasonably stunned by the brilliance of this; the facility, without any conspiracy or shame, to have their agents present at moments like this, punctums, moments of floating emotion, to make a new hatred, to inflect the rot with another rot, to consecrate the cadaver of the huge mammal with the corpse juice of racism. I know now what ghost I'd seen. It was the wraith of colonies, the trace of imperialism's cadaver floating like a Venetian slave galley on the face of the waters.

I vomit. My breakfast on the sand, splashing the feet of the Racist Party activist.

It's all part of the theft of enjoyment.

The racists – and those infected by them – impute to their Other an excessive enjoyment. The mistake they neurotically pursue with fierce glee, is to think a dead refugee child on a beach is in fact a giant whale bloated by the pleasures that a racist never feels. Hence the fascination that so many racists express for those they purport to hate; all those far-right activists with mixed-race partners, who see no contradiction.

I turn and walk away. Ashamed; shamed by my own shame. I set off to the station at Dawlish Warren, pass under The Creep.

There is no train for 50 minutes.

I retrace my steps to savour the huge moulds of clinker among the waste of massive granite pieces protecting the Warren sea wall. Then wander back and into the 'Amusements Centre' to watch the women feeding the machines and listen to the electronic circus music. Finally, on the way up to the platform, passing 'Bedlam Manor' holiday let, a couple emerge from a car. A laconic young man preceded by his grinning girlfriend. "Here, doggie, doggie!" And she beckons at him to follow. "Here, doggie, doggie!" A cloud of cigarette smoke belches from his lips.

I sit and think about the whale. Later, on FB, I see that Dan Harvey has posted about his and Heather Ackroyd's 'Stranded' piece, where they render down a whale corpse and then encrust the bones with crystals.

Wonderful.

But I have had enough.

I abandon thoughts of re-walking Plymouth permanently. I have no stomach for more ghosts.

At times it feels, when walking, no matter how spontaneously or randomly, as if you are dragging a giant squid, and then at other times the jellies lift you up. Though the octopus may drink you alive, that alive is important; despite its violence, it holds out the possibility of extended organisms entangling sustainably. Just the possibility of such things makes the walk onerous and liberating, simultaneously. When, as Karen Barad writes, "[K]nowing is a direct material engagement", that is a huge

336

obligation for how you site imagination, and how, as part of that engagement, by diffraction, "[W]e are not merely differently situated in the world [but] 'each of us' is part of the intra-active ongoing articulation of the world in its differential meaning". We make space, like the Old Ones once made malevolent lanes for Widger. We risk drowning and are lifted up by the jellies, overwhelmed by the ethical responsibilities of a walk to the shops, empowered by its revolutionary and industrial possibilities. By the refusal of a certain kind of expert epistemological 'cut' or separation that defines politics as mediated and democracy as only representative and representational; and that, rather, there is a political everyday which requires us to reposition that 'cut' in order to understand it; not to denounce the field of Trump and Brexit and inanity and Spectacle and 'reality', but to see it for the potent field of post-truth that it is, when we cut it differently, diffractedly; when we stop mirroring it and start messing with it.

But I have failed that opportunity, and I walk away.

I don't even, too late, think of a clever thing to say back to the racist.

I am tired now. The weave has got too tight for me.

As the train pulls away, I notice that wedged against the side of the dull, symmetrical building that has replaced the old station, is a crude plastic replica of *La Bocca della Verità*, the first century manhole cover that stars along with Audrey Hepburn and Gregory Peck in 'Roman Holiday'. Peck, the torn instrument of the Spectacle – later seeking to tear the surface of the Spectacle down to the dark depths of truth in 'Moby Dick' – and Hepburn the victim-celebrity, as fake an icon as a rebel-cop, frightening each other with the threat of zealous lips that bite off the hand of a liar. The two of them terrify each other, and their audience, with the prospect of the dull stone's malevolence; even in a light comedy, Hepburn's scream is real, when Peck pulls out an empty sleeve: he had not warned his co-star.

The threat that the malevolence of the past might be both mythical and bonily real. 'Roman Holiday' is comic only insofar as it allows its journalists to bury a story for the sake of a princess's happiness, but realist enough to end with the separation of all its agents.

The Roman drain lid bears the face of Oceanus, son of Gaia, a deity with horns like crab claws and a serpent's body. Its Dawlish Warren replica, once dispensing printed fortunes, is silent; its fused and rusted mechanism exposed by a perishing of its plastic casing. Its mouth is dull, like the slack jaw of the dead whale.

I have my hand in a mouth of truth. Making subjectivity a crucial battleground means that the scope for self-deception is profound. Imagining what it might feel like, if the old Roman mask were really to close its lips on my wrist and cut through the skin, the arteries, the bones. I lose my appetite for biting off fingers. Better to let all the lying fingers swim in shoals and read their movements instead.

Later, when I have time to read Eileen Buckle's *The Scoriton Mystery* quietly, I grasp the significance of those fields on the edge of the moor and what Arthur Bryant started there; with its assemblage of an anti-self on the way to destruction, narcissism and the willingness to destroy those most dear, a researcher equally committed to putting herself in utopia's way, narratives of *aufhebung* (simultaneously lifting themselves up and abolishing themselves), doctored tapes, a sea of fakes poisoned by authoritative individuals (like Sir Patrick Moore), problems without solutions and mirages: a dis-organised conspiracy against the world, against each other and, in the end most importantly, against truth. Somehow, by a magic trick with algorithms, Arthur Bryant's brain tumour is now in charge; that's what is really stacked against the wall of the rebuilt, *ersatz*, non-railway station.

The sea has receded and the wrecks on the Exe re-emerge. There are mountains of purple cloud over Exmouth and stair rods of light offshore. The water seems familiar now. I feel it swimming around me as it had when I swam in it. The outline of the Warren dunes forms the outlying tress of Dumna's locks; that community, without police or representation, is a model of the mercy of the swell, whether deep in the sea or gushing up from below. Dumna's time is coming again.

As we pass the wreck of the 'South Coaster' I remember again what Steve Mentz says in *Shipwreck Modernity*: how the nostalgia for sail since its replacement by steam and diesel has exaggerated the loss of a connection between sailor and sea, traveller and world, and that in this nostalgia what we miss is "the growth, mostly in the 20th century but with deep historical roots, of swimming as a form of popular recreation and site of cultural meaning. Immersion, not sea travel, is now the dominant way humans engage physically with the ocean. Ocean swimming still awaits its Melville..."

I imagine how I could use Roger Deakin's *Waterlog* as a diving board for leading walks into the sea. I want to be its Melville. I am going back to being the amanuensis for whatever it is that is writing this mythogeography. Just as the supposedly extinct Neanderthals were all along hiding inside half of the world's *homo sapiens*, so there may be a second or third genesis of life hiding within the world's flora and fauna, including us, but they would be undetectable because no one knows how to look for alien. We need to check on things that look ridiculous, shy things that refuse to perform in a petri dish.

The young woman wildlife officer on the beach, earlier, had described how the bloom of tiny micro-organisms, expanding as the Arctic heats up, has led to a baleen whale population explosion, forcing those on the margins of the baleen community further and further afield until they find themselves in absurdity. The ripples of global warming have ended up here, on a Devon beach, beside the Point in View (the Crab Man emails later to say a Humpback Whale has appeared in waters near Dartmouth, and a Crocodile Shark has washed up on a beach nearby), the end in sight, an elephantine anomaly maybe meaning nothing, maybe a bad sign, or a sign of bad signs, a marginality forced to the margins; only the second fin whale stranding in the county in a quarter of a century. This in a coming age of jellies. Oceanus turning acidic and biting us back.

I am inexplicably affected by all this. What do I *care*? I intellectually care. Of course, but why this visceral, peristaltic chill of remorse? Come on! I am the walking stereotype of sentinel sentiment, wicked Diana hunting the hunters, tracking the trackers inside the twinge of my own feelings. There is no simple foe but I had wanted – as I walked quickly through the whiffs of rotting fin whale – to rip off every one of their motor limbs and bring them to their senses. Spiders with no legs, turning in circles. Feeling everything. An establishment without artisans. Rich with no poor. To strip the whole fucking thing of its rottenness – like Ackroyd and Harvey did – and encrust the monster with crystals! Turn this shit into oblique angels!

I close my eyes. Then chase down the trolley man and buy a tea. Sipping its burning brown stew. I am jelly, upheld by tendrils, by the walkers, the floaters, the believers in the recoil, the blooms. The lovely wanders woven together in compromises; for a few days I have experienced a place thick with strangers, 'just popping out for something' and becoming distracted by the world.

"This must be the bones of a fallen angel".

Laurie Anderson has it perfectly. And she walks. In Milan she says: "I suddenly thought maybe I should walk to Paris to mix this. Because walking is a lot like writing a diary... You don't know what's going to happen next..."

Later, on the train, my journey over, I become morose. I cannot console myself. The dancer with a copy of Lepecki's book emails, she had found a loading bay area behind the market and crawled there, while I was eating Thai Pad. That should cheer me up, but does not. I will be haunted all the way up through the West Country and the Midlands by something I had seen some time ago in London, in Whitehall. Along from the statues of "the master of strategy", with his parade stick bent, and of Viscount Slim, accused of outrages against young children in the Australian child migration farms under his control, a large piece of human excrement left beneath his plinth, close by there is a ramshackle set of huts and stands. Almost a village. Their posters and banners are wind-blown and fading to dim traces; their statements incendiary and ignored: wholesale accusations of child abuse against the establishment. Right at the massive gates of Downing Street. A tatty libel that no one is prosecuting, one way or the other, a few volunteers hoarsely repeating slanders to anyone who will listen. Names are named. It could not be a better 'mirage', all the better for being real. It being tolerated is a marker for the 'civilised' attitude of big power to the eccentric, the devolved, the small time, the self-contained.

A few metres further up the road I had wandered into the House of Commons shop where they sell 'Suffragette Coasters', and a model "House of Commons in a box".

I close my eyes and the sea is such a field of grey, sky and sea indeterminable, water like wrinkled steel.

The two women across the table from me chat.

"Thanks heavens we seem to be over all that awful pessimism around CCTV cameras."

"I saw a very funny scene in a film recently..."

"O?"

"Yes. Those women who were protesting about nuclear missiles in Britain ages ago. They chained up the front gates of the air base...."

"Chained themselves?"

"No, chained the gates. They weren't stupid. The missiles were trapped inside the base. The police came with a set of bolt cutters, then a bigger set, then an even bigger set, none could get through the chain. Eventually, all the police got together in a group and charged the gates, the posts gave way and they pushed over the whole bloody fence, and the women streamed onto the base. It was the funniest thing."

"What happened to them?"

"They were all arrested. We didn't have a nuclear war though, did we?"

The other woman laughs at this; she laughs at everything, with a general air of despair.

I close my inner eyes. I try to sleep.

There is no special quality that sets this particular bit of South Devon above the special qualities of anywhere else; that should be clear from its waters. There is nothing to indicate that it sits within any hierarchy of interest; it shares with other places the same tendency to contradiction, absurdity, poetry and eccentricity. Where there are nodes of such connectivity – whether by the generosity of one person to another (like the parishioner in the church to the suicidal man) or by their generosity to things – there is an Anywhere: a set of spaces, with their own meshwork, that are characterised by connectivity. This is where this part of South Devon (like other localities) has its uniqueness. Not in an essentialist 'identity', but in the particular layout of its connectivities; its perverse cartography encouraging the redrawing of its subjects-locales as the means to the pleasure of all its 'others'. It possesses and has possessed numerous asymmetrical hinges, and massive things are rehearsed here: the nuclear bombing of Russian ports, the invention of the computer, Marconi's signals from the Haldon Hills... not uniquely, but connectedly: things are brought to a point here, things are sent out from here.

This is what mythogeography can be, a serious geography, and I will seek to restore it, to finish the job that the originators of the idea left half-cooked. Salmon quoted from the occultist Arthur Machen that "he who cannot find mystery, wonder, awe, the sense of a new world and an undiscovered realm in the places by the Gray's Inn Road will never find those secrets elsewhere, not in the heart of Africa, not in the fabled hidden cities of Tibet". What Salmon and Machen wanted to say was that the local is exotic, there is no hierarchy of wonder, simply a hierarchy in looking and feeling; but what I have found is that there is a post-colonialist undercurrent to this charming thought. What my accidental tourism in South Devon taught me is that there is imagination enough, there is no need for piercing or invasion; instead there is a need to listen, to look, to respect, to think better of, to connect to the existing weaves: from the Palestinian beach attendant sharing his life story to the giant jellyfish washed up dead after an orgy.

Mermaids on a tread mill running against the tide,
An army of instrument makers trying to decide
How deeply they feel about intentions.

The "totality" I heard so much about is not a strategy. Nor is it a legitimate representation of a mythogeography. It is a form for fictional construction and a manifesto. And a mythogeography is both of those, so the totality in a mythogeography, a serious mythogeography of a specific locality, which is what I have, by accident or by bamboozlement, come to make, is divided, real and ghost, immersed and fictional. But, most importantly, accountable and unaccountable. It has the privilege of the stranger and the vulnerability of the local: me and Salmon.

Up till now (as with most people, I suspect) the only journeys I saw were my own, and those of my daughter, my ex-partner, close family members and friends, but it was pretty narrow, colleagues maybe, but not really their journeys, their geographies, and then some very remote ones I picked up from the news, and from fiction: many of them very faint tracks. We see a few very close trajectories and then we leap to a fantasy Middle Earth or a Marvel world or the ins and outs of 'Downton Abbey'; but around all those there is a nomadic totality of field or grounds. This, surely, is what mythogeography is meant to be. Crab Man only walked it in linear routes, he did not weave much, but I had. I had no route, I kept looping and crossing my own path, and I had Salmon with me, who had walked these places repeatedly (he must have), and I had the others – Helen B., the birdman, the storyteller, the psychoswimographers, the rambling women and the rest, with all their journeys weaving into mine and lifting me up from falling down...

I feel wetness around my fingers. The women opposite have stopped talking. The table top is like a mirror, I can see the startled faces of the two women reflected, I begin to slip....

"You're leaking," says the laughing one.

The tea is dripping from a tear in the cup. I take it to a bin and mop up the mess with some notes I no longer have any faith in.

I change at Exeter St David's for a cross-country service up to the North. At St David's Station, Brian Fawcett had caught the last sight of his father, "his tall figure was lost beyond view from the carriage window"; but I am on my way to Yorkshire not Peru, and it is Devon I am leaving behind and I have no expectation that "we should meet again in a few years in South America".

As we pick up speed, I lie back as best I can in my seat and let the landscape flash by at ten times as civilised a pace as any horsewoman, forty times any walker. In my head I log and label the anywheres of my small slice of South Devon: the ruined cave, the stone cadaver, the killing field flint scatter, the pole for dangling from in Funland and the greasy one for climbing up on the Front Lawn at Cockington Court. I could not quite pin them down. They were floating about like the giant Singer and Smith villas, between a mediaeval, clunky, ecclesiastically-focused ordering and a collective proletarian joy, sweet and fatty, the thrill of sham, music hall 'presence', the neo-neo-pagan dream of the Renaissance overleaping Oldway's Pans and Sphinxes, sealed up now, into a theological swill of sentiment and dirty jokes and competing racial inferiorities, a collective reactionary-rebel paroxysm unfettered by empathy, that made this space so dangerous, holiday camps waiting for their guards. The rich were mostly gone. I hardly saw any, but I repeatedly heard their guns outside Exeter and above Dawlish. I passed the gates of large houses. But not much display. 'The System' had been systematised, sex farmed in clubs rather than spread across the sands in 'beauty contests'.

The waters had seemed empty, the rock pools raided and stripped like little Crystal Caves, their denuded ecologies filling up with jellies, liberating spaces in which we might "reimagine the human relationship with the nonhuman environment".

The strange development of the economies here. Nothing textbook. Just as with the missing eras in the cliffs beyond Goodrington, the Industrial Revolution barely happens here. Yes, the technology changes, but there is little forging with its ideas. What Salmon describes instead is a different kind of technology, something much closer to the postmodern economy is created: military, digital, ornamental without being aesthetic, ultra-precise, nostalgic, crafted foods, spectacles for dying Europeans, mass tourism – the refining of gold at Shaldon, the super-skilled industries around Newton Abbot, brief potteries.

The hills and small fields have kept at bay the kinds of monster farms there are in East Anglia. Agriculture, though the machines and feeds may have changed, is not so very different from a hundred years ago, at least in the *shape* of the land. But appearances are deceptive. The chemical structure has been transformed. And minds are wholly different. The Anglican structure has been ripped up – when it was not ripping itself up in sectarian dispute in Exeter's surplice riots and the endless sniping and affray against Puseyism. The martyrs burnt at Livery Dole, the paintings and tapestries burnt on Cathedral Close. The whitewashing of popular mysticism and hallucination. All fed the acceleration of monastic timetables, until now the countryside is a blur.

It strikes me, in that strange way that ideas arrive sideways, that railway carriages are a lot like aquaria. That falling asleep in the carriages at Dawlish Warren, children sank down into deep oceans. How they must miss that! And how it was missed by those who only see, like me, the polymer-fabrication and redistribution of wealth (in the wrong direction) of the Entertainment Centre.

Class was strange here too. Torquay brought over the ruling classes in the late 19th century. The First World War brought thousands of Belgians, but in the end it destroyed the nascent cosmopolitanism beneath the bunting of chauvinism. The democratisation of holiday, well under way, was always accompanied by its militarisation; the selling of a variety of tiny flags for sand castles had by the 21st century been narrowed down to the red and white of St George.

I realise that I have written about the propagandists of race in uncompromising terms, but there is something more insidious about them that I may have missed – many of them were heroes, eccentrics, visionaries, innovators, explorers, discoverers, leaders. That is much the most dangerous thing about this layer of racist fundamentalism; made up not so much of prejudices and unfamiliarity and strangerhood, but of a systematic faith in the violent superiority of one 'race' over another and in the oneness of this 'one race'. Learning nothing from the emergence of modern archaeology – that just as God died in the caves of Windmill Hill, Torbryan and Kent's Cavern, so did Race as any meaningful description of the multiplicities of miscegenations that bring us to the Multiplicity of now, a Multiplicity that includes both variation and reproduction unevenly. Racism is a faith against the facts and findings of what happened; it is a faith that is not at the margins, an unfortunate incomprehension of these modern societies whose living ruins I have been walking through, but fundamental to them. The genius of Heaviside, Blomfield or Mallock is posited on their self-understanding of themselves as elevated by and legitimated in the dehumanisation of others. There is nothing universal about their faith, nothing fundamental even to colonialism (the Romans were not 'racist' in the ideological sense that Heaviside, Blomfield and Mallock were, the Normans were not, probably the Dumnonii were not, given their welcome to traders from the Mediterranean and Africa), but it is fundamental to what emerged after feudal society, after monasticism, sustained by the massive surpluses from a labour force that did not need to be paid, did not need to be educated, did not need to be sustained except in their profitable survival, did not need to be seen.

The wreck of the merchant ship at Church Rocks off Teignmouth is an exceptional event, but despite that it is also emblematic; how many other times did the ship land safely and the slave crew disembark? And then there were the two hundred black grooms arriving at Brixham with King Billy? That such encounters dwindle in the industrial period marks just how its new technologies were used not to broaden transport but to control and narrow and racialise it, until the spaces I have been walking in were bleached and the rest of the world became darkness and distant siege. Then the eccentricity of Heaviside, the aesthetics of Blomfield and the sophisticated adventure of ideas in the young Mallock's *New Republic* could be born and raised in the rape house of the slave fortress on Bunce Island in the Sierra Leone River; and while many knew and some did something about it, mostly these heinous narratives have been sustained. The sufferings taint every penny, every rupee, every dollar of surplus that becomes manifest in statues and monuments and in the fabrics, ornaments and ambience of stately homes, neo-gothic churches, public parks and TV sit-coms. No one alive today is to blame for that wreckage of human lives and its impregnation of the materials of our terrain; unless they choose to celebrate and perpetuate it and behave as if that terrain is not a shared one.

'Fukei-ron' might have been a crude theory of landscape – identifying every terrain, chocolate-box pretty, waste land or postmodern mall, as a spatial representation of a particular form of economic surplus – but my experience of exploring the route of one particular shipwreck of the South West is no less distressingly banal. There was so much more to my route, but without accepting the role of serial killing – at Lidwell Chapel, the graveyard under the Goodrington prom, the galley wreck on Church Rocks – there is no way to understand the proportions, the motion of the layers, what pulls the orbits here.

These thoughts are mixed by the swaying of the train as it passes over points before Taunton. I feel them tugged and repelled by curved theories of spacetime, until the whole orrery comes off its stanchions and floats off. I can feel the hands of others upon it. I have a child to see and another county to go to. I grab it back.

There are the places I knew were out there that I was unable to find: Drake's Leat in a retail park's parking lot; the Old Grotto in the Torbryan caves; the X-Rings garden inside Exeter Prison; the derelict fort run by the Showmen's Guild at Efford; the remnants of the greenhouses of the violet trade; the car park and underpass murals in Exeter made by a mosaicist who trained with Nek Chand; the tap for the once famous bottled-for-London 'Meadfoot Water' that I must have walked right by and missed; the road from the church near Blomfield's village where a young priest had been thrown from an overturning coach, somersaulted, and landed on his feet; the Egyptomaniac catacombs at Exeter and the obelisk nearby for a seditious Jacobin jailed for supporting universal suffrage; the pub where Forbes Julian had his acid baths; Lethbridge's orchard...

There are the walking artists that I knew were out there, but never found: the mathematician walking some Fibonacci sequence; the neo-vitalist group walking with things; the ambulatory architects making imaginary cities; a group making memory theatres; the Heaviside Layer choir singing in (and about) the red mud of the unfinished major road; barnprowlers and *circumcelliones*; a group in wheelchairs working with the idea of time and progressive illness; and a solo walker who walks naked and unseen (appropriate then that I did not find him).

I organise and list the things I have found out about my route, not what Salmon interprets, but what I touched, felt or saw, not sure if this is a kind of finding out that will be of any use to anyone:

I was witness to desperation. So many of the marginalised heritage sites I found were used as inadequate shelters by homeless people: in the same month as my walking four suicides washed up on Torbay beaches, two women were murdered on my route and one of their murderers died in Exeter jail; on just a couple of streets in Torquay and Paignton I felt an aggressive desperation that I did not feel elsewhere.

I met with and repeatedly witnessed civility; almost all motorists looked out for my safety, and when I trespassed or knocked on doors to ask questions about some ornament or whatever, I was surprised by how unthreatened and helpful people were. At the Plymouth Pannier Market and in Exeter's Sidwell Street I thought I detected a tentative 'cosmopolitan canopy' "where the display of public acceptance by all of all is especially intense" (Anderson).

I saw very few insects.

Appearances in the countryside are deceptive. The vista can be breathtakingly aesthetic – the pattern of fields and the use of hedges and trees as windbreaks taken from the idealised landscapes of painters – but get a little closer and the hedges are no longer cut and laid, but slashed back with a mechanical flail and many are failing as hedges and have to be reinforced with metal fences. And those bright green nitrate fields support little more than sheep and cattle.

I was surprised by how many sinister towers there are: from phone masts faked to look like trees, Ashcombe Tower with Hitler's private telephone (stamped with the makers' name: Siemens, still packaging Centrax's turbines made at Newton Abbot), Haldon Belvedere like the Eye of Sauron over the Exe Valley, Langage's gas-fired power station and the shipwreck thievery of Italianate pumping stations and Catholic churches.

This was a far more magical landscape than anyone is noticing: tunnels, arches to nowhere, caves, pits, chapels, cavities, forts, the Roland Levinsky Building, Peter Blundell Jones's 'Round House', the Mount Wise ray-gun viewing platform, the Merritt Flats built with sewing machine profits in Totnes Road, Paignton, with their oddly exposed staircases.

There is a shadow meshwork of sunken routes within the countryside and suburbia; extraordinarily no one knows how they were made or how old they are. They let you walk in mystery.

I saw doorways filled-in everywhere; the final evidence of a once powerful culture of home visiting that has almost died out.

I thought I might have got a very brief insight into a privileged and almost invisible space of wealth when the car park full of 4x4s near Brampford Speke with its tiny sign that I mistook for that of a golf club turned out to be the Duchy Working Gundog Club. That was one of the few times I felt animosity towards my presence.

If power comes by property, then the signs are mixed. There are plenty of footpaths, I never felt excluded much, and most of the folk I encountered on their own property were warm, interested and welcoming to someone with a point to prove and a pilgrimage to complete; the only exceptions were the rich whose properties are heavily gated and fenced, so no connection there; I never got beyond a "hellurgh" and a hasty passing-by, and maybe that was mostly my fault, my prejudice, I don't feel too bad about it, but I never penetrated their tiny world of accumulation and separation.

The other side to the property here is its surplus value. The prices in the windows of estate agents I looked in: silly money, almost London prices, reflecting white flight and speculation. In Plymouth the number of builders and odd-jobbers at work on renovation of old properties suggests that the landlords are buying up the lower end of the market, that rent is the biggest scam around; while those who just managed to get onto the property ladder a generation ago are now floated upwards on the bubble. Those at the bottom are dropping off the last rung. In pretty much every alternative monument or edgelands I had visited there was evidence of rough sleeping, if not the sleepers themselves. In the corners of many fields were caravans. Walking by so many huge houses, the failure of an affluent society to provide a home for all is the scandal of our times; something we were once quite capable of, at a time when we were generally much poorer.

On my walk around outer Exeter I could put together from different sites – meteorological office, metal stag, water tower, old-style housing estate, yew, Waitrose veg section, execution place – my own story of the city. Not my own city, of course. But in a time of the predomination of narratives, the walk has a new kind of re-creational as much as recreational power.

In terms of 'real capital', the one really big factory I passed had just shifted from long-term local family ownership to New York control; the economy is floating on tourism, property speculation, European farming subsidies (oops!), financial and administrative services. The ecology of agriculture and fishing seems fragile.

I never saw a single worm.

Against the declining colonial war machines (red and white flags over tiny domestic territories) and the heritage industry's exploitations of decay as a glue to bind together the hysterical complacency about the past, there stood the magnificent, marginal figure of Oldway Mansion: unstately home, refused by Torquay and its powerful families, industrial, Jewish, subjective and eclectic and a beacon of hopeful decay, already an Ozymandian theme park for those with eyes to see and life memberships of Nationalism-Distrust. Sealed up like a Chernobyl reactor, living out a half-life in Chuckle Brothers virtual reality; keep it sealed as a generator of questions, as a public educational resource! It needs no interpretation; just the nurture of eyes, and the self-restraint to refuse to ever redevelop or 'restore' it. It is glorious in its clothing in what has gone. It is a monument to present ache.

There was very little apparent enforcement. I heard hardly a single police siren. The only cops I saw were in cars. On noticeboards in the villages were the minutes of local council meetings and the marks of a thin, but enduring mesh of support and public service. In the cities there was far less evidence of civil society; yet there was civility. In Plymouth everyone spoke to me; except the people who scared me and I skirted them. There I did see power; the Navy's control of the Sound, but mostly its power was in ruins and relics.

There were signs of public space teetering towards decline; for example, an abandoned Sure Start premises beneath a concrete church; capital sucked directly from public services into the big gated houses with their giant vista-gazes on the quiet lanes.

Given what is coming, I was very unsure if anyone at all was ready for the ecological evacuees.

Cavities were everywhere – passages, tooth extractions, adits, wells, staircases, caves. Not only did this pock-marking undermine any universal efficacy I might have wanted to give to my walking – for when "the fall is towards the center of the earth and not any particular direction... Human feet do not determine the reference point for all directionality" (Woodard) – but it was a constant reminder that I was walking over two very different kinds of ungrounding. Firstly, the worming of worms and gold and uranium miners and imaginary Shoggoths (Lovecraft's living machine-slaves who are barely there in their "shapeless congeries of protoplasmic bubbles" and who constantly dig away at the foundations of anything, longing to hear the sounds of collapse from above); and, secondly, the "deterritorialized digging machines... mov[ing] through space and expand[ing] the yawning spatiality of space itself" (Woodard). This second cavity is the pulsing gap (opening and shutting like a fictional maw under a de-consecrated church) in the land that the birdman and myself were just starting to feel as we circumambulated Denbury Hill; that in the face of an amoral power that seems mostly absent (except when it comes gushing from the Virgin's foot or sucks you down into the deep of the sea), it is possible to shift sideways – away from the ugly geography of division inherent in the phenomenologies of dwelling and home – towards a geo-philosophy in which the materials of the planet (oil, acids, gas) are more clearly in control and respected. This is part of a cosmo-philosophy which grasps and understands that what the cosmos has given, the cosmos will also take away: that "whereas worming regrounds... planet demolishing will unground the grounds" (Woodard). In other words, that it is only by exceeding the sentimental ecology of preserving ourselves that we will grasp the connection between the new civility under the cosmopolitan canopy, the asteroid racing to meet us and the jellies clogging the grills of the Hadera Nuclear Power Station near Tel Aviv, that only by this assemblage will we be able to unground the racialised 'grounds' that have regrounded every space in supremacism. And it works the other way around, too. That without an ethical cosmopolitanism, cosmo-geography is undermined by Shoggoths of resentment and disgruntlement and ends in a Brexit from life and love.

When I was with the void and we came across that water-tank-cum-rocket on the way to Scorriton, I re-remembered the disappointment I felt with my brother's 'Transformers' toys; they were so far from realising the idea that trucks might be biological machines! Then a boyfriend took me to see the 'Transformers' movie (that was the end of him)! I was 21, we were with an audience of kids; they had replaced Lionel Jeffries with Shia LaBeouf and CGI, but they still could not help but trash the seriousness of the idea that "an object is not merely revealed in its actions, connections or networks, but has a vacuum-sealed core that is irreducible" (Woodard).

The water-tank-cum-rocket was like Oldway Mansion, but far scarier; it was the 'thing' which upscaled from marginalisation-by-supremacist-extinction to a more general extinction – or in the words of Timothy Morton, the ecologist and philosopher of massive objects: "the ecological crisis makes us aware of how interdependent everything is. This has resulted in a creepy sensation that there is literally no world anymore"; instead of a world, there is a mesh in which objects have their own life. The challenge of the black rocket is: can we learn to unground the 'grounds' that are encouraging us to destroy each other by meshing together in a cautious accommodation with the rise of slime and reticent things? Soft hands; not grasping at our own survival, but supporting it gently and contingently in a universe of tentacular clubs.

I discovered that Devon was once about to become modern. And that this modernity was purposely crushed. That the making and performing of Devon as a place of rural backwardness is a production of a tourism industry shifting from servicing the elite in cosmopolitan resorts to creating nostalgic destinations for industrial Midlanders. That when Torquay and other towns took in Belgian refugees during the First World War (I found a 'thank you' vase in Teignmouth) no one batted an eyelid; because they had spent two generations hosting European aristocracies on the run from democratic revolutions. In those times, Torquay was a serious venue for bourgeois culture; its municipal symphony orchestra performed new works by now forgotten modern composers like Roger Sacheverell Coke, Susan Spain-Dunk and Gilbert Vintner.

Devon nearly pioneered a new kind of village at Cockington; but it was never built. Also crushed was the modernist communal suburb at Churston Cove. Even in urban Exeter, the planner Thomas Sharp's utilitarian and proto-shock-capitalist vision for the city ("German bombs have already destroyed for us much that we had not had the courage to destroy ourselves. *We* shall have to do even greater destruction") was and, in that case, probably thankfully, sharply curtailed. Equally lost, in terms of regional identity, is the role of South Devon in 19th-century technological innovation and paradigmatic shifts of worldview; all that survives is in fragments, as plaques, old experimental tanks, remnants of laboratories, pamphlets in museums, but as a public narrative of identity it is gone. When, in 1947, planning permission was sought to re-kindle film-making at Watcombe a deputation of councillors visited Ealing Studios and returned, declaring themselves unhappy with what they had seen, concerned by "what went on in the way of noise" and killed the project.

A silent civil war *within* the upper middle class happened in South Devon, (and here I *am* drawing on Salmon), leaving only the results as evidence of it; the cosmopolitan innovators, who often adopted an elitist modernist marginalism and difficulty, were defeated by a powerful petit-bourgeois-like resistance which sustained its positions through nostalgic, rural-inflected popular chauvinism.

Once I was on the road, I expected to find only Wesley and Anglicans, but there were remnants of a last gasp of 20th-century monasticism; and the merest hint of a worrying attempt to raise it again on the back of the New Age movement; yet, having experienced the joys of the fluidity of the lanes, I was also aware again that timetables and routines could provide a skeleton and a torque on fluids without which we give ourselves up to being ruled by a succession of warlord-jesters.

Coming to Devon on the train, and then setting off on my walk, I had always expected to find some evidence of faded empire; what I was not prepared for was just how often architectures and symbols were sustained by a pervasive 'white supremacism', expressed as a science or as a philosophy. Whether it was Heaviside forcing his female relative to sign an agreement never to take a black husband, or the theorising of James Anthony Froude, Bulwer-Lytton's *The Coming Race* or Trevena's dystopian nightmare of miscegenation, this was racism expressed as faith, as science, as existential reality; its pervasiveness in doctrinal form was unrelenting.

Electricity pylons look very different when you know that the criteria for their design includes the antipathy of Sir Reginald Blomfield to the "dull obscenities of negroid Art". Every memorial of a battle or gravestone of a hero that I checked out marked a racist slaughter or an outrage of some kind; though by flipping the gravestones and stone monuments in my head they become markers of anti-colonial rebellion and fightback, like the resistance of Rani Lakshmibai to the 'doctrine of lapse' at Saugor.

Something else I came to understand is that there is an older, but not oldest, history that is emerging about the people who were here before and after the Romans. Romans who not only invaded and occupied, but then dominated the imaginations of those subsequently in power through a variety of neo-classicisms. That what rendered the indigenous people invisible is what should make them so very interesting to us: they were pre-text just as we are becoming post-text, they built no great temples but worshipped at streams and groves and springs, and they lived without centres, in dispersed communities the shape of which endures around West Ogwell and in fainter traces elsewhere. Rather than the myth of 'savagery' inherited from the writings of some Roman militarists, what if these Dumnonii's noted generosity to strangers and their peaceful co-existence with both Roman and Saxons (until Athelstan and his nation-building) speaks of a completely 'other' culture, unimaginable to a modern or hypermodern, but not to a genuinely postmodern and posthuman, mind. A culture of dispersal, de-territorialisation and the facing of darkness.

I could complain about the ignorance, decay and abandonment around this and other marginal heritages; but it does mean that there are many semi-secret (and even some genuinely secret) treasures to be found and savoured: The Old Grotto (even if, for me, it remains only an idea), the quarry sketched by Thomas Moran, the gorsy moor that had been Teignmouth Airfield, the remains of the Crystal Cave, the beautiful water tower of Digby Insane Asylum now illegible between Pizza Hut and KFC.

Or is all this an illusion of understanding – compromised by publication – and does everyone need to go on their own journey to find out for themselves what in this terrain can take them 'somewhere else'? Has all this been more of an experiment in the subjective-placing of oneself – myself – in a terrain?

Which is odd, because I am a Northern lass, this is not my place, and I found few parallels or equivalences to Yorkshire, and yet I still felt as if I was 'here' at last, placed, far from home, away from my girl, I was still in this place, in these lanes, on these streets. In a comfortable 'anywhere'. Wherever I go now this 'anywhere' will be part of who I am, a landscape that walked itself into me just as much as I walked myself into it.

I am not so sure that I thought any great thoughts, but I did attend to how I thought, to how I made thoughts.

I grasped on to fragments of stories far more complex and deeply buried than I had time or energy enough to drag up or dig down to or put together; at times it was as if I was swimming through a sea full of narrative battleships, which were constantly emerging from a Tash-like miasma and crashing into each other. In order to have some, if inadequate, sense of the whole it was necessary to imagine it as a complex shipwreck still grinding around in itself and stirring up the ocean floor.

And I had been helped by those who I had walked with; there was one academic in there, and a swimmer, an ornithologist, a dancer, a student, a storyteller; they all had ideas, but they held them and shared them in the way of autodidacts.

Symbolist theatre had helped me too. Not in a direct way, but it was the myth to my geography. I did not see much theatre on my walk; though of course everything was a performance in some way or other. The symbolist dramas were more spectral in their influence; their journeys and quest stories were running through me, from August Strindberg's *The Great Highway* and *The Road to Damascus*, the journey to and through the castle in Villiers de Lisle-Adam's *Axël*, the march of the villagers in Maeterlinck's *The Intruder* to the quest in Ibsen's *Peer Gynt*. And their locations and architectures seemed to emerge serenely from the places I walked in, loading them with life-changing significance and metaphorical and allegorical references.

Whenever I came to a turning I was at the start of 'The Great Highway' and I was the main character 'The Hunter' unsure whether to go upwards to oblivion and respite or drop down to where my struggles would continue. On a cold night in Plymouth I learned that I must always take the 'low road' to desire and never the 'high' one beyond desire (as Freud wants us); the consequences may be loaded with guilt, discharges and complications, but they will all in time loop around to further opportunities to take the low road back to a new desire.

Other times in quarries I felt I was part of 'The Road to Damascus', where the STRANGER points to a rock formation and says to the LADY, "There's your werewolf from whom I saved you. There he is, in profile, see!", and, as the LADY, I would reply: "Yes, but it's only a rock". To hold in tension the simulacra that appeared – the hill like a beached whale, the plastic bag like a prehistoric reptile – and the vibrancy of their materials.

I was always planning this report in my head, mapping it out, like the LADY crocheting, and the STRANGER would see in my patterns a scene which I would recognise from his description as a real place and – operating like Palfrey and his atomic consciousness – we would go there. So, after noting in my pocketbook "a hill like a beached whale", it was only to be expected that I would find a fin whale on the beach at Langstone Rock.

Ideas are things. They do not 'dwell' in a space above space, but are just as much part of producing and reproducing as a carved stone head or Stumpy Oak, as much about place and displacement as Oldway Mansion. They reveal their meanings by being here and there.

After finding the shining green flying saucer above the valley beside Scorriton Down, as we retraced our steps through Chapel Street in Buckfastleigh, the lights in the old chapel still on and the organ makers still working "to the Glory of God", I was thinking that 'post-truth' had been here for a while in a good way; along this one street some chapels had closed, a new one had opened in a residential house, I doubted if anyone was harassed for their beliefs or if there was much animosity between the different 'houses of God'; that the varieties of belief and the path to atheism possible through Christianity and the working out of Protestantism's dialogic rhetoric that refuses to let God have the last word, has led to stoicism and empathic indifference to those who make the leap to absurdity. Rather than a moral decline, I fancied this represented a moral ascent since the domination by one church matched Anglican church-going with child prostitution as the top two leisure activities of the well-to-do; and that if anything threatened morality it was the anti-clown, anti-Halloween church; that is where the devil gets in very, very easily.

While I have been walking, the world has been changing and mostly I think that people like me think it is much for the worse; but what if this, in the long term, is a return to something more tolerant and early medieval, a time when the authority of priests was less certain and often unheard, not even understood, when belief was far more open to varieties of interpretation and visual multiplicity, inclusive of many experiences and authority was more reserved, more removed. As the authority of the text declines to what it was before the printing press, we are going to have to navigate without the liberal and theoretical certainties we have been accustomed to; what postmodernists preached, we have to practise. It is no longer speculation, and the problem is not a lack of objective truth, but the threat of its return in spectral and chorastic form, the gullibility of a growing minority to such "truth-telling" and "truth-claiming" by a small army of virtual and theatrical charlatans and savvy hate merchants. We need to educate ourselves and the next generation against the translation of marginal disgruntlement and disappointment into a paranoid meta-narrative of establishment conspiracy against each member of the white masses personally.

Symbolism's decadence, anti-textuality, floating free of words from their meanings, anti-utopianism and fatalism are all weapons in our New War. But there are no 'sides'. No collective forces are left to be rolled out or 'got behind'; there will be coalitions of individuals, the arguments will continue, the dust will not settle, we organise in mist, with mist.

What passes for the new idea in 'post-truth' is very old; a mix of the 'rebel cop' with a scaffolding of white-supremacism (or Hindu-supremacism, or whatever-supremacism depending where you are) while its underneath wobbles between state

Keynesianism and rabid neo-liberalism. Nothing new and nothing stable there; which does not mean it cannot last long. If you want a conspiracy, then this is the most perfect realisation of the Okhrana's aims (the mission of the Tsarist secret services, inventors of the 'Protocols of Zion'), to place anti-terrorism and 'conspiracy theory' at the heart of geo-politics, carried on by Stalin and now realised (much to his surprise, probably) by Vladimir Putin, his Trumpuppet and a string of nascent dictatorships. This is very, very old stuff, wholly removed from the lives and interests of those who support it; like that old man in Stoke Canon fantasising about the Chinese invasion of Exeter, in tune with the security forces.

But if we have some confidence in the 'post-truth' of Chapel Street, things can be different and OK. Without texts we can evangelise a deeper, wider gaze, a living in the patterns, a tending to the texture (like those hedges!). Oscillating between geological time on Denbury Hill and the volatility of "rushing water" in Isca, Dumna entangles the two through the springs of Sidwella in the Well Street café and around the feet of the BVM in the Chapel in the Woods, multiply entangled with narratives from Saxony, France, Ireland and the Middle East, here and there simultaneously, deep in this ground and subject to the tidal pulls and volatilities and turbulence of distant gravities. The patterns of a model community, a dispersal rather than a condensing of subjectivities; a lighter and de-monstered Lovecraftian landscape of visiting and open doorways, paths and exchanges, gifts and welcomes; looking into the indifferent faces of the amoral archons, learning to live with the bungled world of the demiurge and being convivial, civil, ready to help the fallen to their feet (if that's what they want) without any need of heaven... that cave, the hill, the graves of the ancestors (even if they are not ours) are enough...

These were the feints I had been throwing for myself, dodges and dreams that allowed my thoughts to get free of the immediate circumstances that were shaping them, allowing them to whirl round in front of my eyes all the anxieties that were being shared with me – the tunnels from Torbryan to Torquay, the emptiness of Exeter, the gap where the car had passed through the railings at Corbyn Head – and in their movements around each other, structured by feelings, helped me see how the air loom was weaving from innocent inferiorities "mind-forg'd manacles". The air loom itself came to look something like a flying jelly out of H. G. Wells. But that was not what it was, because what it was it was making up all the time differently; in feelings. Thanks to Salmon and Villiers de Lisle-Adam, I had been given a peep into the jelly-mechanism of that spongy thinking that brings forth unexpected election results.

Outside, the light has died and the industrial ruins north of Birmingham are just blank patches between city lights.

Often on the lanes of South Devon, or up on the hill forts, I thought I had wandered into the stage directions of a symbolist drama; in the photographic record of the early productions of Symbolist theatre they look so clunkily gothic and representational that it is easy to forget that what they were proposing was the destruction and collapse of more than theatre itself. So when Sara, the renegade Gnostic nun in De L'Isle-Adam's *Axël*, plunges a dagger into a heraldic sign and "the entire mass of the wall section [of the castle] cleaves into a wide, vaulted opening, glides and sinks gradually underground" or when the avalanche at the end of Ibsen's *Brand* sweeps everything away, or when in his *The Master Builder* the steeple is built right up through the ceiling of the theatre, these are not just visual effects, but violent questionings of the very frame of appearance and representation itself. When one interprets the terrain of a walk through such a lens, well... you are sensitised to the responsibility of walking through an ecology under existential threat; and can see that there is not one dagger but many, held in trailing tendrils dangling from the maw of every moto-cross track cut in the hillsides.

And there is another strange shape that recurs in my dreams long after I have returned to the north and to my darling daughter. When lulling her to sleep, lying beside her on her bed and drifting off, in the air below the ceiling an hourglass will appear; the top bulb representing all the reading and preparation I did for the Paignton conference falling down its wide bowl, to the narrow neck where I am on my walk remembered in tiny fragments and momentary scenarios, and then the glass broadens out again to another bulb and I am checking the broken shards of my walk's memory against the wider authorities. In that tiny neck of tube in the middle of the glass I am no expert, I am a stranger... but... and this is what is special here... it is the narrowness itself, having to work with the smallest of samples, by stranger-geography, that if there is any value at all, it is coming from this thin gap... so, if you see or meet a stranger, welcome them; that may be your best geographer.

The hourglass is wrapped around with tentacular thoughts....

Lakshmibai on horseback, clutching her son to her breast, leaping to safety from the ramparts....

I am wearing a jellyfish for a hat...

I cannot explain it. I will have to leave what I have written and hope that the loom is visible in all the writhing of the air...

I am falling asleep now, the light outside is almost gone, the shapes of the folding hills are marbled by the scraps of sunset, I am longing to be out there, sliding down a darkening lane or unfolding novelties on the edge of a city...

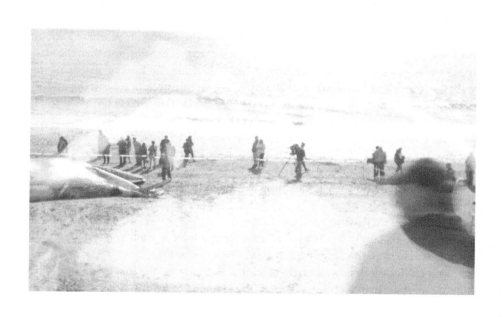

A Mythogeographical Afterword

Although I have written plenty about mythogeography as an experimental approach to the site of the performance of everyday life, a space of multiple layers best understood when in motion, I have never subjected a site to a sustained exploration, analysis and description using mythogeographical principles. Fragments, yes – Queen Street in Exeter, a route through Suffolk – but these projects were limited in terms of the conclusions arrived at or of usable and reusable findings to pass on to others.

Wanting to put the idea of mythogeography to a sterner test, and drawing on almost 20 years of wandering and performance-making across South Devon, I have set out in this book to gather insights, make analyses and write conclusions equivalent to conducting research in cultural geography and publishing it as a book-length study.

In order to write from multiple viewpoints, I adopted two fictional voices: Cecile Oak, a researcher who is a stranger to the area, and A.J. Salmon, who shares my familiarity with the terrain and with some of its histories. Thus I am presenting this work as a hybrid of stranger's and expert's geography. Once settled on my approach, I then began to walk Cecile's route. Some of it I had walked before, but not all, and when I walked I had in mind Cecile's narrative. Using a technique I have described in detail in *The Footbook of Zombie Walking*, I did not pretend to be her, did not pretend to be able to imagine her feelings, but walked with her narrative in mind, thinking about how the terrain might inform her fiction and how her story might work itself out in it.

As with many of my books for Triarchy Press, I hope that, beyond the particular circumstances of South Devon, the techniques of exploration and description can be used by others. I hope that this mythogeography can take its place as a collection of techniques guided by multiple but coherent principles alongside other recognised practices like mobility studies, spatial analysis, nomadology and psychogeography.

Part of the mythogeographical technique is to use lay, expert, specialist and unrespectable materials together. The other side of this coin is that anyone should be able to use mythogeographies like 'Anywhere'. This book is published under a Creative Commons licence, so please use the book to do new things, to change it into something it isn't yet. Use it as a map or handbook or model to be departed from, as a resource for research you haven't even imagined yet. Please use it as a toolkit and a guidebook for making your own journeys in your own 'South Devons'.

Mytho/Crab Man/Phil Smith

Appendix

Four mythogeographical lenses

Layering: an investigative and questioning lens, it adopts Tim Ingold's anti-'global' model of knowledge. According to Ingold, one learns more by an ever closer familiarity and deeper entry into the layers and textures of the world, rather than by uninvolved, cool and elevated examination or distant spectatorship. It seeks to expose the hidden, and to liberate the repressed as if these were especially meaningful; it assumes that there has been organisation rather than coincidence, until proven otherwise. It seeks to illuminate or point to ironies. Its characteristic sites are the archaeological dig, the crime scene and the palimpsest. It seeks to encourage hypersensitivity to the hidden or ignored meanings of the everyday, and to detect evidence for structures through the further dis-assemblage of already fragmenting evidence, seeking meaning in texture, grain, minutiae, details, marginalia and etiquette.

Rhizomatic interweaving: this lens takes from Doreen Massey the idea that space is made up of trajectories rather than boundaries. Its re-assembling of disparate elements and journeys is complementary to the inquisitive dismantling of the Layering lens. Its key tactics include détournement (the re-use of moribund art forms and media through adaptation, juxtaposition and disruption to new ends) and assemblage. The latter, as described by Deleuze and Guattari refers to the collection of divergent forms, practices and objects in ways that continue to maintain their differences within their collectivity. From Deleuze and Guattari this lens also takes its resistance to roots and identity, rather seeking 'being' in the weaving of connections between small groups led by their margins and through spiral distributions and disseminations of small but non-localised behaviours, tasks and provocations.

The making of 'anywheres': despite the resistance of mythogeography to bounded space and identity, it has a constructive agenda for the making of 'anywheres'. These are heterotopias rather than utopias. These are places of interconnectivity and diversity, irony and bricolage rather than conformity to principles. 'anywheres' are domains that are characterised by hybridity and unboundedness and do not conform to state or local boundaries, nor to national, local or sectarian identities (though they are not necessarily always local, small scale or 'human-sized'). They are places where many sites co-exist within a single site (like the 'ambient hubs' of situationist psychogeography). Tim Edensor adds to this another aspect: the fluid chaos of numerous parallel behaviours, characters and compartments in one space, in unordered flux. He sees the potential (or affordance) for this where there are problems in the ordering of space: "weakly classified space[s]... not under the sway of some overarching convention of ordering... have the potential to facilitate imaginings, epistemological dislocations and memories better than others" Such spaces are a socialisation of the idea of 'cosmopolitanism', seeking to transfer the cosmopolitan capacity and ethics – and, in particular, Kwame Anthony Appia's ethics of strangers, which revolve around our responsibility to those beyond any co-identity – from the trajectory of privileged individual to common, public spaces.

The self-mythologising of the activist: mythogeography applies the same principles to persons as to spaces. Through this lens mythogeography seeks a breaking down of identities, social roles and functions while avoiding the development of alternative milieus, adopting The Invisible Committee's critique of such milieus. Mythogeographers disrupt themselves; then, in turn, disrupt this disruption. So mythogeography's self-mythologisation is a limited one; temporary and transferable (it is not unique). This is similar to the adoption by anti-artists of shared pseudonyms such as 'Karen Eliot' or 'Luther Blissett'. The adoption of a limited self-mythologisation attempts to transfer the playfulness of a subversive identity from the mythogeographer to their 'myth'; entangling the performer with the site of their performance.

References

Chapter One
Walking with Fancy (1942) E.L. Grant Watson. Country Life

Chapter Two
Weird Realism: Lovecraft and Philosophy (2012) Graham Harman. Zero Books. p.17
The Landscape of Power (1958) Sylvia Crowe. The Architectural Press. p.44

Chapter Three
The King in Yellow (1895/2010) Robert W. Chambers. Wordsworth Editions. pp.68, 71
Forms: Whole, Rhythm, Hierarchy, Network (2015) Caroline Levine. Princeton University Press

Chapter Four
Shipwreck Modernity: Ecologies of Globalization, 1550-1719 (2015) Steve Mentz. University of Minnesota Press. pp.x, xx, xviii
Sir Constant: Knight of the Great King (1899) W.E. Cule. The Pilgrim Press. pp.34, 35
Crowe, *ibid*, p.55

Chapter Five
Memoirs of Life and Literature (1920) W.H. Mallock. Harpers & Bros. p.28, 210-213
'Ding und Schatten' (1934) Lajos Kardos. In *Zeitschrift für Psychologie*, Er. Bd 23. Translated in Alan Gilchrist's *Seeing Black and White*. OUP: 2006
Modernismus (1934) Reginald Blomfield. Macmillan. p.103
We Wander in The West. (1950) S.P.B. Mais. Ward, Lock & Co. p.5
The New Republic (1877) W. H. Mallock. Chatto & Windus

Chapter Six
Glaucus: or The Wonders of the Shore. (1859) Charles Kingsley. Macmillan
Vibrant Matter. (2010) Jane Bennett. Duke University Press. p. 11
Devon and Its People (1959) W.G. Hoskins. David & Charles
Symbol Sourcebook (1984) Henry Dreyfuss. Van Nostrand Reinhold
World Without Words (2003) Michael Evamy. Lawrence King

Orientalism (1978) Edward Said. Pantheon

'A Game of Cat's Cradle' (1994) Donna Haraway. In *Configurations*, 2 (1), pp.59-71

Dramaturgy and Architecture (2015) Cathy Turner. Palgrave Macmillan

'Walking in London at night' (1979) Celia Fremlin. In *New Society*, 19.4.79

Chapter Seven

'The Soul of Man under Socialism' (1891) Oscar Wilde. In *Fortnightly Review*, Feb 1891

Mentz, *ibid*, p.162

Where the Rainbow Ends (1932) Clifford Mills. Hodder & Stoughton

Places of the Mind (1949) Geoffrey Grigson. Routledge & Kegan Paul. p.120

Chapter Eight

'Black and Blue' (2015) Garnette Cadogan. In *Freeman's Arrival*, ed. John Freeman. Grove Press.

The Art of Walking (2015) Sonia Overall. Shearsman Books

Crow (1970) Ted Hughes. Faber & Faber

Harman, *ibid*, p.17

'At the Mountains of Madness' (1936/2005) H. P. Lovecraft. In *Tales*, Library of America. pp.508-509.

Town Planning (1940) Thomas Sharp. Penguin Books

The Unheimlich Manoeuvre (2016) Tracy Fahey. Bee Books

Reactions in Devon to Invasions (1992) Ross Whitefield et al. The Devonian Assoc.

The Roman Villa in South-West England (1976) K. Branigan. pp.17, 25

Three Men Seeking Monsters (2004) Nick Redfern. Paraview Pocket Books. pp.48-49

Bunyan Calling (1943) Mary P. Willcocks. Allen & Unwin

Levine, *ibid*, p.64

Chapter Nine

Over the Hills (1968) W. Keble Martin. Michael Joseph

The Secret Life of God (2015) Alex Klaushofer. Hermes Books. pp.66-67

A Philosophy of Walking (2014) Frédéric Gros. Verso. p.181

Forgive the Language: Essays on Poets and Poetry (2015) Katy Evans-Bush. Penned in The Margins. p. 19

Chapter Ten

Flying Saucer from Mars (1954) Cedric Allingham. Frederick Muller. p.14

From Cairo to Coffee (2010) Gillian Roberts. Authorhouse. pp.150-151

Grigson, *ibid*, p.107

Secret Invasion (2015) Ed. Tony Eccles. Cygnus Alpha. p.155

Reassembling the Social (2007) Bruno Latour. OUP. p.243

'The Horror of the Heights' (1913/2000) H.G. Wells. In *Tales of Unease*. Wordsworth Classics. p.95

Chapter Eleven
The Reign of the Saints (1911) John Trevena. Altson Rivers
Cadogan, *ibid*, p.142
Vathek (1786/2008) William Beckford. Oxford Paperbacks
Architecture and Ritual. (2016) Peter Blundell Jones. Bloomsbury. p.3
Crowe, *ibid*, p.43

Chapter Twelve
Through the Length of Africa (1927) C.V.A. Peel. Old Royalty Books. pp.111-114
The Ideal Island (1927) C.V.A. Peel. Old Royalty Books
The Way Up (1910) Mary P. Willcocks. John Lane
Britannia Obscura (2015) Joanne Parker. Vintage. p.104, 101
Crowe, *ibid*, p.19
Modernismus (1934) Reginald Blomfield. Macmillan. pp.67, 72, 70, 68, 81, 81, 82, 118, 115, 116

Chapter Thirteen
Mallock, *The New Republic*, p.48
Such Silvery Currents (2002) M. Chisholm. Lutterworth Press. p.175
Sharp, *ibid*, p.36
Meeting the Universe Halfway (2007) Karen Barad. Duke University Press. p.88
The Uprising (2012) Franco 'Bifo' Berardi. semiotexte(e). pp.17, 140, 147
Barad, *ibid*, pp.90-91

Chapter Fourteen
Expedition Fawcett (1953/2001) Lt. Col. P.H. Fawcett. Phoenix Press. p.13

Chapter Fifteen
Astrology: The Evidence of Science (1990) Percy Seymour. Arkana. pp.112, 171, 234
Exhausting Dance (2006) André Lepecki. Routledge
Projected Cities: Cinema and Urban Space (2002) Stephen Barber. Reaktion Books. p.156
Discovering Scarfolk (2014) Richard Littler. Ebury Press
Flâneur: The Art of Wandering the Streets of Paris (2016) Frederico Castigliano. CreateSpace
Flâneuse (2016) Lauren Elkin. Chatto & Windus
New Renaissance (1987) Maurice Ashe. Green Books

Chapter Sixteen

Blomfield, *ibid*, pp.152, 96

Crowe, *ibid*, 11

The Haunting of Toby Jugg (1948) Dennis Wheatley. Hutchison. pp.54, 145, 225, 301, 61

The Mushroom at the End of the World (2015) Anna L. Tsing. Princeton UP. p. 38

The English in the West Indies, or The Bow of Ulysses (1888) James A. Froude. Longman, Green & Co. pp.25, 4

Tsing, *ibid*, p.39

Froude, *ibid*, pp.50, 22, 43, 50

Froudacity: West Indian Fables (1889) John Jacob Thomas. T. Fisher Unwin. p.10

The Scoriton Mystery (1967) Eileen Buckle. Neville Spearman

'Jellyfish Science, Jellyfish Aesthetics'. (2013) Stacy Alaimo. Chapter (pp.139-164) in *Thinking with Water*. McGill-Queen's University Press. p.140

Chapter Seventeen

Atomic Consciousness (1892) James Bathurst. Harris & Haddon

The Last Battle (1956) C.S. Lewis. Bodley Head

Between the Old World and The New (1926/1967) Mary P. Willcocks. Books for Libraries Press

Guy Debord (1999) Anselm Jappe. Trans. Donald Nicholson-Smith. University of California Press. p.142

Barber, *ibid*, pp.160-161

Stung! (2013) Lisa-Ann Gershwin. University of Chicago Press. pp.340-341

Barad, *ibid*, pp.379, 381

The Cosmopolitan Canopy (2011) Elijah Anderson. W.W. Norton & Co. p.3

On an Ungrounded Earth (2013) Bob Woodard. Punctum Books. pp.43, 40, 41, 48

Lovecraft, *ibid*, p.581.

The Ecological Thought (2010) Timothy Morton. Harvard University Press. p.31

Blomfield, *ibid*, p.118

Four mythogeographical lenses

'Globes and spheres: the topology of environmentalism' (1993) Tim Ingold. In *Environmentalism: the view from anthropology*. (ed.) Kay Milton. Routledge. pp.31-42

For Space. (2005) Doreen Massey. Sage Publications. pp.9-15

A Thousand Plateaus. (1987) Gilles Deleuze & Felix Guattari. (trans. Brian Massumi) Continuum. pp.289-290

Industrial Ruins. (2005) Tim Edensor. Berg. p.44

Cosmopolitanism: ethics in a world of strangers. (2007) Kwame A. Appiah. Penguin.

The Coming Insurrection. (2009) The Invisible Committee. semiotexte(e). p.100

About

Triarchy Press is a small, independent publisher of interesting, original and wide/alternative/contextual/radical thinking about:

- organisations and government, financial and social systems – and how to make them work better
- human beings and the ways in which they participate in the world – moving, walking, performing, growing up, suffering and loving.

Triarchy Press has published a number of books about radical, performative or alternative walking (by authors like Roy Bayfield, Claire Hind, Clare Qualmann and Phil Smith). For details of all of them, visit:

www.triarchypress.net/walking

Links to more of Phil Smith's work – on film, in print and online – can be found at:

www.triarchypress.net/smithereens

Additional images associated with each chapter of the book can be found at:

www.triarchypress.net/anyimages